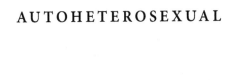

AUTOHETEROSEXUAL

AUTO
HETEROSEXUAL

ATTRACTED TO **BEING** THE OTHER SEX

PHIL ILLY

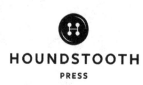

HOUNDSTOOTH
PRESS

AUTOHETEROSEXUAL
Attracted to Being the Other Sex
First Edition

ISBN   978-1-5445-4145-7   *Hardcover*
          978-1-5445-4144-0   *Paperback*
          978-1-5445-4257-7   *Ebook*

For my people—

even those who don't think they are.

I was wanting in only one respect: I could not understand my own condition. I knew that I had feminine inclinations, but believed that I was a man. Yet I doubt whether...I ever admired a woman without wishing I were she; or without asking myself whether I should not like to be the woman, or be in her attire.

—Hungarian physician (c. 1890)

CONTENTS

FOREWORD

As the founder of the adult dating website, *AdultFriendFinder.com,* I've seen a sizable percentage of men join as their feminine sides to socialize and explore their sexuality. Although some of them are full-time transwomen, most, like me, are not.

When I finally encountered the concept of autogynephilia, I was relieved that this phenomenon had a name. But I was also struck by how little formal academic research had been done on the matter: there were a few papers and studies, but there was practically nothing out there.

To combat this dearth of material, I started contacting academic researchers who were interested in the topic. Through this, I met Kevin Hsu, assistant professor of clinical psychology at Penn State University. I decided to join his research and fund an autogynephilia study that, when completed, will be the largest of its kind to date.

Through that sexology work, I was introduced to Phil Illy, who was researching autogynephilia and autoandrophilia for this book. Sharp and methodical, I recognized that he was the ideal person to explain both of these orientations to a wider audience. It is my pleasure to work with Phil in this endeavor.

I want autogynephilic men to know they aren't crazy or perverse, or destined to live a lonely, isolated life. I want them to know that it's completely acceptable to be AGP, and that it's even possible to continue their relationships with their wives or girlfriends without denying who they are. By fostering mutual understanding, this book can help autogynephilic men and their partners adapt to their unique circumstances or even thrive in them.

Through regular contemplation of a woman's perspective, autogynephilic men can develop greater empathy for women. With this enhanced empathy, they can be more thoughtful partners and build stronger relationships with the women they love. Seen in this light, autogynephilia isn't something to be ashamed of. Instead, it can be a personal superpower.

Lastly, I want autogynephilic men to understand that while hormones and surgeries are options, they aren't the only ones. With a vivid imagination and open mind, they can embrace their inner duality in ways that bring greater meaning to their lives and authenticity in their relationships, yet don't rely upon permanent medical interventions.

This book clearly explains what autogynephilia and autoandrophilia are, but it doesn't prescribe a specific course of action. Autoheterosexuals must make these decisions for themselves.

I hope the knowledge in this book steers you toward decisions that bring you greater joy and meaning on your gender path, wherever it leads.

—Andrew Conru

PART 1

AUTOHETEROSEXUALITY AND ITS CONTEXT

1 . 0

STRAIGHT, TURNED INSIDE OUT

There are two known types of transgenderism. One is associated with homosexuality and the other with autoheterosexuality: a sexual attraction to being the other sex.

Autoheterosexuality is straight, turned inside out.

Sexually, this cross-gender attraction manifests as arousal at the thought or image of oneself as the other sex. And just like conventional heterosexuality, autoheterosexuality can lead to profoundly deep attachment—but instead of a romantic desire to be *with* people of the other sex, this erotic empathy drives a heartfelt longing to *be* the other sex in body, mind, behavior, presentation, or identity.

Autoheterosexual cross-gender identity can present as a private, internal way of seeing oneself, an everyday social reality, or something in between. It can also range from occasional to full time, or from mostly sexual to mostly romantic.

It's a truly dynamic orientation with great diversity among the people who have it, which is why autoheterosexuals may ultimately identify as *any* of the letters in the LGBTQ political coalition.

The cross-gender self is constructed through reinforcement over time. It can be so important and meaningful that autoheterosexuals decide to transition to another gender in order to live as a version of themselves that feels more vital and authentic than their original, default-gendered self.

Autoheterosexuals can experience good gender-related feelings when they sense they're embodying the other sex and bad gender-related feelings when they perceive a shortcoming in this embodiment. The desire to feel good gender feelings and avoid bad ones reinforces their cross-gender behavior, steadily nudging them across the gender divide.

These gender feelings predictably alter their sentiments and attitudes about gender. Their natal gender is discounted, while the other increases in value. At its most extreme, their natal gender becomes spiritually devoid of worth, while the other is exalted above all else. Eventually, existing in their natal gender can become absolutely meaningless or excruciating, and crossing over to the desired gender seems like the best path forward.

Only a subset of autoheterosexuals reach such an advanced state of cross-gender development, but the ones who do tend to transition either *medically* (by taking hormones or getting

ALLO**HETEROSEXUAL**
└─ "other" ─┘

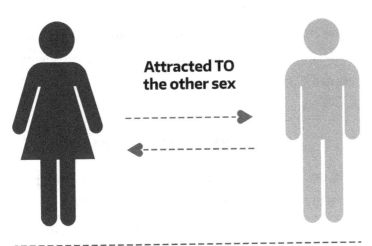

Attracted TO
the other sex

AUTOHETEROSEXUAL
└─ "self" ─┘

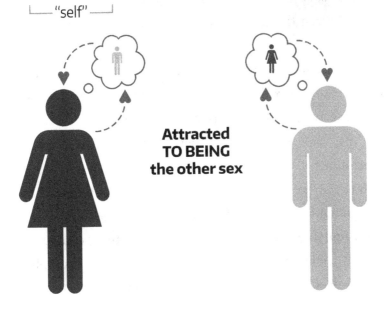

Attracted
TO BEING
the other sex

surgeries), *socially* (by changing their gender presentation, name, and pronouns), or through *identification* (identifying as another gender or as transgender).

Autoheterosexuals who medically transition may identify as *transsexual*, but it's more common for them to identify as *transgender*.

HOMOSEXUAL TRANSGENDERISM

To better understand autoheterosexual transgenderism, it's helpful to understand homosexual transgenderism. In brief, homosexual transgenderism comes about by the following process.

Males and females have different optimal mating strategies because reproduction requires far more effort from females than males, so evolution has led to physical and mental differences between the sexes that support these different reproductive strategies.

Human cultures generally have two gender categories that loosely fit these sex-based differences. People are often expected to behave within the norms of these gender categories, and they may face sanctions for deviating from these gendered expectations.

Many sex-based differences arise in the womb as part of the process that creates either females or males. The development of conventional sexual orientation is a part of this process, and as a result, some homosexuals have a cross-gender psychological shift associated with their sexual orientation.

In some cases, this cross-gender shift in traits can contribute to discomfort with their bodies or social roles, and they may decide that living as another gender will improve their quality of life.

In males, this type of transgenderism goes way back. Some scientists have even proposed that the ancestral form of male homosexuality was its transgendered form[1].

AUTOANDROPHILIA AND AUTOGYNEPHILIA

In the past few decades, sexologists have moved away from referring to trans people as "heterosexual" or "homosexual". Gender transition makes the meaning of these terms uncertain, and because they're anchored to sex rather than gender identity, some people consider them disrespectful. To bypass these issues, sexologists started to name the attractions themselves.

Attraction to adult males became *androphilia* ("love of men"). Attraction to adult females became *gynephilia* ("love of women"). Before transition or after transition, female or male, it didn't matter: the terms remained constant.

Due in part to this linguistic innovation, a sexologist named Ray Blanchard came up with a term for the attraction to being a woman that many of his male gender patients reported. He called it *autogynephilia* ("love of self as woman")[2].

"Auto" means "self"—for example, an airplane with autopilot is self-piloting.

Autogynephilia is a useful term for talking about male auto-heterosexuality. Likewise, *autoandrophilia* ("love of self as man") is a useful term for talking about female autoheterosexuality.

Both autogynephilia and autoandrophilia are *autosexual orientations*: enduring patterns of sexual or romantic self-attraction. Autosexual orientations can also be thought of as enduring patterns of attraction to particular types of embodiment, states of self, or ways of being.

TRANSGENDER DEMOGRAPHICS

Autoheterosexual preferences are about as prevalent as homosexual preferences, but culture influences how often either orientation leads to transgenderism.

Homosexual transgenderism tends to be more common in collectivistic countries. In contrast, autoheterosexual transgenderism is usually more common in Western, individualistic countries.

Thus, the relative prevalence of the two types is an indirect indicator of societal individualism. Societies in which autoheterosexual trans people can live openly as their cross-gender selves tend to be the same societies in which people have more freedom to chart their own course in life and live in alignment with their innermost feelings.

In the United States, about three out of four trans people are autoheterosexual.

SORTING THE TWO TYPES

The two-type model of transgenderism says that all—or virtually all—cases of transgenderism are ultimately caused by homosexuality or autoheterosexuality.

This cause is an *etiology* (pronounced "ee-tee-ology" or "eh-tee-ology"). In discussions of transgenderism, the two orientations that cause it are often referred to as *etiologies*. Get comfy with this word—it's an important one.

Within the two-type model, there is a sorting system known as the *two-type typology of transgenderism*. A typology is a way of classifying things into groups based on shared characteristics.

The two-type transgender typology sorts transgender people into groups based on whether their sexual orientations are homosexual or nonhomosexual with respect to their birth sex. Heterosexual, bisexual, and asexual trans people are all nonhomosexual, so they get sorted into the autoheterosexual group. Homosexual trans people get sorted into the homosexual etiology group. This way of sorting is useful, but it's not perfect.

Some autoheterosexuals only want same-sex partners or only report same-sex attraction, so this sorting method mistakenly sorts them into the homosexual group. And sometimes trans people who don't like the two-type typology will misrepresent their orientations because they don't want to be sorted into the autoheterosexual group.

This categorization system has proven reasonably effective for sorting male-to-female transsexuals, but it hasn't been researched much in female-to-male transsexuals. I anticipate that future research will confirm its utility in both sexes, but that differentiating between the two types will be a little fuzzier for female-to-male transsexuals.

The two-type typology is a powerful method for classifying trans people. It's fast, and with just the smallest scraps of information about them, it's possible to have a strong guess about which etiology they are.

KNOWLEDGE ABOUT AUTOHETEROSEXUALITY IS BEING ACTIVELY SUPPRESSED

Autoheterosexual orientations are about as common as homosexual orientations, but misinformed activists are preventing the public from learning about them. I'll describe a few of the most brazen examples to show what I mean.

At present, Wikipedia pages for "autogynephilia" and "autoandrophilia" don't even exist. Instead, they redirect[3] to "Blanchard's transsexualism typology"[4]—a misdirection that switches the focus away from these sexual orientations and toward a categorization system and a particular scientist instead.

It's not just the world's most influential source of knowledge that has this problem. These lies of omission are also found in the reference materials produced by and for medical professionals.

Thousands of clinicians with transgender patients rely upon the *Standards of Care* document[5] published by the World

Professional Association for Transgender Health, but autogynephilia and autoandrophilia aren't even mentioned in it.

In comparison, the American Psychiatric Association's *Diagnostic and Statistical Manual* does a better job of informing readers about transgenderism. To their credit, both the fifth edition of the DSM (DSM-5) and its text revision (DSM-5-TR) include a single reference to autogynephilia as a "predisposing factor" within the gender dysphoria chapter[6], and both describe developmental trajectories corresponding to the two known transgender etiologies.

Still, these two most recent editions of the DSM don't mention autoandrophilia at all, and one fleeting reference to autogynephilia is hardly enough to make it clear to autogynephilic readers that their sexual orientations are the ultimate source of their gender issues. The unwillingness to outright name the two known types of transgenderism also harms gender dysphoric homosexuals, who often don't realize they have a fundamentally different type of dysphoria.

There are other examples I could cite, but these are enough to show how thorough and pervasive the cover-up is. The appropriate Wikipedia pages don't exist, and professionals who work in transgender health care can't get straightforward information about the causes behind the conditions they are tasked with treating.

This precludes many clinicians from having even a basic, 101-level understanding of transgenderism. But even more importantly, it harms homosexuals and autoheterosexuals who want to accurately interpret their gender feelings and make informed decisions that will optimize their well-being.

This cover-up can't go on forever. It's time to end the lie.

ENDING THE COVER-UP: PRIORITIZING "IS" OVER "OUGHT"

There are a few main reasons for the widespread cover-up of autoheterosexuality:

* It contradicts many trans people's personal narratives about themselves

* It frames gender identity as a product of sexual orientation rather than an independent aspect of oneself, and it's anchored to sex rather than gender identity

* There is concern that if knowledge of autoheterosexuality becomes mainstream, trans people will face discrimination or not be regarded as the gender to which they aspire

These concerns are understandable, but prioritizing political considerations over truth privileges "ought" over "is".

In this book, I aim to describe what *is*. I want people to have mental models that correspond to reality so that they can make accurate predictions (i.e., whether or not they would benefit from gender transition).

I will sometimes suggest an "ought" that's grounded in my liberal humanist outlook. If your moral framework differs and you disagree, that's fine.

But take the two-type model seriously.

There is already ample evidence that homosexual transgenderism and autoheterosexual transgenderism exist in both sexes. The real question is whether there are more than these two main types, not whether multiple distinct types exist in the first place.

WHY THE CONCEPT OF AUTOHETEROSEXUALITY IS SO THREATENING

If someone's deepest, most heartfelt wish was to be the other sex, which of the following explanations for their gender feelings would feel more emotionally satisfying?

They want to be the other sex because:

1. In truth, they are actually more like the other sex in mind and spirit, but a mistake in development led them to have the wrong anatomy

2. They have an autosexual version of heterosexuality that makes them happier when they feel similar to the other sex or embody traits they associate with it

It's a no-brainer, right? The first one is obviously more emotionally satisfying.

This is why hearing about autoheterosexuality is so upsetting to many trans people. It suggests to them that their desire to be the other sex is ultimately because they are not that sex.

Furthermore, their drive to be the other sex comes from a type of heterosexuality—the least queer kind of sexuality.

The autoheterosexual explanation can undermine the hard-earned sense of identity they've painstakingly constructed over years. Many loathe the concepts of autoandrophilia and autogynephilia, as well as the two-type typology that categorizes them as autoheterosexual if they aren't solely same-sex attracted.

However, only a minority of autoheterosexuals transition to live as the other sex.

What about the rest of us? Don't we deserve a fair shot at making sense of our experiences?

WHY I WROTE THIS BOOK

Learning about autogynephilia and accepting that it described me was a pivotal moment in my life. It revealed the continuity between *so many* prior thoughts, feelings, and inclinations that I otherwise couldn't make sense of—things that sometimes made me feel uneasy, or even ashamed.

I finally knew why it hurt to be male and why I wished I were female.

I finally understood what the hell happened at that Lady Gaga concert back in 2013, when a powerful surge of feminine euphoria made me feel as though I had a female soul and left me with a lingering paranoia that I might be transgender.

It finally made sense why I immediately fell in love with hooping and came to dedicate thousands of hours to the art of hooping: the vast majority of hoopers are female. Although hoops are the best flow arts prop, it was their ability to signify femininity that likely kept me coming back (and why I could become sullen or irritable if there were gaps in my practice).

Once I understood myself as autogynephilic, I realized that no matter how hard I tried, my reasoning abilities would never fully extinguish my desire to be the other sex, because my cross-gender wish ultimately came from a sexual orientation. If gay people couldn't change their orientations, then I probably couldn't either.

Repression no longer made sense, so I switched over to wearing women's clothes full time. This seemingly simple change greatly improved my quality of life.

Now that I know *why* maleness can feel unsatisfying and meaningless, it hurts less. Just that change alone—knowing why—has done wonders for me.

I'd previously thought I was conventionally heterosexual, so the realization that I was a different kind of heterosexual was initially uncomfortable. Although it didn't feel nearly as jarring as it would have if I'd thought of myself as a woman, it still felt like a big adjustment at the time.

Prior to this realization, I worked in mechanical engineering. I had to wear men's clothes and sit in a cubicle under fluorescent lights, surrounded by men forty hours a week. I felt that I was dying physically, emotionally, and spiritually every day I was there. I hated it.

I learned about autogynephilia shortly after being laid off. My autistic ability to fixate on a "special interest" kicked into high gear, and I thought constantly about the science pertaining to autogynephilia.

I read most of the influential sexology writings on transgenderism from 1890 to the present day. I ultimately read many of these papers and books several times as I checked them against each other for coherence. I also closely analyzed first-person narratives and found that it didn't matter if the narratives were from the early 1900s or early 2000s—the same themes popped up again and again.

During this process, I found online communities where self-aware autoheterosexuals worked together to better understand our orientation. It was a massive relief to learn that I wasn't alone in pursuing this knowledge.

After roughly a year of full-time investigation, I realized that few people knew as much about autogynephilia as I did. I also realized there was systemic ignorance on the subject within the transgender community, and this ignorance was held in place by an unwritten rule which went something like this:

> You may not speak of autogynephilia, autoandrophilia, or the two-type transgender model in a way that treats them as relevant, accurate, or true.

It was obvious to me that this rule had to go: it prevented autoheterosexuals from fully understanding themselves, and this undermined their ability to give truly informed consent for gender-affirming medical interventions.

Over and over, I saw people recount their experiences in online trans spaces as part of their gender-questioning process, only to be told by transsexuals that what they were describing meant they were probably trans and should therefore transition.

They weren't told that their feelings indicated attraction to being the other sex, and that this sexuality was the most common cause of transgenderism. They weren't told that most people with this orientation don't transition.

I figured if autoheterosexual orientations were about as common as homosexual ones, there were *millions* of people out there privately grappling with confusing gender feelings like I had been. One-on-one interactions wouldn't be enough to reach them.

I needed an indestructible approach that could work on a massive scale.

I needed a book.

LANGUAGE CHOICES

In my first attempt at writing this book, I tried to dance around the imagined audience's gender identities. This corralled my thinking and stilted my language. It didn't work.

Eventually, I accepted that I was going to catch an immense amount of shit, and nothing could save me. People would lie about what I actually wrote, most without reading it. I was going to be insulted, berated, denigrated, canceled, hated, and dehumanized.

I was fucked either way.

This realization freed me to make several language choices that prioritize accuracy, clarity, and brevity.

Throughout this book, I will frequently use the terms "heterosexual", "homosexual", and their variants (i.e., "autoheterosexual", "nonheterosexual", "nonhomosexual"). **When I do this, I am talking about sexual orientation in relation to natal sex, *not* to gender identity.** I do this to be clear and concise, not to invalidate anyone's gender identity.

Although gender identity can change over time, sex is immutable. Humans can change some of their sex traits, but not sex itself. The binary and immutable nature of sex makes it the only stable point of reference for terms like "homosexual" and "autoheterosexual" which define sexuality in relation to the self.

These terms are also needed to explain the two types of transgenderism succinctly. Without them, it takes four comparatively awkward terms to describe the different types of transgenderism.

Since the terms "autoheterosexual" and "autoheterosexuality" are so long and occur so frequently, I will sometimes shorten them to "autohet" to increase readability. Likewise, I will sometimes shorten "autoheterosexuals" to "autohets".

I will refer to the gender associated with someone's sex as their *default* gender[7]. By contrast, the gender that doesn't match their sex will be their *cross* gender. Autoheterosexuals tend to have a default-gender self and a cross-gender self that coexist in an internal union, so it's important to have a name for both of these sides. Additionally, when I speak of something as "gender-affirming", I am specifically referring to affirmation of the cross-gender identity.

I will frequently call upon first-person narratives to demonstrate aspects of autoheterosexuality. Most of the people in these narratives are dead or otherwise inaccessible, so I can't be sure of their preferred pronouns. I will default to honoring their cross-gender self with corresponding pronouns.

Although autoheterosexuality is an atypical form of sexuality, I will never call it a "fetish" or "kink". I strongly recommend against using terms like these when speaking of autoheterosexuality. By conjuring up a narrow image of autoheterosexuality that is restricted to matters of eroticism, these terms fail to capture the true breadth of the autohet experience and its emotional significance to autoheterosexuals.

Instead, I refer to autoheterosexuality as a "sexual orientation" or simply an "orientation". This terminology acknowledges its sexual nature while implicitly recognizing its emotional and sentimental side, which runs deep.

I will often refer to individuals on the male-to-female spectrum as "MTF" or "transfem", and to individuals on the female-to-male spectrum as "FTM" or "transmasc". I use these terms in a broad sense. I'm not here to police who counts as "legitimately trans" based on their identity or state of gender transition.

To stay out of the category war over "woman" and "man", I'll often use "female" and "male" instead. I'll use "female" or "male" instead of "natal female" or "natal male" because they transmit exactly the same information.

I also won't be using phrases like "assigned female", "assigned female at birth", "AFAB", or their male equivalents. These bullshit obfuscations aim to bring biological sex into the realm of social construction, a place it simply doesn't belong.

Biological sex, which I will usually just call "sex", has been around for over a billion years[8]. It exists regardless of how we think, feel, or speak about it. Sex is not a social construction and never has been.

In this book, I aim to characterize a sexual orientation that millions of people have. There is considerable diversity within this group of people, so many things I say will only apply to a subset of them. This fact requires that I frequently hedge my statements with qualifiers such as "many", "tends to", "usually", "often", and "can". Interpret these qualifiers as acknowledgments of diversity.

Lastly, I want to mention a couple unconventional grammar choices I made. Periods mark the boundaries between sentences, so citation superscripts will usually come before the concluding period and fall within the sentence to which they apply. Quotation marks also act as boundaries, so punctuation which is not part of a quote will fall outside of the quoted region.

ARE YOU AUTOHETEROSEXUAL?

Autoheterosexuality has a spectrum of intensity. On the extreme end, it can be so intense that someone isn't even attracted to other people. However, it's most common for it to be mild or moderate in its intensity.

I'm going to present some feelings, thoughts, and experiences that are common in autoheterosexuals, so you can quickly estimate whether you're autoheterosexual—and if so, to what degree.

These aren't exhaustive. They are just a starting point for introspection.

Do you relate to any of these positive gender-related experiences?

* It's comforting when you dress as the other sex—it just feels right. In that clothing, you feel relaxed, excited, or at peace with yourself.

* It's emotionally reassuring or pleasurable to position or move your body in a way that reminds you of the other sex.

* Your heterosexuality directs you toward men with feminine traits or women with masculine traits. These traits may be either mental or physical.

* You long to be "one of the ladies" or "one of the guys". When you socialize in groups of the other sex, it's emotionally rewarding. When they treat you as one of them, it means the world to you. You cherish those validating moments, and they stand out in your memory.

* Your feelings about this cross-gender side of yourself are significant and meaningful. You treasure the positive feelings; they feel like love.

Have you experienced any of these negative gender-related feelings?

* Your physique is normal for your sex, so you feel that your body parts are in the wrong place or just plain wrong. Some body parts are missing. Others you wish were missing.

* Any tissue or physical feature that differs between the sexes can bring displeasure or disconnection. Your bones are the wrong size, the wrong shape. Your fat collects in all the wrong places. Your face and voice feel alien.

* You're disappointed in your appearance because you measure yourself by the standards of the other sex.

* You envy the other sex and sometimes wish you were born that way.

* You resent the social pressure to wear gender-typical clothing or behave a certain way because of your sex.

* You don't like that others see you as your birth sex.

* You feel that it would be easier to relate to yourself, care about yourself, or find meaning in life if you were the other sex.

* You feel that life would be better if you were the other sex. You wish you were born that way.

* If you could press a button and permanently change sex, you would press it without hesitation.

Are any of these relatable?

If so, it doesn't necessarily mean you're autoheterosexual. But these kinds of feelings are common among autoheterosexuals, so if many of them resonate with you, it's worth further introspection.

Now, let's look at some sexual signs of autoheterosexuality. Have you ever had any of these sexual experiences?

* You have become aroused after wearing clothing associated with the other sex.

* During sexual fantasies, you have seen yourself as the other sex or with physical features of the other sex.

* You have fantasized about playing a cross-gender sex role with someone of your sex (i.e., playing a man's sexual role with a woman, or playing a woman's sexual role with a man).

* You have become aroused by being treated as the other sex.

* You have imagined yourself with physical features of the other sex and become aroused.

* You have become aroused after imagining you had the bodily functions of the other sex (i.e., ejaculation, erection, menstruation, or lactation).

* You have switched sex roles during heterosexual sex and found it preferable or especially arousing.

These are all manifestations of autoheterosexuality.

If you've repeatedly had any of these sexual experiences, it's worth considering the degree to which you are autoheterosexual. If erotic cross-gender embodiment is your primary source of sexual arousal, then you are autoheterosexual.

The best way to accurately determine if you are autoheterosexual is to try various forms of cross-gender embodiment in private to see if arousal happens. This is most commonly done through dressing in clothing associated with the other sex (crossdressing) or imagining oneself as the other sex or another gender (*crossdreaming*[9]).

AUTOHETEROSEXUAL READERS: STAY CALM. THINK.

This book proposes a model of transgenderism that is drastically different from the mainstream one.

If you are transgender, it may drastically change your personal narrative about who or what you are and how you came to be that way.

Don't jump to making drastic life changes.

If you have already socially or medically transitioned, stay that way for now. If you haven't transitioned yet, don't rush into it.

Give yourself time to think things through. Don't freak out. It'll be okay.

It's okay to be autoandrophilic or autogynephilic. What you choose to do about your sexual orientation or gender situation is up to you. There is no one right way to do it.

There's also no way to be 100% certain of the best way forward, but if you become informed about autoheterosexuality and give yourself time to think, you increase the odds that your decisions will be the right ones for you.

AUTOHETEROSEXUAL EMBODIMENT SUBTYPES

Autoheterosexuality isn't just one thing. It's complex. It has many aspects.

Research findings suggest that male autoheterosexuality has five known embodiment subtypes[10]. Formal research hasn't yet tested whether females have them as well, but I'll treat them as if they do.

Two of these subtypes concern *bodies* and *bodily functions*. The other three pertain to *clothing*, *behavior*, and *social interactions*:

* *Anatomic*—having the other sex's body or its features
* *Physiologic*—having the bodily functions of the other sex
* *Sartorial*—dressing as the other sex
* *Behavioral*—behaving as the other sex
* *Interpersonal*—socially being the other sex

Autoheterosexuals derive comfort, meaning, or arousal from embodying these aspects of the other sex.

Any given autohet individual may have just one of these subtypes or all of them. Each drives different aspects of cross-gender embodiment. This embodiment operates through association.

Based on their life experience, everyone has their own set of ideas and associations about the other sex. Sometimes these associations align with stereotypes, but that's because stereotypes are often accurate[11].

For autohets, the behavioral and sartorial subtypes of autoheterosexuality are the most attainable aspects of cross-gender embodiment. The interpersonal and anatomic subtypes of autoheterosexuality are most successfully embodied through medical interventions such as hormones or surgeries, so they are bigger contributors to autohet transsexualism.

Autohet transsexualism is also motivated by *core autoheterosexuality*: attraction to the idea of being the other sex. Although it's not technically a subtype, it's useful to have a name for this stripped-down, core essence of autoheterosexuality.

Countless autoheterosexuals have prayed to God or blown out birthday candles with a wish to change sex. Many have fallen in love with this beautiful idea and thought, *I want to be a man* or *I want to be a woman* so often that it left deep grooves in the wagon ruts of their minds.

Although these autohet subtypes are conceptually distinct, in practice they tend to merge into one unified cross-gender expression.

Sartorial Autoheterosexuality

For many autoheterosexuals, sartorial embodiment is the most accessible form of cross-gender embodiment. "Sartorial" means "of or relating to clothing".

Through wearing clothing associated with the other sex, autoheterosexuals symbolically evoke the idea of being that sex. Different clothing articles symbolize different aspects of anatomy.

For autohet females, wearing a jockstrap evokes the idea of having male genitals, and wearing a binder evokes the idea of having a flat, male-typical chest.

For autohet males, wearing a bra evokes the idea of having female breasts, and wearing women's underwear evokes the idea of having female genitals.

Although each piece of clothing can evoke the idea of being the other sex on its own, wearing a complete cross-gender outfit is the most thorough way of doing so.

Traditionally, sartorial autoheterosexuality has been called "transvestism" or "crossdressing". However, these labels can be confusing when describing post-transition autoheterosexuals, and they are completely unfit for describing the cisvestism of *autohomosexuals* (people who are attracted to being their own sex).

To get around these issues, I decided to introduce language that isn't anchored to sex. This brings it in line with the other subtype descriptors, none of which reference sex.

Psyche Autoheterosexuality

Some autoheterosexuals embody the other sex through their state of consciousness. This *psyche autoheterosexuality* is about having the consciousness of the other sex.

Psyche autoheterosexuality creates a tangible feeling of cross-gender identity—a sensation of looking through the eyes of the other sex and having their thoughts, feelings, perceptions, or sensations. Some feel it as a cross-gender soul that dwells inside them.

This compelling, beautiful feeling is a *mental shift*.

At first, mental shifts are transient. Through repetition, mental shifts happen more often and last longer when they do. For some autoheterosexuals, this feeling becomes a permanent feature of their everyday consciousness, which is a form of cross-gender identity.

Cross-gender embodiment can trigger mental shifts, and mental shifts can motivate further cross-gender embodiment. Each reinforces and encourages the other.

Dressing or behaving as the other sex are the most accessible forms of cross-gender embodiment, so they often trigger an autohet person's first mental shifts. Over time, some autoheterosexuals learn how to access the feeling of a mental shift directly, without the need for external triggers.

I suspect that psyche autoheterosexuality is a distinct subtype of autoheterosexuality, but it hasn't been empirically studied yet.

PARTNER PREFERENCES AND META-ATTRACTION

Autoheterosexuals can sexually prefer to be with females, males, both, or neither.

Most autohets are attracted to the other sex. However, their desire for cross-gender embodiment increases their attraction to people of the same sex, as well as people of the other sex who have gender-atypical traits.

Perceiving these attributes in sexual partners helps an autoheterosexual person cultivate a sense of cross-gender embodiment through contrast. When autoheterosexuals are more attracted to someone because that person's traits strengthen a feeling of cross-gender embodiment, it's called *meta-attraction*.

Meta-attraction makes feminine males and masculine women more attractive. Partnering with a feminine man makes it easier for an autoandrophilic female to feel like a man. Alongside a masculine woman, it's easier for an autogynephilic male to feel like a woman.

This attraction through contrast also fuels desire for same-sex partners. This gender-affirming same-sex attraction is *meta-homosexuality*.

With a same-sex partner, autoheterosexuals can play a cross-gender sex role: autoandrophilic females can be a man with a woman, and autogynephilic males can be a woman with a man.

Much of the same-sex behavior seen among autoheterosexuals ultimately originates in meta-homosexuality.

The existence of meta-homosexuality means that some pre-transition autohets are part of the homosexual community. In these instances, autohet males are likely to play a submissive, receptive sex role, and autohet females are likely to play a dominant, assertive sex role.

Post-transition autohets also participate in the homosexual community as gay trans men and trans lesbians. Because these autohets are attracted both *to* the other sex and *to being* the other sex, their heterosexuality is directed *both* externally and internally. Thus, they are *ambiheterosexual* ("ambi" means "both").

Autoheterosexuals who experience meta-attraction to people of the same sex often identify as bisexual. It's common for these autoheterosexuals to be behaviorally bisexual, yet romantically heterosexual.

Autoheterosexuals are often attracted to feminized males or masculinized females. This attraction to people with mixed gender traits is another source of their bisexuality.

Some autohets aren't attracted to other people at all. In theory, this is because their autosexuality is such a big proportion of their sexuality that it overpowers their allosexuality. Autohets like this may identify as asexual.

Altogether, autoheterosexuals vary widely in their sexual partner preferences. They may desire other-sex partners, or they may not. They may desire same-sex partners, or they may not. It all depends on the individual. Therefore, autohets can be behaviorally heterosexual, homosexual, bisexual, or asexual.

Due to this variation in partner choice and their propensity for gender transition, autoheterosexuals can fall anywhere within the LGBTQ political coalition.

SIMPLIFYING THE LGBTQ ALPHABET SOUP: NONHET AND AUTOHET

The LGBTQ coalition is simpler than it seems at first glance.

Most of its members are homosexual, bisexual, or autoheterosexual: they exhibit same-sex sexuality or cross-gender sexuality. In other words, they are nonheterosexual or autoheterosexual (nonhet or autohet).

The "L" and "G" are about preferential same-sex attraction (homosexuality). Preferential homosexuality is usually caused by inborn attraction to the same sex, but it can also be caused by the meta-homosexuality that some autoheterosexuals have.

Of all the letters in the rainbow coalition, the "B" is the most complex. Bisexuality has many causes and manifestations[12]. Bisexual behavior can be caused by attraction to both sexes, meta-homosexuality, attraction to androgyny, an uninhibited disposition toward sexuality, life circumstances, a lack of strict sexual preferences, or other factors. It's unknown exactly how many types of bisexuality there are.

The "T" is about transgenderism. To reiterate, there are two known types: homosexual and autoheterosexual.

The "Q" represents *queer*—an umbrella term for sexualities that fall outside of heterosexual attraction to others (alloheterosexuality). Thus, queer simply means *nonalloheterosexual.* *Queer* is an intentionally ambiguous label indicating that someone belongs within the rainbow coalition, but it doesn't specify where. However, queer-identified people are usually homosexual, bisexual, or autoheterosexual.

Seen in this way, the gender-based, mainstream segment of the political movement for sexual and gender minority rights is simpler than the vast array of letters seemingly implies.

It can be collapsed down to three categories: homosexual, bisexual, and autoheterosexual. Since the former two are both nonheterosexual forms of sexuality, these three categories can be whittled down to just two gender-based sexual proclivities: non-heterosexuality and autoheterosexuality (nonhet and autohet).

WHY "AUTOHETEROSEXUAL"?

Because it's accurate. *Autoheterosexual* describes attraction to self as the other sex. It's simply the right word for the job.

Its abbreviated form, *autohet*, is also short and easy to say.

The autoheterosexual concept is efficient: it packs female autoandrophilia and male autogynephilia into one word. Both rest on equal footing under the autoheterosexual umbrella, giving autoandrophilia the long-overdue recognition it deserves as the female counterpart to male autogynephilia.

Much how lesbians and gay males know they're homosexual, the concept of autoheterosexuality will let autoandrophilic females and autogynephilic males know they're autoheterosexual.

The current conceptual landscape provides ample habitat for the concept of autoheterosexuality to thrive. The adjacent idea of heterosexuality is already firmly etched into people's brains, providing fertile ground in which the autohet concept can take root, welcomed in by familiarity and held in place by association.

Another reason to use *autoheterosexual* is to minimize potential political backlash against trans people after the two-type model enters mainstream awareness. The vast majority of people are heterosexual, so describing attraction to being the other sex as *autoheterosexual* makes it as relatable as possible, to as many people as possible. No orientation is more normalized, acceptable, and mainstream than heterosexuality.

Most people also understand that heterosexuality isn't just about sexual intercourse with someone of the other sex. It's also about companionship, love, family, joy, and all else that flows downstream of that initial sexual spark. Heterosexuality is a source of meaning and guidance that radically alters someone's life path. It's *important*.

Sexuality and romance both play a central role in the emotional well-being of heterosexuals, and heterosexuality is absolutely fundamental to the way they think. The idea of autoheterosexuality allows heterosexuals to understand—as best they can—that some people have the same sort of strong feelings about *being* the other gender that they have *toward* the other gender.

This relatability will prove essential when autoheterosexuality goes mainstream and people inevitably deride it as a "kink" or "fetish" in their political war against transgender people. Accurately describing it as a type of heterosexuality offers the strongest defense against these familiar, sex-negative attacks on legitimacy.

The idea of autoheterosexuality also prepares people to comprehend the two-type model of transgenderism. The general public already knows that homosexual transgenderism exists, even if they don't always have a name for it. Once they understand autoheterosexuality and its associated form of transgenderism, a model of transgenderism with two or more distinct types becomes implicit. They'll *get it*.

The decision to use *autoheterosexual* is also an aesthetic one: *autogynephilia* and *autoandrophilia* both have subpar mouthfeel. These clinical-sounding, awkward terms are often hard for people to remember or say.

Aesthetics matter. Neuroscientist Simon LeVay once proclaimed, "The day someone insists on a friendlier-sounding term than 'autogynephile' will be the day another sexual minority claims a place at the table"[13].

Autoheterosexuals, pull up a chair.

That day has arrived.

SEX, GENDER, AND TRANSGENDER

SETTING THE CONTEXT

It's important to set the context before diving into the specifics of autoheterosexuality. I'll start with sex, without which we wouldn't exist.

Sex, or *biological sex*, is a system of reproduction that combines genes from two different organisms to create a new organism. The genes that each parent contributes are contained in specialized cells called *gametes* (pronounced "gam-eets").

Each gamete contributes half of the genetic information needed to make a new organism. When female and male gametes merge, they create a full genome containing traits from both parents.

Before sexual reproduction appeared, most organisms reproduced asexually by cloning themselves. When sexual reproduction first came about, gametes tended to be the same size. With time, the size of gametes diverged. One type grew larger, and the other smaller.

In mammals, sexually reproducing species have a stable two-type gamete configuration. One is small, numerous, and mobile. The other is large, few in number, and immobile.

The large gametes are optimized to survive after being fertilized. In humans and other mammals, these gametes are called *ova*, or eggs. The sex that makes them is *female*.

The small gametes are optimized to find and fertilize as many of the large gametes as possible. This is why they are small, mobile, and created by the millions. In humans and other mammals, these are called *sperm*. The sex that makes them is *male*.

The size difference between female gametes and male gametes has had enormous repercussions. It's why each sex has a different optimal mating strategy and why most animal species have two different forms based upon sex—a tendency known as *sexual dimorphism*.

Eggs and pregnancies take far more energy to create and maintain than do sperm, so females usually devote more resources toward offspring and are more discerning about who they choose to mate with. For human females, reproduction takes years: nine months of pregnancy and a potentially fatal childbirth, followed by a few years of breastfeeding until the child is weaned off breast milk.

By contrast, males often try to mate with as many females as possible because successful reproduction requires as little as a few *minutes* of effort on their part.

This unequal reproductive effort has left enormous impacts on our sexual psychology. It is why males are more likely to coerce females into sex[1]. It's also why stereotypical males will fuck anything that moves, and stereotypical females will carefully assess their options to see if any meet their standards.

Even though there are plenty of exceptions we could point to, this sexual dynamic in animals is common and it ultimately arose because gametes are different sizes. These size differences are also why animals have different female and male forms.

In humans there are two types of gametes, sperm and egg, so humans have two sexes. People whose bodies developed the type of parts that make and deliver sperm are male. People who developed the types of parts that release eggs are female.

Sperm are created in the testes, and they exit the body through the penis. People who developed testes and a penis are male.

Eggs develop in the ovaries. If an egg is fertilized by a sperm, it starts becoming an embryo and may attach to the lining of the uterus. People who developed ovaries and a uterus are female.

Genitals are highly reliable indicators of a person's sex. Someone with a penis is almost certainly male. Someone with a vulva is almost certainly female.

It's uncommon, but a person can possess ambiguous genitalia at birth that make it harder to discern their sex. Someone like this has historically been called *intersex* because they have sex traits that don't fit binary notions of female or male.

These variations of sexual development are also called *disorders of sexual development* (DSDs)[2]. Depending on how DSDs are defined, somewhere between 0.0018%[3] and 1.7%[4] of people have them.

The fact that DSDs and intersex people exist doesn't mean sex is a spectrum. Sex is a system of biological reproduction based on gametes. In humans, only sperm and egg exist. There is no third type of gamete, so there are only two sexes.

Intersex people don't create a third type of gamete, so they are not a third sex. Treating intersex people as an intermediary (or third) sex conflates sex traits with sex itself.

GENDER

Gender is the social, cultural, and psychological domain of sex. Gender comes from the interaction between sex and culture. If biological sex didn't exist, neither would gender.

Gender can be masculine, feminine, or somewhere in between.

Masculine describes maleness: qualities traditionally associated with males.

Feminine describes femaleness: qualities traditionally associated with females.

Therefore, *gender* describes sexness: qualities traditionally associated with a particular sex.

Depending on the context, *gender* can describe our identities, expressions, social roles, or psychological traits as they pertain to masculinity and femininity. It is how we see ourselves and each other based on the masculinity or femininity of our appearances, behaviors, personalities, and social roles.

Sex existed long before culture. Once human culture came into existence, so did gender.

Gender continually evolves in tandem with culture. It impacts how we see ourselves, how we express ourselves, and the social role we are expected to perform.

Gender identity is a sense of ourselves as masculine, feminine, in between the two, or somewhere outside the gender binary.

Gender expression is how we outwardly embody masculinity and femininity through our appearance or behavior. It's often an external expression of an inner gender identity.

Gender role is a social role associated with either males or females. Almost every culture has a set of expectations and allowable behaviors for people based on whether they are, or appear to be, female or male. The specific aspects of these gender roles vary across cultures.

Sometimes a person's gender identity, preferred gender expression, desired anatomy, or desired gender role are in conflict with their biological sex. Someone like this may develop *gender issues*: a continuous underlying liability toward preference for gender transition[5]. If their gender issues are strong enough, they may transition to a gender that aligns with their nature.

People like this are often called "transgender".

TRANSGENDER

There is no single definition of *transgender* that everyone will agree upon, but there are two criteria frequently used to determine inclusion in the category: *identity* or *transition*.

In the *identity* definition, people are transgender if they identify as transgender, or if they identify as a gender that doesn't correspond to their sex. In the *transition* definition of *transgender*, people are transgender if they transition to live as a gender that doesn't correspond to their sex.

Transition usually indicates either social or medical transition. *Social transition* is when someone changes their name, pronouns, or stated gender identity and starts to live as a gender that doesn't correspond to their sex. *Medical transition* is when someone takes hormones or undergoes surgeries to more closely resemble the other sex (transsexualism).

Desistance is when someone intends to transition but ultimately decides against it before transitioning. People who have done this are *desisters*.

Detransition is when someone who has socially or medically transitioned decides to socially or medically revert to living as their birth sex. People who have done this are *detransitioners*.

When someone identifies as *nonbinary*, they consider themselves to be both masculine and feminine, somewhere between the two, or somewhere outside the masculine–feminine binary altogether. The *genderqueer* identity label has a similar meaning.

Nonbinary is sometimes abbreviated "NB", which is commonly written out as "enby". "Enby" can describe either the nonbinary identity itself or the people who claim it. Enbies often use they/them pronouns. Most enbies are female[6].

Enbies typically have a lesser degree of gender issues than people with binary transgender identities. However, some people identify as both nonbinary and transgender.

WHAT IS A WOMAN? WHAT IS A MAN?

The terms "woman" and "man" have historically been used to describe someone's sex, albeit indirectly.

If someone looked like a woman or had a vulva, they were a woman. If someone looked like a man or had a penis, they were a man.

Recently, awareness of transgenderism and feminism has increased. People have begun to place more significance on gender and less on sex.

The words "woman" and "man" are increasingly used to describe someone's gender role, gender expression, or gender identity, rather than their biological sex. For instance, some young males are told to "man up" when they cry. This usage of "man" is describing a set of behaviors and expectations associated with the male sex, not anatomy itself.

In domains where physical differences between the sexes are the most relevant factor, "woman" and "man" usually denote sex. One prominent example is competitive sports, because male puberty confers many permanent physical changes that improve athletic performance.

Most people continue to use the sex-based definitions of "woman" and "man". In these classic definitions, a man is an adult human male, and a woman is an adult human female.

However, people with gender-based definitions of "woman" and "man" have different criteria for belonging to these categories. They may decide that another person is a "woman" or "man" if they identify as one (identity criteria), live as one (social/medical transition criteria), or appear to be one (passing criteria). These criteria can be used alone or in combination with one another.

Because of these widely varying definitions of "woman" and "man", people often disagree about whether transgender men are men or transgender women are women.

A *transgender man,* or *trans man,* is someone who was born female and 1) identifies as a man (identity criteria); 2) has socially transitioned to live as a man (social transition criteria); or 3) has undergone medical interventions to have a more male-typical appearance (medical transition criteria).

A *transgender woman,* or *trans woman,* is someone who was born male and 1) identifies as a woman (identity criteria); 2) has socially transitioned to live as a woman (social transition criteria); or 3) has undergone medical interventions to have a more female-typical appearance (medical transition criteria).

If a trans person has undergone gender-affirming medical interventions, they can be fairly described as *transsexual.*

Transsexualism is the use of medical interventions to make a person more closely resemble the other sex.

Whether or not people agree that "trans men are men" or "trans women are women" generally comes down to the definitions they use. People who use sex-based definitions tend to think these claims are false, while those who use gender-based definitions tend to think these claims are true.

IN SUM

* Sex is a system of reproduction that combines genetic information from specialized cells—gametes—to create a new organism. The small gametes are known as sperm, and the large gametes are known as ova, or eggs.

* Because each sex has a different optimal mating strategy, evolution has left each sex with different physical and mental traits that correspond to these respective mating strategies. This difference in traits between females and males is known as sexual dimorphism.

* In humans and other mammals, an individual's sex is determined based on whether their bodies developed to produce sperm (male) or eggs (female). Sometimes, a disorder of sexual development makes it hard to discern an individual's sex, but since there are only two

types of gametes and sex is based on gametes, there are still only two sexes.

* In contrast to sex—which refers to female and male—gender refers to femaleness (femininity) and maleness (masculinity). Thus, gender is sexness. Gender is the social, cultural, and psychological domain of sex. It comes from the interaction between sexual dimorphism and human culture. Each culture has gender roles—a set of expectations and condoned behaviors based on whether someone is a woman or a man.

* Transgender people identify as or choose to live as a gender that doesn't correspond to their sex. They may do this through identification, social transition, medical transition, or any combination of these.

SEXUAL ORIENTATION
ENDURING PATTERNS OF ATTRACTION

Many animals have something inside them that compels them to mate with others of their species. This inner drive motivates them to get closer to the object of their affection, court them, and make sexual contact with them.

This motivating force is *sexual orientation*, and it plays a key role in uniting sperm and egg. Without it, the two might never find each other. The most common sexual orientations are *allosexual orientations*, meaning they involve attraction to others ("allo" means "other").

The American Psychological Association has defined sexual orientation as "one's enduring sexual attraction to male partners, female partners, or both"[1]. Likewise, some sexologists have defined it as "relative sexual attraction to men, to women, or to both"[2].

This is the mainstream definition of sexual orientation. When asked about their sexual orientation, most people talk about their attraction to men or women.

The DSM-5 and DSM-5-TR both classify this pattern of attraction as "normophilic", defining it as "sexual interest in genital stimulation or preparatory fondling with phenotypically normal, physically mature, consenting human partners"[3]. It's what most people call "normal", or "vanilla".

But the vast majority of existing sexual orientations are a flavor other than vanilla. When these nonvanilla sexual orientations rival or outshine someone's vanilla side, they fall under the heading of *paraphilia*[4]. "Para-" is a Greek root with many meanings, some of which are "alongside of", "beside", "near", "resembling", "beyond", and "apart from".

These sexual interests are sometimes described as "kinks" or "fetishes", but I won't be using those terms here. Designating a sexual interest as a "kink" or "fetish" makes it seem lesser—less important, less worthy of respect, and less significant overall. This limited erotic framing also underemphasizes the pivotal role that sexuality plays in our emotional lives.

For most people, the object of their affection is an adult human of the other sex. This often leads to love, marriage, and kids, and keeps our species going by starting the cycle anew. But who can say that people with other sexual interests aren't equally justified in pursuing their form of love, provided it doesn't harm others?

Describing the most common forms of love as "sexual orientations" and less common forms of love as "paraphilias" elevates certain sexualities over others in a way that doesn't necessarily apply to our individual lives. When deciding who we are as sexual beings and how we want to structure our lives to accommodate our sexualities, the relative strengths of our various sexual interests often matter more than how common they are.

Therefore, I will use everyday language that makes the same fundamental distinction between "normal" sexuality and all that falls outside of it. Sexuality based on attraction to women, men, or both will be *vanilla*, and everything else will be *nonvanilla*.

I'll also use broad terms that apply no matter what someone is into:

* Sexual interest—a sexually motivated interest in a particular type of entity, embodiment, or method of interaction

* *Sexual orientation*—an enduring pattern of preferential sexual or romantic interest in a particular type of entity, embodiment, or method of interaction

People can be sexually oriented toward other beings based on sex, gender, race, age, health, species, or other attributes. Some are even attracted to nonliving objects[5]. Although some of these types of attraction are uncommon, they are why I use the broad term "entity" in this definition of sexual orientation.

I'm not alone in thinking that the definition of sexual orientation could be broadened. Sexologist Michael Seto proposed a broader conception of sexual orientation, which he defined as "a stable tendency to preferentially orient—in terms of attention, interest, attraction, and genital arousal—to particular classes of sexual stimuli"[6].

These broader definitions of sexual orientation include the elements of *preference* (preferring one thing over other things), *persistence* (stability over time), and an *erotic target* (the type of thing that draws a person's sexual interest).

In short, sexual orientation is a stable sexual preference for particular types of things.

MEASURING SEXUAL ORIENTATION

There is no one perfect way to measure sexual orientation.

If a sexologist is trying to measure someone's sexual preferences, they have two main approaches: they can either ask questions or see how bodies react to stimuli[7].

When conducting such research, they measure up to four aspects of sexual orientation:

1. What a person is attracted to (*sexual attraction*)
2. How they see themselves sexually (*sexual identity*)
3. How they behave sexually (*sexual behavior*)
4. Whether there are signs of physical arousal after exposure to erotic stimuli (*physiologic arousal*)

The first three are measured by asking questions. The last one requires a lab setup, trained technicians, and a lot of man-hours. This is why sexologists usually just ask questions—it's easier, cheaper, and faster.

But relying on self-reports depends on people knowing themselves well and having nothing to hide. A lot of people are uncomfortable with sex in general, so this approach has obvious flaws.

Some people have a tendency to say what they think will portray themselves in a flattering light. This *social desirability bias* can affect how they report on their experience and make the data less accurate than it would otherwise be.

Measuring how people's bodies respond to erotic pictures and videos is important because it's less affected by how well they know themselves or how they want to portray themselves.

Consider the hypothetical situation of a man who arrives at a sexual research facility to get his arousal patterns tested. He says he is only attracted to women, has only been with them, and is heterosexual. But when his genital arousal is measured, his strongest response is to porn depicting men, and he barely responds to porn depicting women.

Based on his self-reported sexual behavior, sexual attraction, and sexual identity, he's straight. But based on his physical arousal pattern, he's gay.

What would you say his sexual orientation is? Is he a straight man who just happens to get most strongly aroused from looking at men, or is he *actually gay*?

I think he's gay, and I suspect this interpretation is common. People often interpret physical arousal as a fairly clear-cut sign of what someone is into. (By the way, this hypothetical scenario wasn't actually hypothetical: it happens sometimes[8]).

This shows one of the pitfalls of relying solely on self-reports when measuring sexual orientation: The way we portray ourselves doesn't always match reality. Sometimes we are wrong about ourselves.

SEXUAL ORIENTATION AND HORMONAL EXPOSURE

Genes and hormone exposure in utero both affect the vanilla sexual orientation that people are likely to have.

The most compelling explanation, the *organizational hypothesis*[9], is that hormonal exposure during critical developmental periods influences the sexual differentiation process.

During human fetal development, males and females experience different levels of testosterone[10]. Males have testes that release testosterone, promoting growth of male genitalia. Females lack testes, so they're exposed to much less testosterone and usually develop female-typical genitalia as a result.

Females and males have different average psychologies[11]. Since hormones influence the sexual differentiation process, hormonal exposure in the womb can shift people's gendered psychology in male-typical or female-typical directions. This shift includes sexual orientation, which is why males tend to be masculine and attracted to women, while females tend to be feminine and attracted to men.

Since sexual orientation and gendered psychological traits tend to develop in tandem, homosexuality is associated with a cross-gender shift in mental traits[12]. On average, homosexual males are more feminine than heterosexual males, and homosexual females are more masculine than heterosexual females[13].

The cross-gender psychological shift associated with homosexuality shows up in childhood behavior, self-rated masculinity and femininity, occupation preferences, and many mental traits[14]. It even shows up in brain structure[15].

The influence of hormones seems to extend to nonvanilla sexualities as well. Most nonvanilla sexual interests are consistently found more often in males[16], which suggests that masculinization is associated with the development of nonvanilla sexual orientations such as autoheterosexuality.

EASIER TO DIFFERENTIATE THE TWO TYPES OF MTFS

By combining these observations that attractions to women and nonvanilla sexualities both seem to be associated with masculinization, it's possible to infer that it can be harder to tell apart the two types of FTMs than the two types of MTFS.

To show what I mean, I'll put a "+" or "-" in parentheses beside traits to indicate positive or negative associations with masculinization:

* Homosexual females are attracted to women (+)
* Autoandrophilic females have an attraction to men (-)
  that is autosexual and therefore nonvanilla (+)

From these associations, we can expect that autoandrophilic females will tend to have an intermediate degree of masculinization which exceeds that of heterosexual females yet falls short of homosexual females.

The situation in males is more straightforward:

* Homosexual males are attracted to men (-)
* Autogynephilic males have an attraction to women (+) that is autosexual and therefore nonvanilla (+)

It follows that we can expect autogynephilic males to usually be about as masculine as typical heterosexual males, or even a bit more so. By contrast, we can expect homosexual males to usually be noticeably more feminine in comparison.

Combining these observations, it seems that the sexualities underlying both types of MTF transgenderism differ far more in terms of associated masculinization than do the sexualities underlying both types of FTM transgenderism. Therefore, it will generally be easier to tell apart the two types of MTFs than the two types of FTMs.

FRATERNAL BIRTH ORDER EFFECT

In addition to genes and hormones, male homosexuality is also affected by birth order. The more older brothers a male has, the more likely that male is to be gay—a phenomenon known as the *fraternal birth order effect* (FBOE).

The FBOE is also particularly associated with gender-atypical homosexuality: feminine homosexual males tend to have more older brothers than masculine homosexual males[17].

The leading explanation for this effect relates to mothers' immune systems[18]. As females, their immune systems are likely to recognize male-related proteins as "other" and form an immune response to them. With each successive male fetus, this immune response grows stronger, which could inhibit one or more male-related proteins involved in male sexual development. The result could be under-masculinization of a male fetus, leading to androphilia and a cross-sex shift in mental traits.

Some scientists hypothesize that a male-related protein called NLGN4Y plays a role. One study found that mothers of homosexual males had more antibodies against this protein than mothers of heterosexual males, and both groups of mothers had more antibodies than mothers without sons[19].

Scientists have estimated that 15–29% of cases of male homosexuality can be attributed to the FBOE[20]. However, research also indicates there's a second type of maternal immune response that contributes to homosexuality in both sexes[21], which suggests the true proportion of homosexual males who owe their orientations to maternal immune factors is likely even higher[22].

These influences of birth order might also influence female homosexuality. Researchers have found evidence suggesting that homosexuality in both sexes is influenced by birth order[23], and that although older brothers raise the odds of homosexuality more than older sisters, older siblings of either sex increase the odds of homosexuality among later-born siblings.

THE "WHERE" AND "WHAT" OF SEXUAL ORIENTATION

Autosexual orientations cause *attractions to being*.

Since autosexual orientations create attractions to being particular types of things, these orientations can also be thought of as attractions to various types of embodiment (e.g., being a particular gender, race, age, or species).

It's theorized that autosexual orientations result when someone's sexuality gets directed toward the self (auto) instead of others (allo). It's a difference of location, not type. The "where" is different, not the "what"[24].

The "what" (woman, man, minor, animal, etc.) is known as an erotic target. The "where" is that erotic target's *location*.

The formal names for sexual orientations usually use Greek roots to describe the *where* and *what of love* by utilizing a "location-type-love" naming structure:

1. Location ("allo-", "auto-", "ambi-")
2. Erotic target or type ("gyne", "andro", "pedo", "zoo", etc.)
3. Love ("-philia")

I'll demonstrate how these location prefixes work with gynephilia, a love of women.

A love of *others* as women is *allogynephilia*. However,

attractions to others are so common that "allo" is often left out for brevity.

A love of *self* as a woman is *auto*gynephilia.

A love of *both* self and others as women is *ambi*gynephilia. Ambigynephilia is co-occurring allogynephilia and autogynephilia.

AUTOSEXUAL TRANS IDENTITIES

Autosexual orientations are the most common cause of *cross-identities* (identities that are incongruent with one's default physical form). These are usually called *trans identities*. "Trans" means "across" or "on the other side of".

Cross-gender identity is the most common type of trans identity, but other types exist too. Autosexual cross-identities take this general form:

> For any dimension of sexual attraction X, autosexual attraction to embodying X can lead to X euphoria, X dysphoria, or a trans-X identity.

I'll use the sexual dimension of race as an example.

Someone with autosexual attraction to being a particular race can have positive feelings (*race euphoria*) in response to perceptions of embodying that race. They can also have negative feelings (*race dysphoria*) when they perceive a shortcoming in their racial embodiment. Working in tandem, these positive and negative race-based feelings influence the development of a *transrace identity*.

People who are autosexual in one dimension of their sexuality are often autosexual in other dimensions of their sexuality. This is why people with rarer types of trans identity are far more likely to be transgender than those who don't have any trans identities at all.

For example, there are people who identify as dragons, werewolves, monsters, or other mythical nonhuman entities. People who identify in this way are *otherkin*. These identities are *transspecies* in nature because they cross in the dimension of species.

Roughly a third of otherkin are transgender. In a sexual context, otherkin usually enjoy being treated as the same type of entity they identify as. They are also likely to be that same type of entity in their sexual fantasies.

This high rate of transgenderism in otherkin and the common underlying interest in erotic cross-embodiment suggests that autosexuality underlies both transgender and transspecies identity.

IN SUM

* Sexual orientation is a motivational system that drives sexual behavior. It originated as a way to unite sperm and egg. People are usually sexually attracted to adult humans of the other sex, but the specific love object can be just about any type of entity.

* In the womb, both genes and hormones influence the development of mental traits and vanilla sexual

orientations. Psychological traits and orientations tend to move together in tandem, so homosexuality is associated with a cross-gender shift in mental traits.

* Some cases of male homosexuality can be attributed to the fraternal birth order effect—the finding that the greater the number of older brothers a male has, the more likely that male is to be gay. Feminine gay males tend to have more older brothers than masculine gay males, which suggests that this cause of male homosexuality may be especially responsible for the kind of gender-atypical male homosexuality that can lead to transgenderism. Some research suggests that birth order also affects the development of homosexuality in females.

* Sexologists usually measure sexual orientation by asking questions about sexual identity, sexual behavior, or sexual attraction. Some sexologists measure physical arousal in the lab to collect data that's less biased by shortcomings of self-knowledge (or the common human tendency to present oneself in a flattering light).

* Formal names for sexual attractions have a "where-what-love" naming structure that describes the "where" and "what" of love. They list the location first (self or other), followed by erotic target (woman, man, child, wolf, etc.), and end with love (-philia). Attraction to others is so

common that the location is often left unmentioned (e.g., "androphilia" instead of "alloandrophilia").

* Autosexual orientations are the most common cause of cross-identities (trans identities). Depending on whether sexual attraction is in the dimension of gender, age, race, or species, it will lead to a different type of trans identity. For any dimension of attraction X, autosexual attraction to embodying X can lead to X euphoria, X dysphoria, or a cross-X identity.

PART 2

MALE AUTOHETEROSEXUALITY

AUTOGYNEPHILIA

"At that time I began to get the idea what I was all about.
Today I know what it is; I know that I was not aroused by
anything physical, that it was not the lover's kiss that caused
my first ejaculation, but rather only the intensive wish to be a
woman, to feel and to think feminine."

—Case 4, from *Transvestites: The Erotic Drive*
to Cross-Dress by Magnus Hirschfeld,
translated by Michael A. Lombardi-Nash

AUTOGYNEPHILIA (AGP)
LOVE OF SELF AS A WOMAN

At its core, autogynephilia is a sexual interest in being a woman.

The DSM-5 defines it as "sexual arousal of a natal male associated with the idea or image of being a woman"[1].

Like conventional heterosexuality, male autoheterosexuality is much more than mere eroticism. Its emotional side impacts sentiments, moods, and even identity. It changes how people think of gender, as well as their place in it.

Autogynephilia drives a desire to embody femininity, and its manifestations vary across individuals: no two people are exactly the same. It also shifts over the course of life.

Just as people vary from being unsentimental horndogs to being true romantics, autogynephilic people range from having primarily sexual feminine embodiment all the way to having a profoundly sentimental longing to simply *be* a woman. Most show a mixture of lust and love.

Depending on the way an autogynephilic person perceives their state of feminine embodiment, their mood can shift up or down. Successful embodiment tends to shift their mood up, and shortcomings of embodiment tend to shift it down. Any stimulus that implies a state of gendered embodiment can lead to these gender-related shifts to mood.

Positive gender-related feelings are *gender euphoria*. Negative gender-related feelings are *gender dysphoria*.

The good feelings associated with femininity attract autogynephilic people, pulling them closer. The bad feelings associated with masculinity repel them, pushing them away from their default gender.

Both good and bad gender feelings work together to shift their gendered sentiments. Over time, femininity rises in importance and masculinity becomes devalued. After years of this dynamic, masculinity can become synonymous with *bad* and femininity with *good*. At this point, autogynephilic people are likely to cherish their feminine traits and regard their masculine traits as aversive or worthless.

It doesn't always start there though.

A stimulus that was exciting or arousing at first will often shift toward feeling nice or comforting as the cross-gender journey progresses. Eventually, doing feminine things just feels right: it's the new normal. At that point, removing the stimulus can feel uncomfortable, as though something is missing.

These gender feelings and the resulting attachment to femininity are the emotional and romantic aspects of autogynephilia. Like conventional romantic feelings, they originate from a sexual orientation but ultimately have wide-ranging effects on behaviors, emotions, and sentiments that go far beyond the lusty eroticism commonly associated with sexuality.

When Ray Blanchard formally introduced the concept of autogynephilia, he noted that it "includes the capacity for pair-bond formation (or something like it)"[2]. The understanding that autogynephilia can foster a romantic attachment to one's feminine side has always been a part of the theory.

The capacity to bond with one's feminine self can grow into a deep familiarity and comfort with feminine embodiment that eventually leads to gender transition. The emotional side of autogynephilia also influences the development of various gender identities.

Think about it: if embodying femininity made you feel better and embodying masculinity made you feel worse, in which direction would your gender identity shift over time?

Toward femininity, right?

It would be weird if it didn't, honestly.

This cross-gender development process can take a while to unfold, which is why it's common for autogynephilic people to take on an intermediary gender identity such as *nonbinary* or *genderqueer* before ultimately arriving at *woman*.

AUTOGYNEPHILIC EMBODIMENT SUBTYPES

Sexologists study sexuality, so they tend to focus on the erotic side of autogynephilia when they write about it. That's their job. It's what they do.

Still, the romantic side of autogynephilia is such a huge part of the autogynephilic experience that focusing solely on eroticism seems misguided or tone-deaf. Those who fixate on eroticism can easily miss the broader emotional picture.

I'll talk about many different autogynephilic interests with the understanding that we are all individuals who experience life in our own unique ways. We don't all have the same interests, and even if we did, we wouldn't all have the same feelings about our experiences.

One person may feel aroused by having breasts, while another just feels reassured by having them. Both want breasts, but their feelings and thoughts about them vary.

For this reason, it can make more sense to categorize based on *interests* themselves, rather than the thoughts and feelings about these interests.

So far, there is evidence that autogynephilic interests fall into five main subtypes[3]. These subtypes represent aspects of life that tend to be different for women and men—bodies, clothing, behaviors, bodily functions, and social experiences:

* Anatomic AGP—having a woman's body
* Sartorial AGP—donning women's fashion

* Behavioral AGP—behaving like a woman
* Physiologic AGP—having a woman's bodily functions
* Interpersonal AGP—socially being a woman

These are the same subtypes I mentioned in the introductory chapter. I will use them as scaffolding to structure the autogynephilia chapters.

Although these categories are helpful conceptual tools for understanding autogynephilia, they're not as useful for attributing motivations to others in everyday life.

Consider the example of an autogynephilic person who is dressed *en femme*. They may not be interested in clothing but instead want to be seen socially as a woman.

Or say that person presents femme at a hair salon. Are they motivated by a desire to get a woman's hairstyle, behave like a woman, or be *one of the ladies*? It's not possible to know for sure through observation alone.

These categories may not be useful for attributing specific motivations to the behavior of others, but they are conceptually useful for making sense of autogynephilia. Autogynephilic people can use these categories to help interpret their own motivations and aid introspection when trying to decide what to do about their gender feelings.

If they want to behave and dress as a woman but have little interest in having a female body or in being treated as if they do, they may reasonably conclude that behaving and dressing as a woman will meet most of their sexual and emotional needs arising from autogynephilia and that gender transition may not help them much.

However, if they want to be seen as a woman and have a feminine body but don't care about clothing, they might conclude that medical interventions are the best way to get what they want.

There's no one-size-fits-all approach to living with autogynephilia, so each autogynephilic person must choose for themself the best way to proceed.

THE IMPORTANCE OF HISTORICAL NARRATIVES

In many places in this book, I'll reference historical narratives of autogynephilia that were first published roughly a century ago.

I prefer older narratives to newer ones because they're far less tainted by received cultural ideas about transgenderism, and they're completely free of modern political considerations.

When writing, these trans people weren't concerned with how their narratives might shape political discourse in the twenty-first century. Nowhere did they mention a fear that what they were writing would affect public perception of them in a way that could harm them.

Their thoughts about their condition came from direct experience to a degree that won't happen again, because people today have preconceived ideas about transgenderism.

Strong societal forces compelled past generations to hide their cross-gender inclinations, which left them isolated. Many went their entire lives without knowingly meeting others like them.

To better understand their condition, they wrote to sexologists or became their patients. Those sexologists then published these firsthand accounts to advance scientific understanding of human sexuality.

In 1890, a male Hungarian physician who felt herself to be a woman shared her extensive account with sexologist Richard von Krafft-Ebing, who included it in his next edition of *Psychopathia Sexualis*.

In 1910, Magnus Hirschfeld presented sixteen new case histories in *Die Transvestiten*, the book that kicked off the "trans" category we know today as "transgender".

A few years later, in 1913, Havelock Ellis published six new cases in an article titled "Sexo-Aesthetic Inversion"[4]. Ellis understood autoheterosexuality well: he regarded the "aesthetic heterosexual inversion"[5] he was seeing as "really a modification of normal hetero-sexuality"[6].

These twenty-three historical accounts of autogynephilia are an important reminder that inborn sexual orientations like autoheterosexuality and homosexuality have appeared across widely varying cultures and times and will continue to do so.

Beauty ideals and fashions can drastically change from one generation to the next, but sexual orientations are perennial.

MODERN AUTOGYNEPHILIC SEXUALITY

Today, autogynephilic people are more likely to be called "transfems" rather than "transvestites", but the underlying erotic predisposition is identical: they want to be women.

Some of them satiate their erotic desire for feminine transformation through *transgender transformation stories*. These stories depict the fantasy of turning into a woman, often by invoking methods of cross-gender transformation that are magical or based in science fiction[7]. Gender transformation also occurs through *forced feminization*, a genre in which women forcibly transform the male protagonist into a beautiful woman.

These stories of gender metamorphosis usually end with the main character permanently transformed into a woman—the autogynephilic version of "happily ever after".

Erotic feminization of males is called *sissification*. Sissification is extremely popular among autogynephilic people. For many, it's their first outlet to express their autogynephilia. Some of them even identify as *sissies*.

A lot of them watch *sissy hypno*, an autogynephilic remix of pornography that rapidly cycles through shots from various pornographic videos while a voice-over speaks directly to the viewer, commanding them to feminize themselves in various ways, many of which involve sexual submission to men. For a lot of autogynephilic people, sissy hypno is their most powerful erotic stimulus.

Quite a few trans women originally realized they wanted to transition after consuming sissy media. Trans woman Andrea Long Chu provocatively admitted, "Sissy porn did make me trans"[8]. She's not alone—thousands have been down that road.

Watching porn depicting "pre-op" MTFs is another way trans women have realized they want to transition. Through continual exposure to erotic imagery of feminized males, some autogynephilic people realize they, too, want to be feminized.

Another genre of erotic media popular with autogynephilic people is *femdom*, which features females or trans women positioned in an assertive, dominant role over a subject, who is usually male. It sometimes involves feminization of the male subject.

Another way that autogynephilic people express their sexuality is through receptive anal penetration, through which they can enact a sex role they associate with being female. *A lot* of autogynephilic people are into getting pegged by women, fucked by men, or even just penetrating themselves.

It's also common for them to shave their body hair, dress up in sexy clothes such as thigh-highs, panties, and bra, or lock their penis in a chastity cage as part of their autoerotic expression.

PSYCHE AUTOGYNEPHILIA, SHIFTING, AND TRANSFEMININE IDENTITY

Autogynephilic people initially feel feminine or like a woman for short spurts, often in association with crossdressing.

This feeling is an *autogynephilic mental shift*—a change toward a mind state associated with women or femininity. I suspect that these mental shifts originate in a desire to have a woman's consciousness, an aspect of autogynephilia I call *psyche autogynephilia*.

Psyche autogynephilia drives a desire to perceive, sense, feel, or think as a woman would. It's about seeing the world through a woman's eyes. It can feel like having a female soul.

Autogynephilia can also create *autogynephilic phantom shifts*, the sensation of having female-typical phantom anatomy such as breasts, a vulva, wide hips, or long hair. Phantom shifts and mental shifts can both contribute to body–mind incongruence.

Any autosexual orientation can lead to mental shifts and phantom shifts. In fact, people who identify as animals created the concept of *shifting* (see Chapter 7.4).

Autogynephilic mental shifts are initially transient and their arrival unexpected. In the beginning, triggers such as cross-dressing tend to induce them, but with practice, some autogyne-philic people learn how to directly will them into being.

Eventually, this feminine mind state may become a perma-nent sensation, at which point it is a form of permanent cross-gender identity. If an autogynephilic person hands the reins to their internal femme self, their default self can become subdued and fade into the background[9].

Males who continually feel feminine or see themselves as women can be considered to have a *transfeminine* gender identity.

Transfeminine (or *transfem*) is an umbrella term for MTF-spectrum people. MTF transvestites, MTF transsexuals, and transgender women all fall under the transfem umbrella.

One of the best early accounts of autogynephilic transfemi-nine identity comes from the middle-aged Hungarian medi-cal doctor whose story appeared in Richard von Krafft-Ebing's *Psychopathia Sexualis*. She had a permanent feeling of femi-ninity that altered her relationship to herself and the world around her. She referred to these autogynephilic mental shifts as "the imperative female feeling"[10], "the imperative feeling of femininity"[11], or "the feeling of being a woman"[12].

The Hungarian physician wrote down her account of auto-gynephilia and mailed it to von Krafft-Ebing. Her account is so compelling and thorough that Hirschfeld reprinted it in *Transvestites*[13]. Over 130 years later, the Hungarian physician's account is still one of the best.

THE HUNGARIAN PHYSICIAN: THE FEMININE IMPERATIVE

When the Hungarian physician wrote her narrative in her forties, she had already developed a strong feminine identity. She hadn't always felt that way though. When she was younger, the feminine feeling was milder and more fleeting. Recalling her high school years, she reported, "Gradually I began to feel like a girl"[14].

By middle age, her mental shifts and phantom shifts had become permanent aspects of everyday life. Every morning, her mental shift into a feminine mindset started within moments of waking and never dissipated[15], and she constantly sensed the presence of phantom anatomy:

"*General feeling:* I feel like a woman in a man's form; and even though I often am sensible of the man's form, yet it is always in a feminine sense. Thus, for example, I feel the penis as clitoris; the urethra and vaginal orifice, which always feels a little wet, even when it is actually dry; the scrotum as *labia majora*; in short, I always feel the vulva. And all that that means one alone can know who feels or has felt so."[16]

In addition to female genitals, the Hungarian physician also felt as though she had female breasts[17] and a female pelvis[18]. Even her waist felt female[19].

She also experienced a type of mental shift known as a *sensory shift* which made her feel as though she had the senses and perception of a woman. Her stomach rebelled against every deviation from a "female diet"[20]. Food that wasn't completely fresh had "a cadaverous odour"[21].

Her skin felt feminine; it had become sensitive to both hot and cold temperatures, as well as direct sunlight[22]. She resented social norms that kept her from using sun parasols to protect her sensitive face skin[23] and took to wearing gloves as much as possible—even while sleeping.

These mental and phantom shifts reinforced each other—her phantom anatomy made her feel like a woman[24], and feeling like a woman reinforced her phantom anatomy[25].

By the time she wrote her account, her feminine identity was dominant, and her default self had already become subordinate to her feminine self:

"It is as if I were robbed of my own skin, and put in a woman's skin that fitted me perfectly, but which felt everything as if it covered a woman; and whose sensations passed through the man's body, and exterminated the masculine element."[26]

"The imperative female feeling remained, and became so strong that I wear only the mask of a man, and in everything else feel like a woman; and gradually I have lost memory of the former individuality."[27]

She was in control now.

IN SUM

* Autogynephilia is a sexual and romantic attraction to being a woman. As with conventional heterosexuality, this form of male autoheterosexuality can range in expression from overt eroticism to romantic sentimentality.

* Autogynephilia can drive progressively larger commitments to feminine embodiment that resemble the escalating commitment of conventional sexual relationships. Through reinforcement from gender-related feelings, the way an autogynephilic person sees themselves can shift over time—usually toward femininity. In some cases, a person who starts out firmly convinced they are a man may ultimately become just as firmly convinced they are a woman.

* Autogynephilia has various subtypes that pertain to having a woman's body, bodily functions, style of dress, behavior, or social treatment. Any given autogynephilic

person may have just one of these aspects of the orientation, or all of them. In its most simple, stripped-down form, autogynephilia presents as a stand-alone interest in having a woman's body. But more commonly, autogynephilic people also want to embody womanly behavior, dress, or social standing.

* Autogynephilic mental shifts create a sense of feminine consciousness, which contributes to the development of a feminine gender identity. Autogynephilic phantom shifts create a sense of having phantom anatomy corresponding to female-typical physical features such as breasts, a vulva, or wide hips. Mental shifts and phantom shifts both contribute to the body–mind incongruence that is so commonly associated with transsexualism.

* Erotic feminization (sissification) is popular among autogynephilic people. Some even identify as sissies. Their preferred erotic media is likely to contain themes of gender transformation, forced feminization, or female domination. They may crossdress, penetrate themselves anally, or wear a chastity cage as part of their autoeroticism.

2 . 1

ANATOMIC AUTOGYNEPHILIA
HAVING A WOMAN'S BODY

Bodies are central to sexuality. The types of bodies people are attracted to usually determine their sexual orientation.

Autoheterosexuality follows a similar pattern: autoheterosexuals usually want the same physical traits they find attractive in people of the other sex. This sexual interest in having a female body—*anatomic autogynephilia*—is likely the most prevalent subtype of autogynephilia[1].

Anatomic AGP commonly includes the desire to have a female face, butt, and vulva as well as breasts. In general, any female traits that autogynephilic people find attractive are traits they would want for themselves.

Maybe they want narrow shoulders, small hands, long legs, small feet, a slender neck, or a big butt. Maybe they wish they were shorter, their jaw was smaller, or their brow ridge jutted out less.

% OF AUTOGYNEPHILIC TRANS WOMEN WHO HAVE EVER BEEN AROUSED BY IMAGINING THEMSELVES WITH:

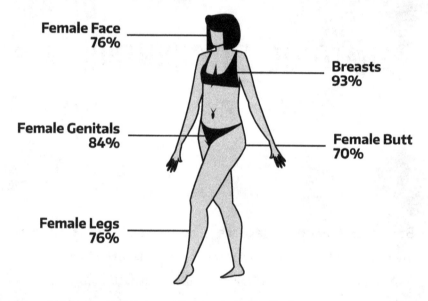

Female Face
76%

Breasts
93%

Female Genitals
84%

Female Butt
70%

Female Legs
76%

Source: Partial versus complete Autogynephilia and gender dysphoria (1993)
Author: Ray Blanchard

Figure 2.1.1: Prior arousal from anatomic autogynephilia among MTFs.

Some autogynephilic people have a strong, selective interest in having a female body, and they don't care about the other feminine stuff. Magnus Hirschfeld described this anatomically inclined subgroup as "congenitally most strongly predisposed"[2]. Havelock Ellis said they were "less common but more complete"[3]. People like this are particularly likely to pursue medical transition.

Effective feminizing technology didn't exist in Hirschfeld's time. Fortunately, autogynephilic people today can attain feminine physical traits by taking hormones and having surgeries.

Still, autogynephilic people who are solely interested in having a female body are in a tough position. Unable to find refuge in women's garb, medical transition is often their best option for satisfying their autogynephilic desires.

ANATOMIC AUTOGYNEPHILIA BEFORE TRANSSEXUALISM

Autogynephilic people are more likely to want female breasts than any other body part[4].

Firsthand narratives from the early 1900s frequently report the desire for breasts[5]. The mammary yearning was real: "I want real breasts very badly indeed"[6], said one transfem.

Transfems whose anatomic interests were strong and persistent were especially likely to experience phantom shifts and feel that they were growing breasts, that their genitals became a vulva, or that they had long hair when their hair was actually short[7].

One of the transfems Ellis profiled suffered from genital dysphoria and only refrained from castrating herself because of the danger of doing so. "I know that I should be immensely happier if my sexual organs were removed"[8], she said. After her wife's death, another transfem made a habit of sleeping with her genitals tucked between her legs, out of view[9].

One of the transfems in Hirschfeld's book memorably reported, "There is something beastly in the boastful exhibition of the male organ"[10].

In these narratives, desire for female anatomy could extend to any physical feature and even to the body as a whole. This desire to see themselves as feminine also shifted their self-perception in that direction[11].

One transfem perceived that her hips were wide like female hips, although in reality, they were only slightly wider than average male hips[12]. Another transfem derived pleasure from perceiving that her small hands and feet were womanly[13].

Another transfem grew excited by her growing corpulence, which she considered to be the "formation of the flesh of the woman"[14]. At age thirty-seven, a transfem reported that her body was becoming more feminine over time[15].

Fueled by a persistent desire to make their bodies more feminine, some transfems used various herbs, oils, or medical salves with the hope of becoming physically feminized[16]. One transfem ordered a product advertised to improve breast size, but it didn't work[17]. Another massaged her breasts with olive oil, hoping it would increase their size[18].

Unfortunately, none of these approaches worked. Effective feminizing technology didn't exist yet.

ANATOMIC AUTOGYNEPHILIA
IN THE AGE OF TRANSSEXUALISM

Once medical technology made hormones and surgeries available, it became possible for more trans people to achieve a cross-gender aesthetic that allowed them to exist in society as their cross-gender self.

Even though this medical technology wasn't nearly as refined as it is today, the advent of transsexualism represented a massive breakthrough for trans people.

The situation is even better now: it's easy to obtain hormones over the internet, and it's becoming easier to get them in person too. As society becomes more aware and accepting of trans people, more medical establishments are offering hormone prescriptions on an informed consent basis.

These *cross-sex hormones* help trans people attain hormone levels more like those of the other sex, which helps them more closely resemble the other sex.

Most trans people refer to these hormones as *hormone replacement therapy*. They have come up with many creative, punny names for these hormones:

"Hormone replacement therapy (HRT) has many nicknames among transfeminine people, including titty pills, titty skittles, smartitties, chicklets, anticistamines, mammary mints, life savers, tit tacs, breast mints, femme&m's, antiboyotics, trans-mission fluid, and the Notorious H.R.T."[19]

Notice a theme? About half of these names allude to female breasts. Having breasts is critically important to many transfems.

It's common for transfems to wear silicone breast forms to temporarily attain a full-chested look. They may also wear a padded bra or choose to stuff a bra. If they don't achieve sufficient breast growth after being on hormones for a few years, they may decide to get breast augmentation surgery.

Transfems who want a vulva may seek *vaginoplasty* (the surgical creation of a neovagina), commonly called "bottom surgery". Over the years, this surgical procedure has also been called "sexual reassignment surgery", "gender reassignment surgery", or "gender confirmation surgery".

To achieve a more feminine facial structure, some transfems undergo a series of surgical procedures collectively referred to as *facial feminization surgery* (FFS). This commonly includes procedures like forehead contouring, jaw contouring, and rhinoplasty (nose job).

Humans usually identify each other by facial recognition, so facial structure is a big part of identity. If part of the face is covered up, we may not recognize someone we already know. When seeing other people's faces, it takes only a fraction of a second to attribute a gender to them[20], which makes FFS a particularly important intervention for transfems who have issues with people gendering them appropriately in everyday life.

Although other procedures exist beyond the ones mentioned here, transsexual women tend to be most consistently interested in surgical interventions in three key areas: face, chest, and genitals.

All these areas have great symbolic value for signifying gender. They are also attractive: gynephilic people are usually attracted to feminine faces, vulvas, and breasts, so autogynephilic people often want those same features for themselves.

IN SUM

* Anatomic autogynephilia often makes autogynephilic people want the same feminine physical features they find attractive in others. They may want a female face, butt, or vulva; breasts; or anything else they deem female-typical. Unsurprisingly, breasts are the single most desired female physical feature.

* Before transsexualism existed, many autogynephilic transfems longed for feminine anatomy in vain because the technology didn't exist yet. But once surgeries and pharmaceutical hormones were developed, a few of them had a chance to more closely resemble the other sex with the help of these technologies.

* Today, many autogynephilic people have access to gender-affirming medical care that previous generations couldn't get. These feminizing hormones and surgeries not only help them feel more comfortable with themselves but also increase the odds that other people will regard them as women.

"The influence which masculine or feminine clothing exerts on the spiritual life of transvestites is uncommonly strong. In the garb of their physical sex...transvestites feel themselves confined, imprisoned, oppressed, they feel that it is something strange, something that does not suit them or belong to them. On the other hand, they cannot find words to describe the feeling of security, restfulness, and exaltation which comes over them in the garb of the opposite sex."

—Magnus Hirschfeld, translated by
Michael A. Lombardi-Nash[1]

SARTORIAL AUTOGYNEPHILIA
DONNING WOMEN'S FASHION

The sartorial pursuit of feminine embodiment through wearing women's clothing is one of the most common manifestations of autogynephilia. It's often the first outward sign of the orientation, which is why autogynephilic people who dressed as the other sex used to be called "transvestites".

After Hirschfeld published *Die Transvestiten* in 1910, "transvestite" described anyone whose clothes didn't match their sex[2]. Female or male, homosexual or autoheterosexual, it didn't matter what kind of trans person was being described: they were all transvestites.

In later decades, sexologists started to use "transvestite" specifically to describe males with a history of erotic crossdressing[3], which continues to be the most common use of the term today. Some contemporary sexologists consider transvestism to be a subtype of autogynephilia and call it "transvestic autogynephilia"[4].

Since it alludes to birth sex, "transvestic autogynephilia" can be a confusing term when talking about people who have already transitioned to live as women. It also doesn't make much sense when describing females who are *autohomosexual* (attracted to being their own sex).

In order to have a term appropriate for both post-transition MTFS and autohomosexual females, I wanted a name for this autogynephilia subtype that didn't allude to birth sex. I settled on "sartorial", which means "of or relating to clothing".

Sartorial autogynephilia is a sexual interest in donning women's fashion. It refers most literally to wearing women's clothing but also includes other body adornments such as wigs, makeup, and perfume. For autogynephilic people, these feminine body adornments "exert their attraction by the impression of their own feminine character"[5].

Dressing in a feminine manner is one of the safest and most accessible ways to embody femininity, so it's where many transfems begin their cross-gender explorations.

Early acts of sartorial embodiment often involve clothes that belong to a female family member, and the crossdressing occurs when other family members are either asleep or outside the home. The fear of getting caught in the act makes these experiences more intense. Intrinsic excitement from crossdressing adds to this intensity, leaving lasting impressions that can be recalled many years later.

It's common to begin with bras or underwear and progressively add more pieces over time. The process can also go the other way: starting with outer layers and then adding underlayers over time.

Eventually, an autogynephilic person who has developed an attachment to wearing women's clothes may want to wear them all the time. If they fear negative social consequences, they may *underdress* by wearing women's clothes beneath men's clothes.

Underdressing is a fairly safe way of wearing women's clothing without much risk of others noticing. Another undercover way to crossdress is by wearing feminine articles that aren't too conspicuous, such as boots or jewelry[6].

In the 1970s and '80s, it took an average of fifteen years of crossdressing before heterosexual transvestites had a complete femme outfit, and twenty-one years before they adopted a femme name[7]. Now that cross-gender expression has been destigmatized in many places, this progression tends to be faster. Kids growing up today find out about transgenderism at a younger age and are more likely to see it portrayed as an acceptable way of life.

Society wasn't always this welcoming to trans people though.

TRANSVESTISM BEFORE TRANSSEXUALISM EXISTED

Before the advent of prescription hormones, the best option for feminization was crossdressing. This is why first-person narratives of autogynephilia from the early 1900s often focus on the act of crossdressing.

This sartorial embodiment wasn't about clothes though; it was about feeling like a woman[8]. The clothes were just the best way of inducing feminine mental shifts. In the unfortunate event that a dressing-induced erection occurred, it was sometimes seen as an unwelcome interruption to dressing[9].

Society was actively hostile to male crossdressing, so transfems had to hide it to the best of their ability. It was socially and legally dangerous for a male to dress as a woman in public, so they often had to make do with underdressing.

One transfem reported wearing stockings and a corset underneath her outer masculine layer in everyday life[10]. As a child, another even thought of joining the priesthood so that she could wear a priest's garb over women's clothing[11].

After the onset of puberty, another transfem felt magnetically drawn to displays of women's clothing in store windows[12]. The urge to dress in a feminine manner could be present from a young age[13] and intensify over time[14].

In these classic narratives of autogynephilia, the desire for women's clothing was extensive. It applied to *anything* that was for women—no detail was too small to overlook. Hirschfeld insightfully noted that "the transvestic drive directs itself toward the whole costume to the very last detail"[15].

The emotional rewards from crossdressing could even supplant transfems' need for friends and socializing[16].

If transfems could not crossdress, their mood would sour.

An inner unrest would build up and take away their ability to feel pleasure in any aspect of life. Unable to dress, one transfem reported that everyday pleasures lost their charm—even food didn't taste good[17].

In the depths of this depression, they sometimes thought of suicide. One said, "May God have mercy on me and help me with my dresses or call me out of this world, because I feel that, if I am not helped, I shall perish"[18].

Sometimes, they *did* kill themselves[19].

The strict gender rules around clothing hurt transfems constantly[20]. Due to these fashion restrictions, they had to hide the most cherished side of themselves from a society that was actively hostile to them. They had "no peace except in pinafores"[21].

Transfems with families often had to sequester their feminine dressing to the rare times they were home alone or could travel. If they were lucky, their wives begrudgingly tolerated or even accepted their nature[22].

WOMEN'S CLOTHING FEEDS TRANSFEM IDENTITY

More often than not, the transfems whose experiences were immortalized in sexology books believed that their interest in women's clothing didn't originate in sexuality. From their perspective, wearing women's clothing was an expression of their femme identity[23], and the clothing itself served to help that true self emerge[24].

Women's clothing had a powerful effect on their identity.

"Dressed as a girl I seem actually to become one"[25], one of Ellis's cases reported. She also referred to her first crossdressing experience as her "change of sex"[26] and for the rest of her life considered herself to be not fully male. Ellis described her attraction to wearing women's garb as merely "the outward symbols of the inner spiritual state"[27].

Many transfems loathed the men's clothing that society forced upon them and only felt at peace in the evening when they could dress in a way that expressed their gender identity. One said, "When evening came, I breathed easier, because I then let fall the burdensome mask, and I felt myself completely a woman"[28].

For many transfems, home was their refuge. Wrapped in women's garb, they found a precious, fleeting peace that eluded them during the day. One of them captured this sartorial sense of safety when she said, "Skirts are a sanctuary to me"[29].

A transfem who had successfully lived as a woman multiple times, R. L., found that afterward, simply dressing as one had lost its allure. R. L. kept her clothing nearby but didn't see the point in wearing it unless she could do so "as a woman"[30]. She desired to be a woman, not to dress like one[31]. "Simply to 'dress up' has never satisfied me", she lamented[32].

Although wearing women's clothing was enjoyable at first, in the end it became an irritating reminder of what she wanted more than anything else: to be a woman.

TACTILE SENSATIONS: CORSETS, SOFTNESS, AND LACE

When dressing as a woman, autogynephilic people often like soft materials, fine lace, or the constriction of corsets. Tactile sensations play a powerful role in sartorial embodiment.

Transfems of the past were no different: they got sensual enjoyment and emotional reassurance from feeling women's clothing on their skin. Seeing the clothes or hearing them rustle also added to the overall effect. This sensory feedback cultivated femme feelings and brightened their moods.

R. L. poetically captured how this worked:

"Dressing is a sort of ritual; I am really 'in the spirit' and see and feel myself to be a woman; it is pleasing to put on the clothes, especially the touch of a pretty blouse on bare arms and shoulders. The soft comfort of underwear, and clasp of corsets, the caress of petticoats around silk-stockinged legs, the smartness of shoes, together with the delightful sensation from the graceful movements, and happy frame of mind, all combine to cause the most delicious aesthetic feelings of happiness and content."[33]

Quotes like this are why R. L.'s firsthand narrative is one of my favorites. Her account is memorable and thorough, and its contents indicate that she was thoroughly autogynephilic. For these reasons, I will refer to her by name and call upon her testimony several times.

Other transfems reported similar enjoyment from feeling women's clothing on their bodies. Soft, silky, or lacy fabrics were particularly appealing.

Transfems of the past loved the gentle touch of soft materials[34] and the comfort of soft fur[35]. They longed to be wrapped in soft slips[36] and cradled by soft underwear[37].

Although softness is inherently pleasurable to some extent, part of their enjoyment came about because they associated softness with women. They thought that women had soft bodies[38], soft skin[39], soft voices[40], and soft hair[41], so they aspired to softness and wore soft clothing to help them embody it.

Silk and Lace

Silk was a popular material for embodying this softness.

Transfems were likely to enjoy wearing silk dresses[42], silk scarves[43], silk underwear[44], or silk stockings[45]. They enjoyed being ensconced in "elegant silk shoes"[46] or "rustling silk underwear"[47].

The sweet song of rustling silk could even bring upon sartorial euphoria[48]: "again and again a wonderful feeling penetrated me when the silk skirts rustled around me", reported one transfem[49].

Transfems of the past also enjoyed lace in many forms. Both its appearance and texture were appealing. They wore lace slips[50], lace underwear[51], and lace petticoats[52], and they sometimes carried perfumed lace handkerchiefs[53].

One transfem even described an attractive dress as "so delicate, so fragrant, like a poem translated into lace"[54].

Corsets: "Corsetted and Laced to the Last Gasp"

As much as transfems of the past enjoyed softness, silk, and lace, *corsets were next level*. They absolutely adored the constriction of corsets.

The consistent firm embrace of a corset induced and maintained feminine mental shifts, making it a powerful tool for cross-gender embodiment.

Corsets could provide "exquisite physical pleasure"[55], especially when they were "corsetted and laced to the last gasp"[56].

But sometimes the power of corsets was too great. When trying on a corset for the first time, one transfem had her first erection. This startled her, so she quickly took it off and was left "deeply dissatisfied with the whole process" because she wanted to keep wearing the corset[57].

While trying on a corset for a theatrical role, another transfem got a "vigorous erection". Soon after, she "sallied forth for a promenade in Piccadilly" to procure a corset of her own[58].

Whether it was the soft caress of silk or the prolonged hug of a corset, being wrapped in feminine garb conjured up femme feelings and brought emotional comfort to autogynephilic people of past generations. The act of putting on women's clothing brought forth feminine mental shifts, and the sight, sound, and feel of the clothing added to the overall effect.

IN SUM

* Sartorial autogynephilia is a sexual interest in donning women's fashion. This most obvious and striking example

of feminine embodiment is why transvestite was the term that began the gender-related category of trans that we usually call transgender in the present day.

* Like other aspects of autogynephilia, sartorial autogynephilia goes beyond eroticism and enters the realm of emotions and sentiments. Over time, an autogynephilic person may become emotionally attached to wearing women's clothing. If they aren't comfortable wearing it publicly, they may decide to wear it underneath their men's clothing while in public—a practice known as underdressing.

* Wearing women's clothing has the potential to shift an autogynephilic person's gender identity across the gender divide. Prior to the recent destigmatization of gender nonconformity, it often took decades of crossdressing before a solid feminine gender identity emerged.

* Dressing in women's clothing is one of the safest and most accessible ways for an autogynephilic person to tap into and express their feminine side.

* Feeling, hearing, and seeing themselves in women's clothing all contribute to an autogynephilic person's sense of feminine embodiment, which makes tight, soft, or richly textured garments especially appealing.

BEHAVIORAL AUTOGYNEPHILIA
BEHAVING LIKE A WOMAN

In 2019, a trans woman named Mia Mulder made a tongue-in-cheek tweet that resonated among transfems:

> "Trans women transition for one single, depraved sexual reason: 'Dress go spinny.'"[1]

Since then, "dress go spinny" and "skirt go spinny" have become popular memes in online trans culture[2]. Mulder's tweet became popular because it humorously tapped into something real: spinning one's skirt or dress is a common source of joy among transfems, and this inclination is ultimately an outgrowth of sexuality.

This innocuous behavior is a manifestation of *behavioral autogynephilia*, a sexual interest in behaving like a woman. Any behavior that autogynephilic people code as feminine can fall within this admittedly broad category.

The behavior-sculpting power of behavioral autogynephilia can impact how they walk, sit, stand, or lay. It can even change the way they speak.

Moving in a feminine manner and speaking with a feminine voice are common manifestations of behavioral AGP. Although these feminine mannerisms ultimately arise because of a sexual orientation, they are more likely to provide emotional reassurance or provide a bit of cheer than they are to cause noticeable arousal.

It's common for autogynephilic people to enjoy walking in a way that accentuates hip movement, stand with hips shifted off-center to accentuate their hips, or sit with legs crossed rather than spread.

Any body positioning or movements that signify femininity can bring joy. Thanks to *proprioception*, the sense of body position and movement, people can feel where their body is and where it's moving without having to see it. When autogynephilic people get proprioceptive feedback that their bodies are positioned or moving in a feminine way, they may experience positive, reassuring feelings. These feelings, in turn, reinforce the behaviors that led to them.

Over time, reinforced feminine behaviors happen more frequently and become ingrained habits that occur without any conscious effort. The warm fuzzy feelings may be long gone, but the behaviors remain.

BEHAVIORAL AUTOGYNEPHILIA IN THE PAST

Behavioral autogynephilia has existed throughout the generations. In the classic autogynephilia narratives from the early 1900s, some transfems reported behaving like girls from a very young age. For a few, it was one of their earliest memories.

R. L. recalled dressing in girls' clothes as a child and going to the bathroom not because she needed to, but because she wanted to do it as a girl would[3]. Another transfem tried to copy the gait of girls and hoped that others might see her as a girl in boy's clothing[4].

Sewing and playing with dolls could be part of the behavior too. After seeing her mom and sister crochet, one transfem developed a "zeal for needlework"[5] that later extended to knitting. She even made two-dimensional dollhouses by gluing pictures of people and furniture into a notebook[6].

Could these transfems have exhibited such childhood behaviors even if they weren't autogynephilic? Of course.

But they faced strong social pressure to conform to masculinity, and these memories stood out to them to such a degree that, in their thirties and forties, they included them in the retrospective accounts they wrote about their gender experiences.

As adults, the act of crossdressing put transfems in a feminine headspace and facilitated feminine behavior. In a princess dress, one transfem felt "totally feminine" in her movements[7]. While in the embrace of a corset, another transfem breathed with her chest and considered it womanly[8].

Every little feminine movement could bring pleasure and comfort.

R. L. was like this—she treasured "the delightful sensation from the graceful movements"[9]. For her, *any* feminine behavior could bring joy, no matter how small:

"Every trivial action, such as using a dainty and perfumed handkerchief, placing articles down gently, acknowledging the trivial courtesies generally received by women with a smile and soft 'Thank you,' all gave me as much pleasure as the opposite would give pain."[10]

When these transfems lived with females, their behavioral autogynephilia could benefit the women they lived with.

One married transfem boasted: "I treat my wife very well, because I take care of almost all of the housework"[11]. As a child, another transfem delighted in caring for her baby sister[12], which eased the burden on her mother.

Another transfem looked after her roommate's kid like a nanny would. During this four-year period, her libido took a back seat to her role as caretaker. "Bringing up and caring for children is my greatest joy", she reported[13].

Many transfems back then put serious work into developing a femme voice[14]. They lived before they could benefit from modern voice feminization techniques, so they spoke in falsetto. But even if their voice was deep, they might perceive it as soft and high anyway[15].

PLAYING THE SUCCUBUS (BEING A BOTTOM)

In the classic narratives of autogynephilia, one sexual tendency shows up especially often: wanting to enact a feminine role during sexual activities.

"I always wanted to be the womanish, passive partner in love-making"[16], one transfem characteristically reported.

Almost all of them wanted to be the passive, receptive partner during sex. They wanted to be the one on bottom, lying on their back, and for their partner to have an energetic vigor that complemented their passivity.

They reported this so many times[17] that Hirschfeld gave it a name: "As regards the activities they tended toward, almost all of the persons explored preferred the position of *succumbentes*, i.e., 'those lying underneath' or 'those who yield'"[18].

Almost all of them wanted to play the role of *succubus*. They wanted to be with an energetic woman and be ravished by her[19].

Being in a masculine sexual role was not interesting to them. One reported that if she could physically pull it off, it was "merely as a performance of the body"[20]. Today, we might call someone like this a *bottom*, in the broad sense of being the submissive or receptive partner.

The inclination to behave like a woman could also lead transfems to masturbate with anal penetration[21], which enabled them to enact the fantasy of being penetrated. As the Hungarian physician reported, "the anus feels feminine"[22].

In the old narratives, anal masturbation didn't come up nearly as often as it would today—it must have been quite taboo at the time. However, the widespread prevalence of anal play among contemporary autogynephilic people suggests that transfems of the past almost certainly tried it or were at least tempted by the idea.

MODERN BEHAVIORAL AGP

Technology and culture have changed, but behavioral autogynephilia continues to present similarly. Modern-day autogynephilic people still tend to be submissive, receptive partners in sexual contexts.

During penis-in-vagina intercourse, they are likely to prefer lying on their back and may even mentally switch places with their partner, imagining that their partner has the penis and is penetrating them.

Since most females are attracted to men and are thus likely to perform fellatio as part of heterosexual relationships, some autogynephilic people like to perform fellatio on dildos as part of their autoerotic activities.

Chastity cages and butt plugs are also popular among autogynephilic people. By locking their penis into chastity, they symbolically demasculinize themselves. By wearing butt plugs, they make themselves ready for penetration and have a constant reminder of their penetrability.

The destigmatization of anal sex has also made it more likely that autogynephilic people will engage in anal masturbation or receptive anal intercourse. If they're dating a woman, they might want her to wear a strap-on and peg them. During anal masturbation, it's common for them to anally penetrate themselves using a dildo—which itself may be hand-powered, wall-mounted, or attached to the business end of a fucking machine.

IN SUM

* Behavioral autogynephilia drives a desire to enact feminine behavior. Over time, everyday behaviors such as speaking, walking, standing, or sitting may all become more feminine due to emotional reinforcement from behavioral autogynephilia.

* Behavioral AGP often shows up as a desire to bottom sexually. It's very common for autogynephilic people to want to be made love to—to be the passive, receptive partner during sex. During penis-in-vagina intercourse, they are likely to prefer lying on their back and may even mentally switch places with their partner, imagining that their partner has the penis and is penetrating them.

* The symbolic power of penetrability makes receiving anal penetration especially appealing to autogynephilic people. Many engage in receptive anal intercourse with males, females with strap-ons, or on their own. They may also perform fellatio on dildos or penises.

PHYSIOLOGIC AUTOGYNEPHILIA
HAVING FEMALE BODILY FUNCTIONS

Each sex has specific bodily functions that support its reproductive strategy. Males ejaculate semen. Females menstruate,
lactate, and become pregnant.

Sexual interest in having these female bodily functions is
physiologic autogynephilia.

Just like any other aspect of autogynephilia, physiologic autogynephilia can occur in the realm of emotions and underlie a
wistful longing to become pregnant, give birth, or breastfeed.
For some, this longing is experienced as a desire for motherhood
rather than an interest in having the bodily functions themselves.

Physiologic autogynephilia can even cause psychosomatic
period symptoms such as abdominal cramping or headaches.

It's unlikely that these symptoms are caused by hormones: auto-gynephilic people reported having these symptoms before synthetic hormones even existed.

Writing four decades before scientists isolated and named various forms of estrogen, the Hungarian physician alluded to her monthly period symptoms when she spoke of her molimen:

> "Every four weeks, at the time of the full moon, I have the molimen of a woman for five days, physically and mentally, only I do not bleed; but I have the feeling of a loss of fluid; a feeling that the genitals and abdomen are (internally) swollen."[1]

The full moon served as a timing cue for her psychosomatic period symptoms. After the permanent onset of her cross-gender identity, this "periodicity of the monthly molimina"[2] was a regular feature of her life.

Twenty years later, another case of period symptoms in a male appeared in the sexology literature[3]. According to Ellis, this "man...desired to be a woman and in his day-dreams imagined himself physically changed to a woman. There was a tendency to identification with his mother, and, like her, he had attacks of headache every month which he called his 'periods'"[4].

During this patient's childhood, her mother suffered from headaches accompanying menstruation which left her overly sensitive to any stimulus and unable to do much of anything for a few days at a time. After her mother's passing, this patient experienced headaches every four weeks. Each one lasted three to four days, one or two of which were spent in bed, unable to work[5]. The calendar likely served as the timing cue for her symptoms.

PREGNANCY TRANSVESTITES

In classic sexology narratives from the early 1900s, many auto-gynephilic transfems wanted to become pregnant or give birth. These feelings were often intense and held close to their hearts. Although they longed to be women, they particularly wanted to be *mothers*.

Hirschfeld called this *pregnancy transvestism*[6]. It came up in first-person narratives much more than other physiologic interests. These *pregnancy transvestites* were particularly prone to envy when their wives became pregnant and gave birth—a reaction Hirschfeld described as "very characteristic"[7].

One transfem even described her feelings about her wife giving birth as "the most acute suffering I ever felt in my life"[8]. Another teared up when recalling her first gender euphoria experience at the idea of having a child:

"There came a day when I felt that I wanted to have a child! The feeling was beautiful! I can write no more now for I am crying. The feeling came one evening, when I was in bed with influenza. The sensation began in my penis and then it was only a feeling in my heart, I *will* have a child! I *will* have a child!…That evening I cried terribly…I was 11 or 12 at the time."[9] [emphasis in original]

The bodily sensation that started in her penis and made its way to her heart is reminiscent of autogynephilic feelings in general: an initial sexual spark can develop into a profoundly deep attachment to feminine embodiment or the idea of being a woman.

After that first experience, this transfem dressed up as though she were pregnant, gazed at her reflection in the mirror, and had "the most blissful feeling"[10]. She repeated this behavior hundreds of times.

Another transfem felt "hopeful and joyful" when she had the impression of being a pregnant woman[11]. For another, dreaming of being pregnant and giving birth was the only time she was truly happy[12]. Even though waking up was a disappointment, she was thankful for the dream experience nonetheless: it was the closest she could get to what she wanted.

When recounting her earlier sexual experiences with an energetic woman, a transvestite reported that she "had the burning wish to become a mother by her"[13]. Another felt crazy because of her "burning desire to be pregnant"[14].

The Hungarian physician wanted to get pregnant too. She was plagued with thoughts of pregnancy and even had psychosomatic symptoms:

"For about three years I had a feeling as if the prostate were enlarged—a bearing-down feeling, as if giving birth to something; and also pain in the hips, constant pain in the back, and the like. Yet, with the strength of despair, I fought against these complaints, which impressed me as being female or effeminate."[15]

Perhaps because of her medical knowledge, she also felt another kind of female bodily function: female ejaculation during intercourse[16].

In these historical narratives, the thought of becoming pregnant and giving birth had great emotional significance. The feelings expressed about pregnancy ranged from great euphoric heights all the way down to the darkest depths of dysphoria. It *moved* them.

I focus on the strength of these emotions because it's easy for non-autogynephilic people to be squicked out by these interests in periods and pregnancy, or to deride them as simple fetishes, but the truth is more complex.

Female bodily functions are powerful signifiers of womanhood. The ability to get pregnant and give birth drastically alters the lives of females and the role they play in society, so some autogynephilic people attach great emotional significance to the idea of having the female bodily functions that allow that possibility.

LACTATION AND BREASTFEEDING

It wasn't common, but a few historical narratives mentioned an interest in lactation or breastfeeding. Like other aspects of autogynephilia, these functions carried an emotional weight that transcended eroticism.

Some transfems found breastfeeding appealing because of its association with motherhood. "The acme of physical human happiness often appears to me to be a woman suckling a healthy child"[17], reported one such transfem. After seeing a mother breastfeeding her child, another transfem lamented, "If only I had such breasts and could give milk!"[18].

One of Hirschfeld's transfems was downright *obsessed* with the idea of lactation and thought about it for much of her life. At around ten years of age, she had a powerful experience while simulating lactation: "I...took out a teaspoon of milk, and let it fall in drops over my teats to lead myself to the illusion of being a soothing mother. This brought on a strong feeling, naturally without ejaculation"[19].

Unfortunately for her, she died before medical technology allowed males to lactate.

MODERN PHYSIOLOGIC AUTOGYNEPHILIA

Scientific advances in medicine have allowed trans women to induce lactation if they really want to and can afford to pay for it.

The first case report of induced lactation in a trans woman was summarized in a *New York Times* article[20] that brought the news to a mainstream audience. In that case report, the study's authors reported a peak output of eight ounces per day and enough overall milk production to be the sole source of nourishment for a newborn's first six weeks[21]. A second case study reported a peak output of three to five ounces per day[22].

While the desire to lactate among trans women isn't the norm, it's prevalent enough that about a third of clinicians surveyed at a major transgender health conference reported encountering trans women who expressed interest in inducing lactation[23]. Approximately one in five of these clinicians knew of places that would help trans women induce lactation[24].

One trans woman who induced lactation in her late fifties reported that it gave her strong personal satisfaction because it affirmed her womanhood[25]. Once she was confident in her ability to lactate, she stopped trying to do so: she had already succeeded at her goal of reinforcing her womanhood.

Some trans women claim to have period symptoms such as mood swings, food cravings, headaches, and bloating[26]. In response to perceiving being on their period, some have experienced feelings they describe as "gender euphoria", "strangely validating", and "wonderful"[27]. One trans woman reported that before she awakened to being transgender, she obsessed over the idea of having periods because it symbolized the ability to get pregnant and give birth[28].

Trans women who feel they are experiencing symptoms on a somewhat regular basis may be getting a timing cue from their environment—perhaps from using a period tracker app or from syncing up with a female they live with.

It's common for trans women to attribute these feelings to feminizing hormones, but old sexology narratives reveal that hormones aren't needed for these feelings to occur. And besides, estrogen taken at consistent intervals is unlikely to create a monthly hormonal cycle like that of females.

IN SUM

* Physiologic autogynephilia is a sexual interest in having a woman's bodily functions. Since bodily functions that differ between the sexes pertain to sexual reproduction, physiologic autogynephilia may drive interest in menstruating, becoming pregnant, giving birth, or lactating. It may also lead to interest in having female ejaculation.

* The desire to have female bodily functions can lead to psychosomatic period symptoms. Autogynephilic people who experience these at regular intervals may be getting a timing cue from their environment.

* Some trans women receive medical help to induce lactation because they see the ability to lactate as a symbolically important part of being a female or mother. If they succeed at lactating, it is a powerful validation of their womanhood.

INTERPERSONAL AUTOGYNEPHILIA

SOCIALLY BEING A WOMAN

In order to coordinate behavior and complete necessary tasks, cultures tend to develop sex-based social roles that prescribe the range of acceptable behaviors and the expected responsibilities of people based on their apparent sex.

Men do *this*; women do *that*.

Men and women are seen and treated differently in social situations, so autogynephilic people often want to be in the gender role associated with females. This desire is associated with *interpersonal autogynephilia*, a sexual interest in socially being a woman.

Interpersonal autogynephilia is about being seen and treated as a woman by others. It commonly includes the desire to be admired as a woman, to pass and be treated as a woman, or to attract men as a woman.

The way others treat us has an outsized impact on how we see ourselves[1], so feminine reinforcement from interpersonal AGP is an especially strong contributor to cross-gender identity formation.

Just being in a group where everyone else is a woman can be emotionally rewarding for autogynephilic people, even if they aren't being explicitly treated as one of them. When they are treated as one of the ladies, however, it can be a big deal[2].

BEING A WOMAN AMONG WOMEN

Plenty of transfems in old sexology narratives expressed a desire to be accepted into the world of women.

Their narratives suggest that this interest wasn't consciously sexual to them. Instead, it was a powerful source of emotional validation. After all, who else has the standing to decide who counts as a woman other than women themselves?

This interest wasn't limited to overt acceptance by women. Just talking with women about feminine things brought satisfaction to some transfems. To some extent, being the only male in a group of women could also satisfy the desire to be a woman among women (surrounded by women, it's easier to feel like one of them).

Magnus Hirschfeld remarked on this desire to be a woman among women because he saw it often: "It is even more striking that many times there is the wish to be in the company of women when dressed like this, as one of them says, 'Above all, I like to appear in the company of ladies as a lady'"[3].

Hirschfeld knew how important this symbolic inclusion in womanhood was to his transfeminine patients, so he arranged for one of them to spend a vacation under the guidance of a woman who was willing to support her efforts to socially present as a woman.

She spent the most memorable evening in the company of women, cracking nuts and listening to poetry together. The patient said of this experience, "From the bottom of my heart I felt so comfortable in their midst", and "at no other time had I ever wanted to be a lady so much as this evening"[4].

Her language is unambiguous: it was enormously meaningful to her to be considered a woman by women and to be able to socialize with them in that role. The lasting memory of this experience alleviated her depression for a long time afterward[5].

Another transfem remarked that even though she'd had sex with plenty of women, she preferred to talk to them about womanly things like clothing and jewelry. On the odd occasion when women noticed her pierced ears and placed one of their earrings in it, it was a "moment of the greatest pleasure"[6].

Other transfems said they felt most comfortable among women or that they felt magnetically drawn to their company[7]. "I should like to be a woman in order to enter utterly into their lives as one of themselves", shared one transfem[8].

This interest in being a woman among women didn't seem to stem from a desire to have sexual access to women. If anything, experiencing sexual attraction to women would interfere with their aims.

R. L. acknowledged that although she wanted to be "admitted to the inner sanctuary of a woman's life", she didn't want to "intrude or wish to be subject to temptation as a man by being in a woman's bedroom"[9].

Being sexually attracted to women at these times would actively interfere with their goal of being a woman among women, so these autogynephilic transfems explicitly did not want to feel amorous toward women in women's spaces. The powerful emotional validation of being included as a woman was much more important to them. Regular heterosexuality was contrary to their goals and a distant concern in comparison to the emotional rewards they sought from inclusion in womanhood.

AMBIGYNEPHILIA AND AUTOGYNEPHILIC META-ATTRACTION

Autogynephilia can shift sexual partner preferences toward masculinity because a partner's masculinity helps the autogynephilic person embody femininity in comparison. The more masculine their partner is, the easier it is to feel feminine. The more feminine their partner is, the harder it is to feel feminine in contrast.

This gender-affirming sexual attraction, *meta-attraction*, is an increased attraction to others based on what that person's traits imply about oneself. Autogynephilic meta-attraction increases sexual interest in men, masculine women, and lesbians.

Autogynephilic people who are simultaneously attracted to women and to being one are *ambigynephilic*. Their gynephilia is bidirectional, pointing both internally and externally at the same time.

For an ambigynephilic person, a woman with masculine traits can appeal to both sides of their gynephilia. Her female body appeals to their allogynephilia (attraction to others as women), and any of her physical or mental traits they interpret as masculine play into their autogynephilic meta-attraction. Women who are energetic, confident, assertive, strong, competent, dominant, or intelligent tend to be especially attractive in this way.

Autogynephilic meta-attraction also makes lesbians more appealing, but not necessarily because lesbians are typically more masculine than heterosexual women. More importantly, their sexual identity as lesbians implies that people who are with them sexually are women, or at least feminine enough to attract a lesbian.

NARRATIVES OF META-ATTRACTION TO WOMEN

In Hirschfeld's day, homosexuality was heavily stigmatized, so most of his transfeminine patients stuck to relationships with women. The women they sought had a consistent type: "The majority of male transvestites feel attracted to women though as a rule they prefer the mannish type of woman who is more masculine in her mental than in her physical make-up"[10].

The more masculine a woman was, the more attractive she became to these transfems. Hirschfeld noted that they desired "a woman with contrasting characteristics to the ones they themselves possessed"[11]. This desire for gender affirmation through contrast is the heart of autohet meta-attraction.

"Strong, manly women were always my ideal lovers. They always make me feel like a woman", explained one transfem[12]. She knew exactly what she wanted: an "energetic, strong woman who would impress me mentally and physically"—one who would "make the first move" and ideally have "a very small moustache"[13].

One transfem described her wife as "an energetic, educated lady"[14], while another transfem described her ideal woman as "physically, totally a woman; yet emotionally strongly developed, an intellectual"[15].

Meta-attraction could even influence how they saw their wives. One transfem's wife found intercourse painful, so they stopped having it. After this, she started to perceive "the male element in the energetic and…stubborn character" of her wife[16].

Sometimes transfems enacted their desire for a masculine sexual partner through sexual role play in which their partners would dress as a man or seduce them like one[17]. For instance, one of Ellis's cases, C. T., reported, "One night I got my wife to dress in a suit of mine. The result was that I was almost mad with desire to be a girl and to love her as a boy"[18].

The Hungarian physician "married an energetic, amiable lady, of a family in which female government was rampant"[19]. She felt that their love was an "*amor lesbicus*" and that their marriage was "like two women living together, one of whom regards herself as in the mask of a man"[20].

She wasn't the only one who identified with lesbians. One transfem said that she felt "attracted as a woman to women"[21] and that if she were a woman, she'd still want to be with women. When another transfem saw two women being close, intimate friends, she "immediately wanted to be one of the two". After she learned about lesbianism, such scenes could even make her feel envious[22].

With few exceptions, these autogynephilic transfems sought masculine, energetic women with strong intellects or dominant personalities. In relation to this female masculinity, they could feel more feminine in contrast.

META-ANDROPHILIA: GENDER-AFFIRMING ATTRACTION TO MEN

For some autogynephilic people, the erotic impulse to feel feminine in contrast with a partner's masculinity can also make them have sexual fantasies about playing a female sexual role with a man. This sexual interest, *meta-androphilia*, is an attraction to being a woman with a man.

Meta-androphilia is unlike the direct attraction to male bodies that a gay male or straight female experiences. Instead, it's more about being in the sexual role of a woman and the validation that comes from feeling attractive to men.

In meta-androphilic sexual fantasies, the men are often faceless[23]. Some autogynephilic people have reported that when they actually tried to live out the fantasy, they found it to be a letdown or even disgusting[24]. Others have reported that they enjoy sex with men but can only fall in love with women[25].

This attraction to men is contingent upon being a woman, so autogynephilic trans women frequently report that their sexual orientation shifted after undergoing gender transition[26]. Some autogynephilic trans women have even concluded in retrospect that they were actually attracted to men their whole lives, but internalized homophobia held them back from realizing their true orientation[27].

Understandably, fantasies of having sex with men as a woman can make an autogynephilic person confused about their sexual orientation. It can also lead them to identify as bisexual or gay.

Bisexual identity and behavior are both uncommonly prevalent in autogynephilic people. A population-representative study of Swedish men found that those who had ever been aroused by crossdressing were eight times as likely to have ever had sex with another male[28]. Likewise, an online study found that among males who reported any sexual interest in behaving or dressing as women, about 30% identified as bisexual[29]. In comparison, only about 5% of American males report bisexual attractions (see Chapter 5.0).

I suspect that meta-androphilia and attraction to androgyny are the autogynephilia-associated phenomena that contribute to male bisexuality the most—both make males more likely to have sexual interest in other males.

Blanchard found that among trans women, the bisexual ones tended to be the most sexually interested in interpersonal autogynephilia[30]. He also found that attraction to men was significantly related to interpersonal autogynephilia[31], which suggested that meta-androphilia was behind this increased attraction to men.

Meta-androphilia can be so influential on an autogynephilic person's sexuality that prior to gender transition they may even identify as gay men if meta-androphilia is their primary source of sexual interest in others.

From the inside, it can be hard to discern the difference between meta-androphilia and conventional androphilia. It is likely even harder to tell the difference for autogynephilic people who lack sexual interest in women yet are meta-attracted to men: without a conventional sexual attraction for comparison purposes, how can they know the attraction they're experiencing is different from conventional attraction to men?

PREFERENTIAL ANDROPHILIA IN AUTOGYNEPHILIC PEOPLE

Assuming that sexual arousal from crossdressing is a valid indicator of autogynephilia, it seems that some MTFS who sexually prefer men are also autogynephilic.

Blanchard's first typology study found that 15% of androphilic MTFS reported past arousal from crossdressing[32]. A similar study found that 23% of their androphilic MTFS reported past arousal from crossdressing[33].

Data on males who identify as crossdressers also suggests that some pre-transition autogynephilic people prefer to be with men.

The crossdresser identity is typically adopted by heterosexual males and the drag queen identity is typically adopted by homosexual males[34]. However, in the two largest surveys of trans people conducted to date, 9%[35] and 13%[36] of male crossdressers seemingly preferred men as sexual partners.

These numbers strongly suggest that autogynephilic people can have strictly androphilic partner preferences, even though much of the attraction seemingly originates in autoheterosexuality rather than homosexuality.

META-ANDROPHILIA: A CONTENTIOUS CONCEPT

Since meta-androphilia is a downstream effect of autogynephilia, the concept of meta-androphilia is sometimes perceived as offensive or invalidating by bisexual trans women.

To complicate matters, sexologists have sometimes used terms like "pseudobisexuality"[37] or "pseudo-androphilia"[38] which seem to imply that this attraction to men is not a real attraction or is somehow less legitimate than conventional androphilia.

But regardless of which words people use to describe it, meta-androphilia definitely exists—it's been a known phenomenon for over a century at this point.

HISTORICAL NARRATIVES OF META-ANDROPHILIA

It didn't take long for sexologists to notice that meta-androphilia was obviously different from conventional androphilia.

The big dawgs of early transgender science—Magnus Hirschfeld and Havelock Ellis—both clearly articulated that the crossdressing males they studied weren't into men in the same way that homosexuals were.

In fact, when Ellis wrote about the differences between *sexual inversion* (homosexuality) and *eonism* (transgenderism), he got so close to the insight that there are two types of MTF transgenderism:

> "Sexual inversion when it appears in Eonism would appear to be merely a secondary result of the aesthetically inverted psychic state. Eonism, when it appears in homosexual persons, is perhaps merely a secondary result of the sexually inverted psychic state."[39]

Ellis knew that the interest in men shown by the transfems he studied was different than conventional homosexuality. So did Hirschfeld.

As a gay man and the world's foremost expert on both homosexuality and transvestism, Hirschfeld could easily suss out that meta-androphilia was distinct from homosexuality:

> "It had the appearance of being only 'episodic' and accidental in character. It was either a matter of an undesired interlude...or as a desired experiment, but which was soon given up as being an unsatisfying and depressing experience. Number 2 clearly brings the basic core of these relationships

to expression when he observes, 'I have never felt an inclination toward men; only dressed as a lady did I enjoy flirting
with them, because I was greatly flattered when I was thought
to be a lady.'"[40]

Writing twenty years earlier, the Hungarian physician
described her meta-androphilia in ways that don't resemble conventional androphilia at all. She described it as "female desire,
though not directed to any particular man"[41] and said it was
"more a longing to be possessed than a wish for coitus"[42]. Her
erotic dreamworld contained two core aspects of meta-androphilic fantasy—being a woman and there being at least one penis
present: "When erotic dreams or ideas occur, I see myself in the
form I have as a woman, and see erected organs presenting"[43].

Not only were the men in her dreams faceless, they also might
not have been much more than disembodied penises.

Although homosexuality has been greatly destigmatized in
the present day, and it has become more common for autogynephilic people to act upon their meta-androphilic impulses,
homophobia was rampant when these narratives were written.
When transvestites fantasized about men, it could be alarming
to their sense of self.

One transfem, whom Ellis described as having "a profound
repugnance to homosexual relationships"[44], thought that acting on
her meta-androphilia would be a step too far, and actively resisted
her desire to be with a man: "I become absolutely intoxicated with
the exquisite femininity of my feelings and I feel that the next

development of wanting a male lover would be actual madness and so must be resisted with all the means in my power"[45].

Although it was uncommon, one of Hirschfeld's transvestites actually acted upon her interest in men at least once. Perhaps out of caution, she did this when she was far away from home. Hirschfeld reported, "At 21, on vacation in the Orient, he consented to anal intercourse by Arabians"[46].

One transfem even reported experiencing meta-androphilia in the realm of emotions as a child: after she developed feelings for a male teacher, she wanted to be his wife[47].

Another transfem fantasized about being a prostitute with a "strapping young fellow" who would be forceful and sexually dominant[48], while another could clearly tell that she wasn't legitimately attracted to men but enjoyed receiving their flirtations anyways[49].

Overall, it seems that meta-androphilia is an attraction to being a woman with a man rather than a direct attraction to male bodies.

IN SUM

* Interpersonal autogynephilia is a sexual interest in socially being a woman. It can drive a desire to be treated as a woman, admired as a woman, seen as a woman, or accepted as a woman by women. In short, it is about being perceived as a woman by others.

* This desire to have one's femininity validated by others opens the possibility of meta-attraction: attraction to others based on what their traits imply about oneself. Through autogynephilic meta-attraction, interpersonal autogynephilia plays an outsized role in determining the sexual partner preferences of autogynephilic people. It alters taste in women by making masculine women and lesbians more attractive. It also creates gender-affirming sexual interest in men (meta-androphilia).

* Although meta-androphilia usually leads to bisexuality, it can make autogynephilic people prefer men as sexual partners to the point that they have little to no interest in women, and therefore lead to preferential homosexuality. Transgender typology studies have found that there are some MTFs in the "homosexual" group who report prior crossdressing arousal, which suggests that sorting based on the two-type typology underestimates the true proportion of autoheterosexuals among trans people.

PART 3

FEMALE AUTOHETEROSEXUALITY

AUTOANDROPHILIA

DEAR READER

I wrote these autoandrophilia chapters so that autoandrophilic readers can have a section that directly applies to
them: their existence has been ignored or downplayed for
far too long.

Since autoandrophilia is similar to autogynephilia, I will
describe it similarly. Pay attention to the parts that seem to
repeat. These thematic overlaps illuminate the general form
of autosexual orientations.

3 . 0

AUTOANDROPHILIA (AAP)
LOVE OF SELF AS A MAN

The "love of self as a man" that autohet females experience is *autoandrophilia* (AAP). Autoandrophilia is a sexual or romantic interest in being a man. Sexually, it manifests as arousal by the thought or image of oneself as a man (or as manly).

Autoandrophilia can drive a desire to have a man's body, wear men's clothing, behave like a man, or be treated like one. Like conventional heterosexuality, autoandrophilia can cultivate attachments, alter moods, and shape how people view sex and gender—both personally and socially.

Autoandrophilia can manifest in ways that are overtly sexual or in ways that are predominantly emotional or romantic. Some autoandrophilic people have a deep emotional yearning to be the other sex, while others find the idea to be a huge turn-on. Most feel some combination of the two.

As with autogynephilia, autoandrophilia causes both positive and negative gender-related feelings in response to perceptions of gendered embodiment.

When autoandrophilic people perceive that they're embodying masculinity or manhood, they may feel joy, comfort, relaxation, excitement, a sense of well-being, or a feeling of rightness. This upward shift in mood is *gender euphoria*.

At first, gender euphoria can have the giddy excitement of new love. Over time, these warm fuzzies tend to develop into feelings of comfort resembling the companionate love of long-term partnership. The experience goes from "Netflix and chill" to Netflix and literally chilling. Either way, it's enjoyable and meaningful.

Perceiving shortcomings in their masculine embodiment can cause autoandrophilic people's moods to drop. This gender dysphoria is the negative side of gender-related feelings. It may frustrate autoandrophilic people, make them feel alienated from their bodies, or plunge them into depressive moods.

Together, autoandrophilic euphoria and dysphoria put on a good cop/bad cop routine that makes cooperation with the inner masculine self more likely. These feelings elevate the worth of masculinity and devalue femininity. Eventually, masculinity can become synonymous with *good* and femininity with *bad*. As this process continues, the urge to undergo gender transition and live as a man may intensify.

Some autoandrophilic people choose to undergo gender transition and become trans men. After transition, they'll commonly identify as gay or bisexual men. They might also identify using newer, more ambiguous labels such as *queer* or *pansexual*. Autoandrophilic people who lack sexual interest in others tend to identify as asexual.

However, the cross-gender journey doesn't start with the decision to transition. Instead, it usually starts with intermittent mental shifts into a masculine mind state and grows from there.

AUTOANDROPHILIC MENTAL SHIFTS AND GENDER IDENTITY

Autoandrophilia motivates people to think of themselves as male or masculine. Doing so is intrinsically rewarding, so it can become their default way of seeing themselves.

Autoandrophilia enables people to experience mental shifts into a masculine headspace in response to stimuli that reinforce their sense of masculinity or manhood. This experience of feeling like a man is an *autoandrophilic mental shift*.

Initially, autoandrophilic mental shifts tend to be short-lived. They often first arise through crossdressing, being "one of the guys", or imagining being a boy—all of which may lead to feeling confident, strong, or self-assured.

With continued reinforcement over time, autoandrophilic mental shifts can happen more often and last longer when they do. Eventually, as the gaps between these experiences become smaller and less frequent, the feeling of being a man (or wanting to be one) can become more or less continuous.

At this point, a *transmasculine* gender identity has crystallized.

Transmasculine (or *transmasc*) is an umbrella term that can describe a female who identifies with masculinity, identifies as a man, transitions to live as a man, or has a masculine gender expression. It's another way of saying someone is on the female-to-male (FTM) spectrum.

The process of developing a solid transmasculine identity takes years and only happens to a subset of autoandrophilic people. When it does, this masculine self often supplants their default, feminine self.

AUTOANDROPHILIC EMBODIMENT SUBTYPES

There haven't been any studies investigating whether autoandrophilia has subtypes that are analogous to the five subtypes of autogynephilia, but I'll apply those ideas anyway—they are conceptually useful.

After all, the two sexes *are* different in terms of their bodies and their functions. And people usually behave differently, dress differently, and get treated differently in social situations based on their sex.

* Anatomic AAP—having a man's body
* Sartorial AAP—donning men's fashion
* Behavioral AAP—behaving like a man

* Physiologic AAP—having a man's bodily functions
* Interpersonal AAP—socially being a man

These interests are strictly a sexual turn-on for some people, while others pursue surgeries or take testosterone to meet their emotional yearning for masculine embodiment.

Most autoandrophilic people fall somewhere in the middle of these two extremes. Sometimes the orientation is mostly emotional, and other times it's mostly sexual. Depending on the circumstances and the person, it's varying degrees of both.

The same caveats I gave about autogynephilia subtypes apply to autoandrophilia as well: it isn't always possible to discern someone's motivations based on their behavior or appearance. However, these autoandrophilic subtypes are useful concepts that can guide autoandrophilic people's decisions about how they want to manage their gender feelings.

If getting a short haircut, dressing as a guy, and behaving like one would meet most of their needs, then medical transition may not be the right way to go.

On the other hand, if they want masculine physical features and to be socially seen as a man, medical transition will have stronger appeal—especially if they want to embody masculinity and manhood to the greatest degree possible.

The attachment principle of sexual orientation applies here too. If there's something about being a man that a person thinks about regularly, finds particularly arousing, or places on a pedestal, it's possible to get progressively more attached to the idea over time.

Stimuli that initially provide strong gender euphoria can quickly become the new normal, which often leads to a desire for more. When autoandrophilic people can't embody manhood to their satisfaction, they may feel gender dysphoria.

If you're autoandrophilic, whether or not you transition might be the most significant decision you'll ever make. And if you decide to go for it, there's still much to figure out: *when* to transition, *how* to do it, and *how far*.

Knowing that autoandrophilia is behind your desire to be a man can clarify this decision-making process. Rather than wondering if you are trans, you can instead start with the premise that you're autoandrophilic and then decide how you want to incorporate it into your life.

THE LIMITED YET SUFFICIENT FORMAL EVIDENCE FOR AUTOANDROPHILIA

Historically, female sexuality has been studied far less than male sexuality. Strong autoheterosexuality is also less common in females[1]. For these and other reasons, there isn't much about autoandrophilia in the sexology literature. However, people who fit the profile have received occasional mention since the early days of sexology.

For example, all the way back in 1910, Hirschfeld wrote about masculine females who were extremely attracted to feminine men and felt themselves to be gay men[2]. He compared them to male transvestites who loved masculine women and felt themselves to be lesbians.

Even though the sexology literature is limited when it comes to autoandrophilia, there's enough to work with. Combining older papers on female transvestism with newer ones on the sexuality of gay and bisexual trans men gives a clear enough picture.

However, the single best firsthand account of autoandrophilia can be found in Lou Sullivan's diaries[3], which are truly special and offer deep insight into the psychology of autoandrophilia. For example, a couple years before he transitioned, he wrote:

"Just spent the afternoon in a long masturbation session, just like I'd done nearly all last summer. Imagining I'm a boy and masturbating endlessly."[4]

His diaries have plenty of entries that eroticized the idea of being male. He was attracted to the idea of having a flat chest[5] and a male voice[6]. Years before he transitioned, he identified as a female transvestite.

Lou Sullivan was a gay trans man who spread awareness of gay trans men to researchers, clinicians, and trans people. Before his advocacy, many scientists doubted that his kind existed—or that they were legitimate recipients of gender-affirming medical care.

In the previous chapter, I explained the general form of autogynephilic interests, using classical firsthand narratives. I will use a similar approach for autoandrophilia. In addition to Sullivan's diaries, there are two other extensive accounts that I'll draw upon.

The oldest one is of Elsa B., whose account was first published in 1923. He was sexually aroused by transvestism, greatly desired to have a penis, and felt "spiritually male"[7]. He longed to live as a man and suffered immensely because of his inability to do so.

The other lengthy account is truly fascinating. He was one of Robert Stoller's patients. Stoller wrote a book-length case study about him titled *Splitting: A Case of Female Masculinity*[8]. Stoller referred to this patient as "Mrs. G", but he'll be "Mr. G" here.

From his earliest memories, Mr. G had a phantom penis and a masculine entity in his mind that he communicated with. He was also sexually aroused by wearing Levi's jeans and took pleasure in teaching men how to do manly things like hotwiring cars or robbing gas stations.

All three accounts of autoandrophilia demonstrate an interest in having a male body, so let's start with that.

ANATOMIC AUTOANDROPHILIA

People who are androphilic (attracted to men) are attracted to men's bodies. They like men's muscles, height, broad shoulders, penises, deep voices, facial hair, and other masculine features. When that attraction is turned inside out, it drives a desire to have those same physical features.

This attraction to having a man's body is *anatomic auto-androphilia.*

People with anatomic autoandrophilia often want to have a penis, flat chest, facial hair, strong muscles, or body hair. If these desires are strong enough, autoandrophilic people may take testosterone or have surgeries, resulting in autoandrophilic transsexualism. These physical changes help them attain some of the same traits that they admire in others.

Testosterone can redistribute their body fat, thicken facial hair, and masculinize their face. Their larynx can grow, lowering their vocal pitch. If they get a double mastectomy, their chest will have a flat contour. If they undergo phalloplasty (surgical construction of a phallus), they will have masculine genitals.

Autoandrophilic transsexuals are likely to find some of these changes arousing. This might be why a prominent trans man named Jamison Green once noted that "many transmen experience erotic stimulation by observing their own bodies in transition"[9].

Autoandrophilic trans men may subjectively experience these changes as arousal, gender euphoria, or a mixture of the two. Both are usually appreciated. By contrast, the inability to achieve male-typical body features to their satisfaction can fuel gender dysphoria.

Over time, autoandrophilic trans men will continue to derive satisfaction and comfort from their masculinized bodies. Masculine features affirm the masculine self and allow them to better see themselves in the way they want—as men.

Having a Penis

Penises are powerfully symbolic of manhood, so the idea of having a penis is erotically and emotionally appealing to many autoandrophilic people.

In the earliest thorough account of female transvestism in the sexology literature, Elsa B.'s desire for a penis of his own was obvious. The first time he saw one, he realized it was what separated him from the boys, so he immediately thought about cutting it off and taking it for himself[10].

Elsa B. repeatedly dreamed about having a penis[11] and got pleasure from dreaming that he had a large one[12]. When he hit puberty and realized he wouldn't be growing one, he fell into a deep depression.

The autoandrophilic yearning for male anatomy can even lead to *autoandrophilic phantom shifts,* which create the sensation of having phantom male anatomy such as a penis. These phantom penises may be either flaccid or erect.

Prior experience with phantom penises is probably common among autoandrophilic transsexuals: one survey of twenty-nine transsexual men found that 62% reported feeling phantom penises and phantom erections[13].

Mr. G experienced both phantom shifts and mental shifts starting from a young age. His phantom penis began to appear at age four, after he saw a boy peeing and became envious of his penis. His internal masculine self, "Charlie", also appeared around this same time[14].

Mr. G's penis was a huge part of his identity. When asked what would happen if he were to lose it, he said, "I wouldn't be anything. My penis is what I am"[15]. For him, a penis signified strength[16]. He needed it because it made him strong[17].

Depending on the erotic situation at hand, Mr. G.'s phantom penis would move wherever the situation demanded. While masturbating, it was inside his vagina. During sex with men, it was in his abdomen. With women, it was out front[18].

Lou Sullivan's manual for female-to-male transvestites and transsexuals includes testimony from a female transvestite who liked to fantasize about having a penis and penetrating a woman with it[19]. But Sullivan himself fantasized about having a penis and penetrating a man with it[20]. He later pursued surgeries to enhance the size of his phallus and implant prosthetic testicles.

A Man's Flat Chest

When autoandrophilic people have breasts, they often compress them with a breast binder to create the flat look they desire. If they don't have a binder, they might use tape. One creative trans-masc even used a corset to flatten his chest[21].

With a flat chest, autoandrophilic people have a higher chance of being able to look downward without being immediately reminded of their birth sex. To get that flat look permanently, many trans men undergo double mastectomies.

Afterward, they don't have to worry about hiding breasts or put mental effort into pretending they aren't there. Much to their relief, they can go around shirtless like any other guy.

For years, Sullivan bound his breasts and endured chest dysphoria until he finally got them removed. It bothered him to look down and see breasts[22], while the idea of having a flat chest was a big turn-on: "If I had a mastectomy I'd have to beat off 24 hours a day because I'd be so turned on by myself"[23].

He frequently fantasized about having a flat chest[24]. He wanted to get a mastectomy for years and was comforted by the thought of getting one[25]. For example, once when he was going through emotional turmoil because his partner slept with a woman, his first thought was to get a mastectomy because somehow he'd be able to handle it better that way[26].

Manly Hair: Short Hairstyles and Facial Hair

Autoandrophilic people often want to have their hair cut short into a men's style and are sometimes excited by the idea of having a mustache, beard, or body hair.

When Elsa B.'s hair was long, it would send him into "fits of rage", so he kept his hair short[27]. Mr. G and Lou Sullivan kept their hair short too.

One transmasc's crossdressing started with the purchase of a mustache. Wearing it felt erotic, and when he fellated his partner while wearing it, he felt himself to be a gay male[28].

Sullivan became enthralled when he first noticed that dark hair was growing on his upper lip. He wrote in his journal, "God, I'm shaking with ecstasy"[29]. True to form, he then imagined his mustached self kissing a man and got excited by that too.

SARTORIAL AUTOANDROPHILIA: DRESSING AS A MAN

By wearing men's clothing, autoandrophilic people can cultivate a sense of maleness that confers feelings of comfort, empowerment, or arousal.

Those emotions and arousal stem from *sartorial autoandrophilia*, a sexual interest in donning men's fashion. Traditionally, this cross-gender embodiment via clothing was called transvestism.

For many autoandrophilic people, men's clothing just starts to feel "right" over time. It also helps build up a masculine cross-gender identity and feels like a natural outgrowth of that identity.

Among autohet trans people, erotic transvestism is less common among trans men than trans women. For instance, a study on gay and bisexual trans men found that only a third of them had become aroused by dressing in men's clothing[30], which is less than half the rate that Blanchard found in his studies of trans women.

In the past, some leading sexologists even thought that female transvestites didn't exist or that they were exceedingly rare[31]. They were wrong about that though.

Female transvestites definitely exist.

Reports of Transvestism

Elsa B. got sexual arousal from dressing as a man. He even had his first orgasm while wearing a suit[32] and became aroused by dreaming about transvestism[33]. He was willing to forego sexual intercourse, but not transvestism—it was far more pleasurable to him than any intercourse could be[34].

His thirst for men's clothing started around puberty and never went away. He struggled against the feminine clothing that his family insisted upon[35]. When he had to wear it, he felt like "a dressed-up monkey"[36]. On the other hand, he reported that "a great oppression leaves me" when wrapped in men's garb and that he felt "free and easy"[37].

Another transmasc got erotic pleasure from dressing as a man in public—a feeling so strong that he "could barely avoid shaking". He considered his tendency to be "definitely erotic", and he reported that in the men's clothing department, his feeling was "one of fetishism"[38].

One married transmasc reported that he enjoyed dressing up in his husband's clothing, and even went so far as to place a tampon in his vagina so it poked through the slit in his husband's underwear. He imagined that he was his husband during the act, which sexually excited him[39].

Although manly boots helped Mr. G cultivate a feeling of masculinity, they weren't erotic for him[40]. His transvestism revolved around blue denim Levi's jeans, which were his favorite source of erotic pleasure:

> "There is no sensation comparable, and that is probably because the peak of this sensation involves a large range of feelings, including impossible-to-repress sexual excitement. I feel emotionally strengthened, assertive, confident, and totally unafraid. When I put on [a] pair of levis it's as though I shed the neurotic crap that plagues me constantly, all of that stuff that makes me hate being a female, or all of that stuff that keeps me afraid of being feminine."[41]

Wrapped in his jeans, Mr. G's gender dysphoria faded into the background. In his masculine element, he felt strong, secure, powerful, and superior to males around him.

Lou Sullivan was heavily influenced by his clothing as well. Wearing his first leather jacket gave him gender euphoria and a "strange identity feeling"[42]. In contrast, when he wore a skirt during sex because his partner asked him to, it stopped him from being aroused because it made him think of himself as a girl[43]. He also reported that when he didn't have a man available to meet his sexual and romantic needs, he could get some solace from wearing his partner's underwear, which made him feel less alone[44].

Why Is Transvestism in Females Reported Less Frequently?

We don't yet know why females are less likely to report arousal in response to crossdressing, but there are some differences between the sexes and their societal roles that likely contribute to this state of affairs.

Culturally, men are less commonly eroticized than women, and their clothing reflects that. Men's clothing is looser and less brightly colored, and it tends to conceal more of their body. In comparison, women's clothing is more form-fitting and revealing, and it has a greater variety of colors, cuts, materials, and styles.

Males also tend to have more interest in things rather than people. By contrast, females are more interested in people and less interested in things[45]. This "people versus things" personality trait helps explain why nurses, social workers, and teachers tend to be female, while construction workers, programmers, and engineers tend to be male. It's one of the biggest psychological sex differences and has even been detected in babies who are just a few days old[46].

Different reported rates of transvestism might also come down to a difference in sexuality. Males are more likely to have object-related sexual interests such as transvestism and sexual fetishism (a sexual interest in objects, materials, or specific non-genital body parts)[47].

All of these factors potentially contribute to lower reported rates of female transvestism. Aside from these obvious and well-established sex differences, there could be other factors too.

PHYSIOLOGIC AUTOANDROPHILIA

When Mr. G orgasmed with women, he felt his phantom penis ejaculate[48].

Like Mr. G, Elsa B. also envisioned himself ejaculating. In his narrative, it came in a dream where he was having sex with a woman who was his wife:

> "I am married and have a wife. I am having intercourse with her and am happy at the size of my penis and the male form of my chest. Then ejaculation and following that an orgasm which lasted for minutes."[49]

Penile erections and ejaculating semen are physiological functions specific to males that pertain to reproduction, so fantasies about them are arguably examples of *physiologic autoandrophilia*, a sexual interest in having a man's bodily functions.

Those bodily functions are unambiguous signs of male arousal and feature prominently in male sexuality—of course some autoandrophilic people are attracted to having those functions themselves. But is a sexual interest in having erections or ejaculating semen the autoandrophilic equivalent to an autogynephilic person's interest in having female-typical bodily functions such as menstruation, lactation, and pregnancy?

Ultimately, we don't know yet. Answering this question will require further study.

BEHAVIORAL AUTOANDROPHILIA

Autoandrophilic people often take pleasure in behaving like men. For instance, they may walk with a confident male strut, urinate while standing, or intentionally lower the pitch of their voice while speaking.

These are manifestations of *behavioral autoandrophilia*—a sexual interest in behaving like a man.

Like other aspects of autoandrophilia, sometimes it influences everyday behaviors that don't have any apparent eroticism, and other times the eroticism is obvious. Behavioral autoandrophilia can influence behavior even prior to puberty, but it's less likely to feel overtly sexual before then.

For example, Elsa B. used to play only with boy's toys as a kid. He felt ashamed to play with girl's toys, and if he received any, he had a habit of throwing them into the fire[50].

As an adult, he peed standing up, had a masculine strut with long steps, and worked hard even during his period[51]. He would also masturbate while lying on his stomach and "making the movements of a male in coitus"[52].

A different transmasc person recalled that as a kid, they had a lot of toy guns and would play cowboys with the neighborhood boys. When one of those boys peed standing up, they got the idea to try it themselves[53].

As a kid, Lou Sullivan had a habit of pretending he was a boy. In a letter to Blanchard, he recounted a childhood game, "playing boys", that he and his sisters played together. Sullivan wrote, "We took boys' names, dressed as boys, mimicked a male voice and spent the entire day pretending we were boys"[54]. He liked the idea of being a boy so much that he would pretend he was a boy even when he was alone or dressed as a girl.

Masculine Sexual Behavior

In sexual matters, autoandrophilic people often want to play a man's role.

During receptive vaginal intercourse, they may fantasize about being penetrated anally[55]. They might also prefer anal intercourse because it doesn't conflict with their masculine self-image in the way that vaginal penetration does.

One trans man reported that pre-transition, he'd prepare for sex by getting "rat-assed drunk". During sex, he felt alienated from his female body: "Somebody was sticking something in me when I was supposed to be sticking something in them"[56].

Other trans men have a similar desire to be the penetrating partner. In a case study of two androphilic trans men, both of them had the same favorite sexual position: kneeling behind their partner while rubbing their genitals against their backside and stroking their penis. During this, they would imagine that they were anally penetrating their partners[57].

Like those other trans men, Lou Sullivan also fantasized about penetrating another man with his penis. He wanted "to fuck a boy, and to be on top and inside"[58].

Mr. G: A True Bad Boy

Mr. G took pleasure in being better than men at their own activities and aspired to embody the type of aggressive, powerful masculinity that gets men placed in the "bad boy" category. In Mr. G's world, women were fragile and men were invulnerable, strong, and powerful[59].

Mr. G associated driving with men and said he "could drive better than any man on the road"[60]. He learned to drive at fourteen and got a trophy from winning a Powder Puff Derby that same year. The first time he drove a car alone, it was one he stole.

Around age eighteen, Mr. G intentionally drove a motorcycle over an old man[61]. While drag racing, he got pulled over by a cop and proceeded to back into his car[62]. Another time, he shot a cop in the ass[63]. He robbed half a dozen gas stations "for kicks"[64], and he put five bullets into a man who slept with his girlfriend[65].

Mr. G constantly behaved in ways that would be described today as "toxic masculinity". His violence was mostly directed toward men because he didn't think men could be hurt. The actions described here are a small fraction of the total mayhem he caused.

As mentioned previously, he took pride in teaching men how to rob gas stations and steal cars[66], and the way he talked about all of these escapades made his gendered motivations clear:

> "Those boys and those men respected me for my knowledge and my ability to do things that most men do. How many women do you know that go around hot-wiring cars? Not very many."[67]

Being respected by men was gratifying to him. Even if he couldn't be a guy, he could still validate his masculinity by being even more manly than the men around him.

This desire to occupy a man's social role and be seen as masculine by others is similar to behavioral autoandrophilia, but instead of being based on the behaviors of the autoandrophilic person themselves, it's based on the actions, perceptions, and behaviors of other people.

This social dimension of autoandrophilia—interpersonal auto-androphilia—is where we'll go next.

IN SUM

* Autoandrophilia (AAP) is a sexual interest in being a man. This sexual attraction to embodying masculinity is how autoheterosexuality manifests in females.

* An autoandrophilic person is likely to see masculine embodiment as emotionally rewarding and feel

uncomfortable when they perceive shortcomings of masculine embodiment. These positive and negative feelings shape their gender identity over time and tend to increase their overall commitment to masculinity.

* Although scientists haven't yet empirically verified that there are at least five subtypes of autoandrophilia as they have for autogynephilia, there are firsthand accounts in the sexology literature that indicate autoandrophilic people can have sexual interest in embodying masculinity through their bodies, bodily functions, behavior, dress, or social standing.

* Autoandrophilic trans identity forms over time through reinforcement. At first, autoandrophilic mental shifts create a temporary sensation of having a masculine headspace. With time, they tend to happen more often and last longer when they do. Eventually, this masculine mind state can become a solidified masculine identity.

* Anatomic autoandrophilia drives a desire to have a man's body. Autoandrophilic people often want to have a flat chest, facial hair, or a penis. It's common for them to wear a binder to flatten their chest or use prosthetic genitals to create the feeling of having these masculine traits.

* Sartorial autoandrophilia drives a desire to wear men's clothes. Dressing as a man can initially be erotic, but over time it may simply feel comfortable or reassuring. Although erotic transvestism seems to be less common in females, it has still been reported plenty of times. Female transvestism definitely exists.

* Behavioral autoandrophilia drives a desire to behave like a man. It can motivate an autoandrophilic person to walk with a confident male strut, pee standing up, or speak with a low voice. It can also make them want to be the active, insertive partner during sexual intercourse.

INTERPERSONAL AUTOANDROPHILIA

SOCIALLY BEING A MAN

Across a wide variety of societies and cultures, women and men are seen and treated differently. Depending on whether someone is seen as female or male, they generally face expectations to behave and express themselves accordingly "as men" or "as women".

As a result, autoandrophilic people often want to occupy the social role associated with males. This social aspect of autoandrophilia—*interpersonal autoandrophilia*—is a sexual interest in being treated as a man.

Interpersonal AAP might entail passing as a man, attracting women as a man, or being accepted by other men as one of them. In a broad sense, it's about being seen and treated by others as a man.

This social aspect of autoandrophilia can also shift partner preferences toward feminine or androphilic partners because those traits help an autoandrophilic person feel masculine in contrast.

For autoandrophilic people, being seen as a man by others has social and emotional significance. Even without passing, just embodying a man's social role can be gratifying.

The first few times that Lou Sullivan passed as a boy, he became absolutely ecstatic. While waiting to checkout at a grocery store, an older woman referred to Sullivan as "him", and he "skyrocketed to Cloud 9"[1]. A week later, someone couldn't tell if he was a boy or girl. Once again, he "skyrocketed to heaven"[2].

He also fantasized about picking up gay men while passing as a guy. While thinking about this, he wrote in his diary, "I'm getting the hots to get back into some serious passing"[3].

When autoandrophilic people deeply desire to pass as men and still get perceived as women despite their best efforts, it stings. One transmasc in this situation reported that "each failure cuts into me anew"[4].

Even without passing, however, being in a man's social role can be gratifying for autoandrophilic people.

When Sullivan was still living as a woman, he worked with his guy friends to fix up a car, which reminded him of "playing boys" as a kid. He got a lot of pleasure from "working with the guys as a guy", even though his friends didn't necessarily see him as a man at the time[5].

Elsa B. fantasized about being the father of a family and caring for his wife and children[6]. He approximated this fantasy by living with a woman who took care of the household while he played the role of breadwinner.

One transmasc's favorite fantasy was about male bonding through a sort of circle jerk. The fantasy began with talking to a guy about their mutual turn-ons. Then the conversation would progress to watching porn, and he'd float the idea of masturbating themselves, together. Once it got to that point, "He would take out his dick and I would take out my dildo and we would give them a working over"[7].

AUTOANDROPHILIC META-ATTRACTION

Autoandrophilic people are likely to see femininity in their sexual partners as a bonus. The more feminine their partners are, the easier it is to feel masculine in comparison. The reverse is also true: the more masculine their partners are, the harder it can be to feel masculine in contrast.

This shift in partner preferences is the result of *meta-attraction*: increased attraction to others based on what their traits imply about you.

Autoandrophilic meta-attraction increases attraction to others whose traits help an autoandrophilic person feel masculine by comparison. For autoandrophilic meta-attraction, other people's gendered traits and sexual orientation are the most relevant traits to consider. The more androphilic and feminine they are, the more potential there is to feel like a man in relation to them.

As a result, autoandrophilic meta-attraction can increase sexual interest in feminine straight women, feminine men, and gay men. Straight women and gay men are attracted to men, so being with them signals to an autoandrophilic person that they're a man, and femininity in sexual partners makes it easier to feel masculine in contrast.

Meta-Gynephilia: Attraction to Being a Man with a Woman

Over fifty years ago, a doctor writing about an FTM patient noted that his "erotic play with girls…was to demonstrate that [he] was a boy…not because [he] felt gratification in fondling and kissing"[8].

Likewise, Lou Sullivan's manual for FTMs quotes a transmasc who said, "I like to imagine what it would be like to have a penis like a guy and have sex with a girl"[9].

This attraction to being a man with a woman is *meta-gyne-philia*. It is more about being a guy with a girl than it is a direct attraction to the female form. The more feminine, straight, and small a woman is, the easier it is to feel like a man in relation to her.

In Sullivan's diaries, he sometimes contemplated hooking up with women, but it always hinged upon him being a man in relation to them. He wrote about a particularly petite woman more than once; her smallness made him feel big, which led him to think that he could be her boyfriend[10].

A few years later, Sullivan still hadn't picked up a woman. When he thought about doing so, he had no idea how he would do it as a woman, but he felt he could pursue a woman as a man[11]. After becoming a transsexual man, he reported that women started to look better to him because he didn't have to be a woman anymore[12].

However, it doesn't seem like he translated these fleeting thoughts into action. Eight years into his transition, he had hooked up with a transsexual woman once, but he hadn't otherwise been with women[13].

Mr. G acted on his meta-gynephilia often, and his pursuit of women obviously stemmed from his attraction to being a man. His logic was clear as can be. He asked, "How could I have a penis and not want a female?"[14]

While wearing his Levi's jeans, his sexual fantasies always involved a woman[15]. The women he preferred were feminine, virginal, young, and pretty with long hair[16]. They also had to be strictly heterosexual[17].

He was appalled by the idea that having sex with women made him a homosexual[18]. Although male homosexuality was acceptable to him, female homosexuality was absolutely abhorrent[19].

After seducing women, Mr. G felt powerful like a man. During sex with women, he always took men's sexual positions and took pride in his ability to satisfy women better than any man could[20]. And when he orgasmed with them, he felt his phantom penis ejaculate[21].

Ambiandrophilia and Meta-Attraction to Feminine Men

In general, a sexual partner's femininity helps an autoandrophilic person feel more masculine by comparison.

As a result, autoandrophilic meta-attraction enhances sexual interest in feminine men. With a feminine man as a sexual partner, an autoandrophilic person who is attracted to men can satisfy both sides of their attraction at the same time.

Autoandrophilic people who are simultaneously attracted *to* men and to *being* a man are *ambiandrophilic*: their androphilia is bidirectional, pointing both internally and externally at the same time.

It's common for ambiandrophilic people to have pondered the classic "do/be" question: "do I want to *do* him or *be* him?".

For ambiandrophilic people, a feminine male body appeals to their alloandrophilia. If their male partner is gay, bi, or has mental or physical traits that seem feminine, these contribute to autoandrophilic meta-attraction.

Men who are sensitive, submissive, vulnerable, gentle, or empathetic can be especially attractive in this way. The particular desirable traits vary from person to person, but any mental or behavioral traits seen as feminine can contribute to autoandrophilic meta-attraction.

This interest in feminine men shows up in case reports of androphilic trans men. For instance, one wanted a "loving sensitive man whose femininity would complement the maleness in me"[22]. Another wanted "slender, feminine-appearing men"[23]. Blanchard himself highlighted a case in which a trans man was especially into "gentler, nonmacho gay men" that enabled him to feel masculine in contrast[24].

This attraction to feminine men can be turned inward too. One transmasc admitted, "One perversity, perhaps, is that I like the idea of looking like a rather feminine male"[25].

Attraction to Gay Men

Many autoandrophilic people *love* gay men and long to be in a gay relationship of their own. Among autoandrophilic trans men, the partner preference for gay men is especially common.

On one level, it just makes sense. They are erotically interested in men *and* in being one, so it's no surprise they're attracted to gay men.

There's more to it than that though. There is something special about gay relationships in particular that appeal to them.

One aspect is the even playing field—in a gay relationship, it's one man with another. With gay men, there's less of a need to navigate the power differences that disadvantage females in heterosexual relationships. For example, a trans man who'd recently had his first gay sex reported that "it felt like sex between equals for once" and that it "made all other relationships pale by comparison"[26].

Autoandrophilic meta-attraction also contributes to this infatuation with gay men. Gay men are specifically into men, which implies that the person pairing up with them is a man too.

The enthusiasm for being a gay man and having gay male sex among autoandrophilic people is so common that Blanchard uses the term "autohomoerotic gender dysphoria" to describe the gender dysphoria of FTMS who want to participate in gay male sex[27]. When seen as a manifestation of autoandrophilia, however, this "autohomoerotic" dysphoria is simply the interpersonal aspect of autoandrophilic gender dysphoria. Regardless of which conception is best, however, there is obviously a subset of trans men who are sexually attracted to being gay men.

Lou Sullivan was one of them. He wrote in his diary, "As long as I remember I've had to think of myself as a guy making love to another guy to have an orgasm"[28].

Sullivan's diaries were chock-full of references to gay men. From a young age, he longed to be one, greatly admired them, and wanted to be a part of their world. He read their literature, joined their organizations, and pursued them sexually. He saw himself as a gay man too.

When Sullivan explained it, the reason for his attraction to gay men seemed obvious:

"What made gay men more sexually attractive than straight men? Simply the fact that they were aroused by other men. All kinds of gay men appeal(ed) to me romantically and sexually—old, young, leather and muscle types, lithe femmy queens, clean-cut men in business suits. If they loved men, I loved them!"[29]

For Sullivan, gay men's attraction to men was *the* defining characteristic that made them attractive to him. Their gayness increased his attraction because it signified that he was a gay man himself. If men weren't bisexual at the very least, he wasn't interested in them.

A different autoandrophilic person reported that he was specifically attracted to depictions of gay male sex, fantasized about participating in it, and sought a submissive man so that he could play the masculine role. He wanted to exist socially as a gay man so that he could take part in their social world, and he also made sure to specify that he was "not a fag hag"[30]. (A "fag hag" is a straight woman who enjoys or prefers the company of gay men).

When a straight man pursues an autoandrophilic FTM, his straightness might be a deal-breaker: "what's missing is how they're relating to you", a gay trans man explained[31].

This is why relationships between autoandrophilic FTMs and conventionally heterosexual males are often fundamentally incompatible and why gay men are far more appealing. Gay men are attracted to men, so they're intrinsically motivated to see their partners as men. Being with a gay man is an ideal outcome for many autoandrophilic people because there's less second-guessing about whether or not their partner actually sees them as a man.

Unsurprisingly, a study of trans men found that androphilic-leaning trans men were significantly more attracted to gay men than they were to straight men, straight women, or lesbians[32].

CHANGES TO SEXUAL ORIENTATION AFTER FTM TRANSITION

Trans men often report a change in sexual orientation after transitioning.

After becoming more confident in their masculinized body, it's common for autoandrophilic trans men to become comfortable with a wider array of sexual partners and modes of sexual interaction. Some even become comfortable with vaginal penetration[33].

A study of approximately 500 trans men found that 40% of them reported shifts to their sexual partner preferences after transitioning[34]. Most of those preference shifts were toward men.

Similarly, a clinical study on orientation changes found that after two years of gender transition, trans men were more likely to have a male partner and fantasize about men than before transitioning. This rise in attraction to men and drop in attraction to women happened at the same time that many of them started to revert to a female identity in their fantasies[35], which suggests that meta-attraction influenced these changes. I explore this study in greater detail in Chapter 5.3.

In an influential book on female sexual fluidity[36], both of the transmasculine people it featured said that after transitioning, they were more attracted to men than before, and it was gay men in particular who caught their eye. One said he was unusually attracted to gay men[37], and the other started to notice all the attractive gay men in his neighborhood after going on testosterone[38].

HOMOEROTIC MEDIA

Many autoandrophilic people first realize their attraction to being a gay man through media depicting romantic love between men. This media is often categorized as *mlm* ("male loves male").

A popular form of mlm is "slash fanfiction", also known as "m/m slash" or simply "slash". Slash fanfiction depicts male characters from popular media franchises in romantic or erotic situations.

Slash gained momentum as a stand-alone genre when female fans of the original *Star Trek* began to write romantic and erotic stories about Kirk and Spock[39]. Over time, slash fanfiction spread to fans of other media franchises.

Today, media franchises like *Harry Potter*, *Supernatural*, *Naruto*, and *Twilight* are popular in slash fanfiction. Millions of these stories can be found on *fanfiction.net*[40].

Another popular type of homoerotic media is "BL", which is short for "boy's love". BL originated in Japan and commonly comes in the form of manga, anime, and books.

One popular subgenre of BL is *yaoi*, which centers young, beautiful male characters called *bishōnen* ("beautiful boy"). They tend to have slender bodies, stylish hair, and somewhat feminine faces. As a result, some female fans of yaoi who feel themselves to be gay bishōnen seek relationships with others like them[41].

Female fans of yaoi are sometimes called *fujoshi* ("rotten girl"). Originally used as an insult, many yaoi fans have since reclaimed it as an identity.

It's likely that many fans of yaoi are autoandrophilic. Yaoi author Shihomi Sakakibara has argued that the genre is specifically for females who, like him, feel themselves to be men but also love men[42]. Accordingly, some yaoi fans consider themselves to be a sexual minority[43].

The way that one BL fan described sex with their husband also suggested the presence of autoandrophilia:

"Until a few years ago, I could not really recognize sex with my husband as a male-female act. In my mind, I transformed what I was doing to the male-male act in the BL fictions."[44]

Since many autoandrophilic people want to be gay men and find the idea of having gay male sex arousing, it's no surprise that the idealized gay male relationships found in slash fanfiction and yaoi are especially appealing to them.

From One Kind of Gay to Another

When an autoandrophilic trans man comes out as gay, they might be "coming out for a third time"[45]. First, they identify as a lesbian or bisexual woman. Then, after transitioning, as a trans man. Not long after, they realize they're mostly into men and identify as a gay man.

Prior to transition, many autoandrophilic people prefer to have sex with women. Many go through a period of identifying as lesbians[46]. Some even suppress their attraction to men before transitioning because they know that men are attracted to women. One explained his thinking like this:

"It was only as I began to live as a man that I realized my attractions toward other men. Prior to that, I firmly denied any trace of attraction to anything but women. I think I feared that attractions to men would make me less of a man."[47]

They can find men attractive; they just don't like being put into the role of girl or woman[48].

After transitioning, one trans guy finally realized why he was dissatisfied with his pre-transition relationship with a man: "It wasn't about not wanting to be with a guy; it was about not wanting to be the girl"[49].

Before transitioning, being with a woman offers the best odds of having a masculine sex role in sexual exchanges, so many autoandrophilic people choose to date women or even conclude that they're a lesbian before undergoing gender transition.

Even while still dating women, some trans men inwardly identify as gay men. For instance, one said, "I've always identified as a fag even when I dated women"[50], and another described his pre-transition self as "a faggot and a dyke trying to share the same body"[51].

After transitioning, trans men may come out a second time—this time as transgender men.

This new personal and social identity changes their relationship to themselves and others, which can open them up to the possibility of being with men. And if they masculinize their body with testosterone (or otherwise become more secure in their body and identity), sex with men no longer threatens their identity in the way it used to.

Now that they look like men, these trans men attract men who are into men, so they don't have to worry as much that men are attracted to them as women. And if they're lucky enough to draw the interest of gay men, it's a clear sign of passing that can strongly validate their sense of manhood[52].

At this point, they may realize they're far more attracted to men than they ever were toward women. Or that they're completely into men and not actually into women at all.

If so, they come out for a third time—this time, as gay men.

IN SUM

* Interpersonal autoandrophilia is a sexual interest in socially being a man. This subtype of autoandrophilia makes it more likely that an autoandrophilic person will want to be seen and treated as a man by others.

* Autoandrophilic meta-attraction shifts a person's sexual partner preferences toward people whose traits are gender-affirming. This meta-attraction increases attraction to feminine men and gay men and can also create attraction to enacting a man's sexual role with a woman (meta-gynephilia).

* It's particularly common for autoandrophilic people to prefer gay men as sexual partners. With a gay man, they can be sure that their partners are attracted to them as

men and also be intrinsically attracted to their partner's bodies. This dynamic may explain why it's common for autoandrophilic people to enjoy erotic media that focuses on male-male romance, such as slash fanfiction or other mlm.

* It's somewhat common for autoandrophilic trans men to ultimately come out multiple times. Before transition, they are likely to come out as bisexual or lesbian. After transition, they may come out again, this time as transgender. After settling into their masculine identity, they may realize they're mostly attracted to men and decide to come out as gay trans men.

PART 4

ADJACENT PHENOMENA

ATTRACTION TO ANDROGYNY AND MENTAL DISORDERS

ARE TRAPS GAY?

A SERIOUS ANSWER TO A SILLY QUESTION

On the internet, one question animates discussion more than almost any other:

"Are traps gay?"

This irreverent, nonsensical question is one of the most entertaining ways to have conversations about sex, gender, sexuality, and the connections among them. The answers to it are usually as silly as the question itself.

Trap is a slang term for a feminized male with an intact penis. It can refer to MTF transvestites, "pre-op" trans women, and those in between. The term implies a level of passing that would make their birth sex come as a surprise.

Some trans people identify as traps. Others aspire to the level of passing that "trap" implies. But the mainstream view among trans people is that "trap" is a pejorative term.

People usually interpret the question "Are traps gay?" in one of three ways:

1. Are feminized males sexually attracted to men?
2. If a male is inadvertently attracted to a feminized male, is that attraction homosexual in nature?
3. If a male is consciously or particularly attracted to feminized males, does that attraction mean he is homosexual?

The answers, in brief, are:

1. Most of the time, no.
2. No.
3. No.

Let's take these one at a time.

ARE FEMINIZED MALES ATTRACTED TO MEN?

Are some feminized males attracted to men? Yes, some are. But they're in the minority.

Most MTFs in Western, individualistic countries are autogynephilic rather than homosexual (see Chapter 5.3).

Recall that autogynephilia often drives an attraction to being a woman with a man. This contextual attraction to men—*meta-androphilia*—is based in cross-gender embodiment rather than a direct, conventional attraction to the male form.

When meta-androphilia makes a male attracted to being a woman with a man, even if apparently homosexual behavior results, the underlying psychology differs from conventional homosexuality.

In a behavioral sense, it's gay. But psychologically, it's not. If a male is predominantly attracted to men because it allows them to play a feminine sex role, is it *really* gay?

IS IT GAY FOR A MALE TO BE INADVERTENTLY ATTRACTED TO A FEMINIZED MALE?

If a male is inadvertently attracted to someone because they appear female or feminine, that attraction is connected to their interest in women.

Some may argue that even though such a male initially thought they were attracted to someone of the female sex, the fact that the object of attraction was biologically male is evidence that they are technically gay—at least a little bit. After all, they are both of the same sex, which makes the attraction homosexual, right?

Not really. At most, it's only incidentally gay.

Male homosexual attraction involves straightforward sexual attraction to men and male bodies, so an otherwise heterosexual male being attracted to someone of the same sex who appeals to their interest in women and femininity hardly fits the bill.

IS IT GAY FOR A MALE TO BE PARTICULARLY ATTRACTED TO A FEMINIZED MALE?

What about the case where a male is specifically attracted to feminized males?

They are aware that the other person is a male with an intact penis, so surely this situation counts as homosexual attraction, right?

Probably not. Studies suggest that this kind of attraction is a variant of heterosexuality[1].

When trans-attracted males had their genital blood flow measured in the lab, they were mostly aroused by females and MTFs and far less so by males[2]. This result indicates that these trans-attracted males were likely attracted to the feminized aspects of feminized males; it wasn't the maleness itself that drew their attention.

Autogynephilic male crossdressers showed a similar pattern to trans-attracted males when they were tested in the lab[3]. They were into females and feminized males but less interested in men. This pattern suggests that autogynephilia and trans-attraction might be related.

Overall, the evidence suggests that when males are especially attracted to MTFs, it's likely a form of heterosexuality, not homosexuality.

Although trans-attracted males like the mix of female and male sex traits that MTFS have, the female-typical traits usually need to be present for trans-attracted males to be attracted to MTFS.

SO...ARE TRAPS GAY?

No.

Most traps became traps because they are autoheterosexual, so traps themselves are usually not gay.

Males who are attracted to traps are typically much more interested in women than men. In addition, attraction to traps is associated with autoheterosexuality. Therefore, males who are attracted to traps are unlikely to be homosexual.

In short, traps are not gay.

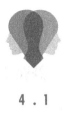

GYNANDROMORPHOPHILIA (GAMP)

ATTRACTION TO FEMINIZED MALES

Some males are *really* into MTFs.

Trans women tend to call these men "chasers", which is short for "tranny chaser". These days, the "tranny" part is usually left out, yet "chaser" remains.

The term "chaser" is often seen as pejorative by those it describes, so many males attracted to MTFs prefer to describe themselves as "trans-attracted", "transfan", "trans-oriented", "transamorous", or "trans-admirer"[1].

The technical term for this nonvanilla attraction is *gynandro-morphophilia*[2], but it's easier to use the acronym GAMP, which rhymes with "camp".

GAMP PREVALENCE

Even though GAMP is fairly common as far as atypical sexual interests go, it hasn't been studied much.

One study that surveyed men about their sexual fantasies found that 4.2% had an MTF in their favorite sexual fantasy, and 6.1% imagined being anally penetrated either by an MTF or a woman with a strap-on in their favorite sexual fantasy[3]. Not coincidentally, internet searches using terms associated with erotic MTF media are highly correlated with searches for strap-ons[4].

Other sexologists found that 5.3% of the heterosexual men they studied were attracted to MTFS[5]. Sexologist Justin Lehmiller surveyed almost four thousand Americans and found that 2% of females and 7% of males surveyed often fantasized about sex with a trans partner[6]. Porn-viewing stats also back up the idea that GAMP is a common interest: the "transgender" category was the fifteenth most-viewed category on Pornhub in 2019[7].

Overall, it seems that about 5% of males are particularly attracted to MTFS.

THE NU GAMP SURVEY

A few years ago, researchers at Northwestern University conducted the largest study of GAMP men to date[8]. It had hundreds of GAMP males and included a straight male control group for comparison. Throughout this chapter, I will refer to this study as "the NU GAMP survey". It's a good one.

Researchers found that GAMPs were most attracted to MTFS whose faces, bodies, voices, and mannerisms were highly feminine[9]. On the other hand, the size of an MTF's genitals and breasts didn't matter as much[10].

The NU GAMP survey found that if GAMPs had to choose just one sexual partner, a bit over half would choose a female and about a third would choose an MTF[11]. Similarly, about a third would "definitely" consider a permanent relationship with an MTF[12].

The GAMPs in this study were twenty-five times as likely as the heterosexual control group to have past experiences with MTFS[13], which suggests that the men who sexually pursue MTFS are almost always specifically attracted to them.

However, it seems that most GAMPs don't have romantic experience with actual, real-life trans women. Approximately seven in eight GAMP males in the NU GAMP survey discovered their attractions to trans women through pornography rather than in person[14], and only about a fifth had been romantically involved with an MTF.

GAMPs are usually attracted to MTFs because they're attracted to women and femininity. Although they like the presence of a penis alongside those feminine traits, the feminine cues generally need to be present to draw their attention.

GYNANDROMORPHOPHILIA AFFECTS SEXUAL IDENTITY

Since MTFS have a mixture of male- and female-typical characteristics, attraction to them complicates traditional notions of sexual orientation.

If a man is attracted to a "pre-op" trans woman, is his attraction straight because of the overall feminine aesthetic, gay because there's another penis in the picture, or bisexual because traits associated with both sexes are present?

A gynandromorphophilic Japanese man pondered his attraction to MTFS ("kama") and came to the following conclusion about his sexual orientation:

"I am neither pure heterosexual nor homosexual. Am I bisexual?...I guess I am a kama lover. So, I'm a 'kamasexual.'"[15]

In other words, he wasn't straight, gay, or bi—he was GAMP.

The NU GAMP survey found that it's common for GAMP men to identify as bisexual because of their attraction to MTFS, or for het-identified GAMPs to have wondered if they were bi or gay because of their attraction to MTFS[16]. In addition, the bi-identified GAMPs were more autogynephilic than the het-identified GAMPs, which suggests that autogynephilia contributed to their interest in men[17]. Even among GAMPs as a whole, autogynephilia was positively associated with sexual interest in men[18].

Sociologists have also observed a relationship between the details of men's sexual interest in MTFs and their sexual identity[19]. They found that the straight-identified men they spoke with were most attracted to the over-the-top feminine presentation and sexual forwardness of some trans women, while the bisexual-identified men were especially attracted to the fact that trans women have both breasts and a penis[20].

Many of these bisexual men would perform fellatio on trans women. "If they can pull a cock out in my face, I'm in ecstasy", reported one such man[21].

Given that bisexual GAMPs are more likely to be autogynephilic, and autogynephilia often creates a desire to sexually interact with penises, it may be the case that bisexual GAMPs are motivated by autogynephilia.

GAMP AND AGP: TWO SIDES OF THE SAME COIN?

Gynandromorphophilia and autogynephilia are related. A male who is GAMP is also likely to have some degree of AGP, and vice versa.

Autogynephilia drives many males to feminize themselves. Since MTFs directly embody that gender transformation, some men's attraction to them could represent an allosexual manifestation of the autogynephilic wish to be feminized.

GAMP and AGP both "stand on the same common root"[22]. For example, some GAMPs want to be feminized themselves but aren't able to do so for social, constitutional, financial, or other reasons and instead satisfy their need for feminization vicariously through their attraction to feminized males[23]. Others start as admirers and later switch to crossdressing themselves.

As one trans woman explained, men who pursue trans women often fantasize about bottoming or being penetrated:

"A lot of men...when they approach a transgender woman... a lot of them are looking for the experience of...bottoming, or being penetrated either anally or orally by a transgender woman. That is kind of what they want."[24]

This desire is so common that it's arguably the norm in males who are attracted to trans women.

In the NU GAMP survey, fantasies of penetrating MTFs were popular, but fantasies of being penetrated by MTFs were even more so[25]. In addition, about a tenth of study participants fantasized about being with an MTF as a woman[26].

This apparent relationship between GAMP and autogynephilia also shows up in Brazil. *Travestis* (effeminate homosexual males who commonly work as prostitutes) report that one of the most common requests from male clients is to be anally penetrated[27]. While being penetrated, those clients often ask to be described as sexy and addressed with feminine names[28].

Almost 60% of GAMPs in the NU GAMP survey answered affirmatively to at least one question on the Core Autogynephilia Scale[29], a scale created by Blanchard to measure prior arousal to the thought of having female anatomy or being female[30]. A solid 34% of GAMPs scored higher than the average of the highest-scoring MTF group in Blanchard's iconic "concept of autogyne-philia" study[31]. By comparison, only 6% of the heterosexual male control group scored that high.

This difference between GAMP males and heterosexual males was especially clear when they were asked about crossdress-ing and questioning their gender identity. GAMPs were sixteen times as likely as conventional heterosexual males to have ever crossdressed[32]. GAMPs were also seventeen times as likely to have ever questioned their gender identity[33]. Among GAMPs who questioned their gender identity, about a quarter gave rea-sons emphasizing an aspect of autogynephilia, and about a tenth said they wanted to become an MTF[34].

The degree of self-reported femininity among GAMPs was strongly correlated with their autogynephilia and transvestism, suggesting that the fantasy of being a woman influenced the amount of femininity they reported[35].

Phallometric data also supports the notion that AGP and GAMP are related (see Figure 4.1.1). When autogynephilic males and GAMP males had their genital arousal measured in the lab, both groups responded most strongly to MTFs, slightly less to females, and far less to males[36]. In fact, the autogynephilic group was so GAMP that there weren't even enough non-GAMP autogynephilic males to determine if they had distinct arousal patterns[37].

These phallometry studies also showed that it didn't matter whether participants were thinking with their little heads or

AUTOHETEROSEXUAL MALES AND GAMP MALES <u>REPORT</u> SIMILAR AROUSAL PATTERNS

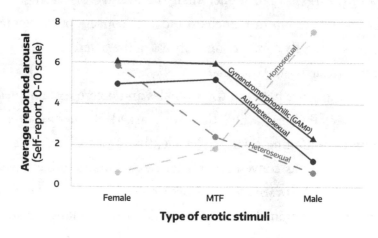

AUTOHETEROSEXUAL MALES AND GAMP MALES <u>HAVE</u> SIMILAR AROUSAL PATTERNS

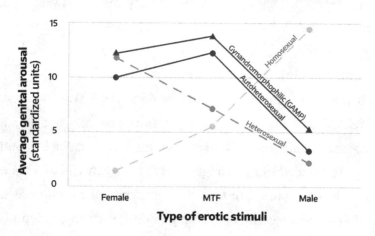

Source: Sexual Arousal Patterns of Autogynephilic Male Cross-Dressers (2016)
Authors: Kevin J. Hsu, A. M. Rosenthal, David I. Miller, and J. Michael Bailey
Note: Sexual orientations are in relation to birth sex

Figure 4.1.1

their big heads: as with the genital arousal data, autogynephilic males and GAMP males both self-reported high arousal
to media depicting females or MTFs, and low arousal to media
depicting males[38]. This pattern of self-reported arousal also
matched the self-reported arousal patterns of GAMPs in the NU
GAMP survey[39].

SAMOAN MEN'S ATTRACTION TO EFFEMINATE MALES

Far out in the Pacific Ocean, inhabitants of the secluded island
nation of Samoa recognize a "third gender" category for effeminate males known as *fa'afafine* (pronounced "fah-fah-fee-neh").
Fa'afafine are often raised as girls, learn to exist within a gender
role similar to the one expected of females, and are valued members of Samoan society known for being helpful and contributing to family life[40].

In Samoa, it's common for men to have sexual interactions
with fa'afafine. These are often one-time interactions[41], but they
aren't seen as gay like they might be in some Western countries.
However, fa'afafine are almost all androphilic (attracted to men).
As with Western populations, they also show the fraternal birth
order effect—the more older brothers a male has, the more likely
that male is to be homosexual[42].

In recent years, scientists have been researching fa'afafine
and men's attraction to them in order to learn more about male
sexual orientation[43]. Due to cultural differences between Samoa
and Western countries, these scientists use nonpornographic

imagery along with equipment that tracks eye movement in order to infer the sexual preferences of study participants.

In studies that track viewing patterns, looking longer at a certain type of person tends to indicate attraction to that type of person[44]. For example, if participants view images of women longer than men, it indicates greater sexual attraction to women.

When scientists tracked the viewing patterns of Samoan men with sexual interest in fa'afafine, their viewing times suggested they were similarly attracted to feminine males and women—or maybe even *more* attracted to feminine males than women[45]. This finding mirrored the pattern of GAMP genital arousal revealed in previous studies[46].

Other studies of Samoan men found that those who had sex with fa'afafine leaned more bisexual than those who only had sex with women, and that bisexuality among fa'afafine-attracted men related to the sexual acts they engaged in with fa'afafine[47]. Prior experience with performing fellatio or being anally penetrated was associated with being more bisexual and less strictly gynephilic[48]. This pattern showed up in their viewing patterns as well as their self-reported sexual behavior and attractions.

Men who received fellatio but didn't perform it themselves were much less likely to have a sexual history with men than were men who had performed fellatio on fa'afafine[49]. The men who had performed fellatio on fa'afafine also had more bisexual viewing patterns[50] and self-reported attractions[51] (although they still leaned slightly toward attraction to women).

The situation with insertive versus receptive anal intercourse was similar: men who only played the insertive role during anal sex with fa'afafine had less sexual history with men[52], less bisexual viewing patterns[53], and reported less bisexual attractions than the men who had engaged in receptive anal sex with fa'afafine.

Among Samoan men, there seems to be a pattern whereby men who have performed oral sex on fa'afafine or been anally penetrated by them show comparatively more interest in men than those who don't. Similarly, American sociologists found that bisexual-identified men showed greater interest in interacting with a trans woman's penis than heterosexual-identified men did[54].

This overall pattern accords with the relationship between autogynephilia and bisexuality found in the NU GAMP survey. There, researchers found that autogynephilia was fairly common in GAMPs and was associated with more attraction to men. Accordingly, bisexual-identified GAMPs were comparatively more autogynephilic than heterosexual-identified GAMPs[55].

Interestingly, almost half of the autogynephilic males in one phallometry study said their ideal female self would have a penis[56]. This autosexual interest in being a woman with a penis is fairly common among autogynephilic males. It represents an overlap between AGP and GAMP.

AUTOGYNANDROMORPHOPHILIA (AGAMP)

If some GAMP males find women with penises more attractive than women with vulvas, and if gynandromorphophilia frequently co-occurs with an autosexual attraction to being a woman (autogynephilia), then some GAMP males will have an autosexual attraction to being a woman with a penis.

An attraction to being a woman with a penis is *autogynandromorphophilia* (AGAMP). This term is atrociously long, so if you talk about it in real life, it's probably easiest to call it "autoGAMP".

Blanchard had quite a few patients who were especially attracted to MTFs and wanted to become one. Those patients still had intense gender dysphoria and wanted access to feminizing medical interventions, but they didn't want vaginoplasty. He called this orientation "partial autogynephilia"[57].

One of Blanchard's patients was so gender dysphoric that she'd previously tried to cut off her penis. But once she encountered MTF pornography, she realized that's what she wanted to be. Although she considered women's bodies the most beautiful thing in existence, Blanchard quoted her as saying, "They haven't got the right thing down there"[58]. Eventually, she hoped to become an MTF herself and date other MTFs.

Blanchard also found evidence that prior arousal from picturing oneself with a vulva was associated with gender dysphoria[59]. This is potentially useful information: if autogynephilic males have a penis in their fantasies instead of a vulva, they may be less susceptible to genital dysphoria.

USING LANGUAGE THAT TREATS TRANS ATTRACTIONS AS WORTHY

As a culture, if we want romantic relationships with trans people to be treated with the same respect that we afford heterosexual and homosexual relationships, then it needs to become normal and acceptable for people to be out about their trans attractions.

To that end, it would help if there were widely recognized sexual identity labels for the following types of attraction:

1. Attraction to feminized males (MTFS)
2. Attraction to masculinized females (FTMS)
3. Attraction to androgynous or nonbinary people
4. Attraction to gender-variant/trans people

The first two would be useful to describe people who like either FTMS or MTFS, but not both. The third would be useful for people who don't prefer any specific genitals or biological sex but specifically like a mixture of female- and male-typical traits. The fourth would be useful as an umbrella term and would include the first three underneath it.

Currently, the most popular label for people who are attracted to trans people is "[tranny] chaser", which has negative connotations both inside and outside the gender community. If "chaser" remains the dominant term for people who are attracted to trans people, then it's unlikely that a truly sex-positive outlook toward attraction to trans people can develop within the gender community, let alone outside of it[60].

How are trans people supposed to be confident in their sexual worth if trans-attracted people are denigrated for being attracted to them—especially when *trans people themselves* use that same unflattering language?

It implies that trans people aren't worth being attracted to, which is bullshit. There are plenty of trans people who are worth dating, marrying, or hooking up with.

Currently, only a small percentage of the broader population would be willing to date a trans person[61]. For evolutionary reasons, it's unlikely that trans people will ever attract as much of the population as people who aren't trans. However, I suspect that trans people innately appeal to a broader subset of the population than current cultural norms allow people to act upon.

As part of creating a culture that allows for transgender relationships to flourish, it would help to have new, sex-positive language that could help trans people and their admirers find each other and have more mutual understanding when they do.

RESEARCHING TRANS-ATTRACTIONS AND INCLUDING THEM IN THE LGBTQ COALITION

The language and cultural approach to trans attractions aren't the only problems; our lack of empirical knowledge about them is too.

* How many people are into trans women and trans men?
* How many people are specifically into an androgynous or nonbinary appearance?
* Which traits (or mixture of traits) make trans people attractive to others?
* How much does stigma factor into people's willingness to date trans people?

The answers to these questions are still largely unknown because they haven't been adequately studied yet.

Even the most studied trans attraction, gynandromorphophilia, is still largely a mystery. This ignorance about trans attractions harms both trans people and the people attracted to them.

Heterosexual men who are attracted to MTFS commonly feel confused or ashamed by their attraction. They may wonder if liking a woman with a penis makes them gay, or if they should instead think of themselves as bisexual. Sexual identities like *straight*, *bi*, or *gay* don't really get to the heart of their desires.

If more GAMP males knew that their attraction to trans women was likely a by-product of their attraction to females, fewer would have these inner conflicts around sexual identity[62]. Fewer would feel confusion and shame about their sexual tastes, and more would be able to open up about their sexual interests.

With greater self-understanding, GAMP males could feel more comfortable with their sexuality, leave their sexual shame in the past, and realize they likely belong in the LGBTQ political coalition.

After all, gynandromorphophilia can motivate males to take on nonheterosexual identities such as bisexual, pansexual, or queer. GAMP also frequently co-occurs alongside the single most common cause of transgenderism, autoheterosexuality, which itself can motivate someone to identify with *any* of the letters in the LGBTQ coalition.

IN SUM

* Gynandromorphophilia (GAMP) is an attraction to feminized males/MTFS. It's a sexual interest in a "woman with a penis" aesthetic.

* Gynandromorphophilia and autogynephilia are both nonvanilla variants of heterosexuality. It's quite common for autogynephilic people to also be gynandromorphophilic, and vice versa. This frequent co-occurrence may be why GAMP males are far more likely to have crossdressed or questioned their gender identity than conventionally heterosexual males.

* GAMP males who want to bottom for feminized males are more likely to identify as bisexual or show interest in men than those who only want to top. They're also more likely to be autogynephilic. Studies of Samoan men who have sex with fa'afafine suggest that this association between

attraction to men and interest in bottoming may arise independently of culture.

* Autogynandromorphophilia (AGAMP) is an attraction to being a feminized male. Although AGAMP can drive a desire for gender transition, that transition is unlikely to include vaginoplasty. It's common for an autogynephilic male's idealized female self to have a penis.

* GAMP males used to be called "tranny chasers", but now they're simply called "chasers". Still, this term suggests this attraction is somehow less valid than other forms of attraction. This negative connotation is a problem because treating gynandromorphophilia as a worthy attraction is necessary to create a sex-positive politics of transgenderism.

* Gynandromorphophilic males belong in the political coalition that advocates for the rights of sexual minorities. GAMPs often have a nonheterosexual identity, and many of them are also autogynephilic—either of which qualifies them for inclusion in the LGBTQ coalition.

MENTAL HEALTH AND TRANSGENDERISM

BEING TRANS AIN'T EASY

Trans people are more likely to have mental health problems than people who aren't trans. They're also more likely to show suicidal behaviors.

Where does this difference come from? Is it societal? Genetic? Both?

In LGBTQ advocacy, it's common to fixate on societal mistreatment and its connection to negative mental health outcomes instead of considering inborn factors that may also contribute to poor mental health.

For now, it's easier to change society than it is to change our genes, so this approach has a certain pragmatic logic to it. Through socially constructing a more perfect society, conditions can improve for sexual and gender minorities (or so the thinking goes).

Among social constructionists, there's a popular school of thought called *minority stress theory* which holds that people in nondominant groups experience greater stress due to perceived prejudice, stigma, and discrimination, and that the stress associated with these perceived discriminatory experiences can cause adverse health effects[1].

At face value, this argument seems rather intuitive. It doesn't take much imagination to see that being part of a nondominant group in society might confer some level of stress or insecurity and perhaps lead to mistreatment.

In my early forays into cross-gender expression, I definitely experienced stress, paranoia, and intense self-consciousness while out in public. Even now, if I go somewhere outside my cozy liberal bubble, I'm usually a little more vigilant about my surroundings.

Perhaps there *is* reason to worry. A recent study examined signs of minority stress among three generations of American sexual minorities and found that even as society supposedly got more welcoming to LGBTQ people, that cultural change didn't seem to translate into fewer minority stressors. Younger sexual minorities were more likely to have previously attempted suicide than older ones, and they also reported more psychological distress and everyday discrimination[2].

Overall, researchers found that little had changed in the metrics they measured. They attributed the overall lack of change to "the endurance of cultural ideologies such as homophobia and heterosexism and accompanying rejection of and violence toward sexual minorities"[3].

But cultural attitudes toward sexual minorities have gotten *way* better in the last few generations! If social and cultural influences are the biggest influence on mental health outcomes among sexual minorities, the finding that not much has changed is certainly surprising. If genes play a greater role than culture in mental health outcomes, however, these findings are to be expected.

Genes change very little from generation to generation. Perhaps these researchers found that reported stressors haven't changed much over the past few generations because genes are actually the primary contributor to mental health outcomes in sexual minorities.

For the genetic explanation to make sense, there would have to be shared genetic contributors to adverse mental health outcomes and nonheterosexual or autoheterosexual orientations. The science is young, but there is some preliminary evidence for this conclusion.

The researchers who wrote the paper referenced above are sociologists, so they didn't explore the possibility that genes contribute to mental health outcomes of sexual minorities. However, I will.

But first, a little math lesson.

BEFRIENDING NUMBERS

In this chapter, I'll present a lot of statistics. If you and numbers don't get along, feel free to gloss over them and not worry about the details too much.

Even if you don't quite know what the numbers mean, you'll probably pick up on the general idea that the bigger the numbers are, the stronger the connection is between the things that are being compared.

Most commonly, I'll compare things using *odds ratios* and *correlations*.

Odds ratios are simple: they express the odds of a particular outcome by comparing study participants who have a trait against those who lack that trait. For example, one study showed that trans people are four to six times as likely to have an autism diagnosis compared to people who aren't trans[4].

Easy, right?

Correlations are pretty simple to understand too. The symbol for a correlation is r. It's always a number whose magnitude is between zero and one. The r says how much one thing moves in relation to another thing—it's a measure of how much two things are in sync and whether or not they move in the same direction (+) or opposite direction (-).

If r is positive, the two things move up and down in relation to each other. If r is negative, as one thing goes up, the other goes down.

For example, if the correlation between two things is $r=0.2$, it means that if one thing moves, the other thing tends to move along with it, but only a fifth as much as the first thing moved. The bigger r is, the more in sync the two things are.

If two variables have a correlation of $r=0.2$, the relationship between them is fairly mild. However, small correlations like these are common in sociology research.

MINORITY STRESS THEORY: MUCH ADO ABOUT MILD EFFECTS

Studies that provide supporting evidence for minority stress theory typically find fairly modest effects. For example, the correlations between perceived discrimination and various health outcomes in one meta-analysis were quite small, ranging from $r=0.11$ to $r=0.18$[5].

Although the small correlations in the minority stress model are usually presented as the result of perceived prejudice and discrimination causing mental health problems, some of this small effect could just as well be from the reverse: preexisting mental traits could contribute to more perceived (or experienced) prejudice and discrimination[6]. Researchers have not yet established the direction of causality in the minority stress model[7].

To put the smallness of these effects in context, a review of fifty years of twin studies found that psychiatric traits between identical twins had a correlation of $r=0.55$, and fraternal twins had a correlation of $r=0.31$[8]. In fact, for traits in general, identical twins had a correlation of $r=0.64$[9].

Notice how all these numbers are bigger than the ones from the minority stress study?

Genes are important—the role they play is too big to ignore. At birth, much of our physical and mental destiny has already been determined by our DNA.

MENTAL TRAITS ARE HIGHLY HERITABLE

Our genes play a massive role in the types of psychological traits and mental disorders we end up with. They affect our personalities, our general intelligence, and even our politics.

A common measure of how much genes affect traits is called *heritability*.

Heritability indicates how much the variation in a trait within a population can be attributed to variation in genetic factors rather than to the environment or random chance. To estimate heritability, scientists often compare identical twins to fraternal twins to see how their traits vary in order to figure out how much of their similarity comes from genes and how much from the environment[10].

Every behavioral trait is heritable[11]. General psychological traits such as the Big Five (openness to experience, conscientiousness, extroversion, agreeableness, and neuroticism) are approximately 50% heritable, meaning that about half their variance in a population is due to variance in genes[12]. Even social attitudes such as conservatism and authoritarianism are a little over half heritable[13], as is self-control[14]. General intelligence (IQ) in adults is roughly 80% heritable[15].

Genetic factors are probably the single biggest contributor to mental traits. This also applies to many mental disorders.

One of the least heritable mental disorders is depression, but 30–40% of variation in depression can still be attributed to genetic factors[16]. The heritability of anxiety is similar. Anxiety symptoms and generalized anxiety disorder are about 30% heritable, while panic disorder is around 40% heritable[17]. Similarly, obsessive-compulsive disorder and total anxiety sensitivity are both almost 50% heritable[18].

Other mental disorders are even more strongly determined by genes. For example, Cluster B personality disorders such as antisocial, borderline, and narcissistic personality disorders are estimated to be 67–71% heritable[19]. Autism spectrum disorder is somewhere around 80% heritable[20], as is bipolar disorder[21]. Psychotic disorders like schizophrenia and mania are both estimated to be at least 80% heritable[22], as is ADHD[23].

Gender-related traits are heritable, but the estimates vary widely. Childhood gender dysphoria has been estimated to be anywhere from 14–84% heritable, and childhood gender-related behaviors have been estimated to be 25–77% heritable[24].

In other words, genes play an absolutely massive role in shaping psychology and behavior. Those who overlook the role of genes will miss the single largest contributor to mental traits and mental disorders.

NONHETEROSEXUALITY AND DEPRESSION
HAVE SHARED GENETIC FACTORS

A couple studies have looked into potential genetic connections between same-sex sexuality and depression, and they found a solid association between the two.

An Australian twin study estimated that shared genetic causes accounted for 60% of the shared variance between sexual orientation and depression in nonheterosexuals[25]. They also found that childhood sex abuse and risky family environment accounted for approximately 9% and 8% of the depression variance, respectively, showing that the social environment had an impact on depression as well[26]. Still, the impact of genes was clearly dominant.

In 2019, a massive genome-wide association study that compared nearly half a million human genomes found associations between same-sex behavior and genes associated with mental traits that tend to worsen mental health outcomes[27].

In males, same-sex sexual behavior was genetically correlated with ADHD ($r=0.27$), neuroticism ($r=0.15$), and depression ($r=0.33$)[28].

In females, same-sex sexual behavior was genetically correlated with ADHD ($r=0.25$), anxiety ($r=0.25$), bipolar disorder ($r=0.34$), autism ($r=0.21$), neuroticism ($r=0.22$), and depression ($r=0.43$)[29].

These relationships suggest that being nonheterosexual can make life more difficult—and that some of this increased difficulty stems from genes rather than culture.

While there is certainly more work to be done on the cultural front to make life better for sexual minorities, trying to achieve better outcomes solely through cultural means will inevitably fall short of the utopic goal of equal outcomes. Until genetic technologies are sufficiently advanced and made available to everyone, there will be genetic barriers to equal outcomes between groups of people whose genetic differences lead to consequential differences in mental traits.

As with nonheterosexuals, trans people also have a much higher rate of mental disorders than the broader population. And since genes are major contributors to mental disorders, it stands to reason that societal discrimination can't account for all of the mental health difficulties that trans people face.

I want to be clear: by bringing up the influence of genetics, I'm not denying that cultural changes can make life better for sexual minorities or gender minorities. There are meaningful solutions outside of gene editing.

Societal discrimination against sexual and gender minorities is a real, well-documented problem. The social environment certainly contributes to the difficulties of being transgender, and I sincerely hope that the cultural project to better incorporate sexual and gender minorities into society will continue to improve our lot in life. Such change is a good thing, and long overdue.

But if culture and society are only part of the picture, then approaches to helping sexual and gender minorities that rely on cultural engineering and unshakeable faith in the power of social construction will inevitably fall short of their goals.

Any realistic analysis must include the contribution of genes. They're too important to ignore.

TRANS PEOPLE HAVE HIGH RATES OF MENTAL DISORDERS

Transgender people are more likely to have previous diagnoses for psychiatric disorders than people who aren't transgender. *Much* more likely.

When researchers studied inpatient hospital encounters in the US, transgender patients were found to be eight times as likely as nontransgender patients to have been diagnosed with any psychiatric disorder in the past[30]. Previous mental health diagnoses in trans patients were almost four times as likely for anxiety, about 1.5 times as likely for depression, and about 2.5 times as likely for psychosis.

Data from large questionnaire databases has also revealed elevated rates of prior psychiatric diagnoses in trans people. For instance, one study found that in trans people, prior diagnoses were two to five times as likely for ADHD, four times as likely for depression, two to five times as likely for bipolar disorder, and two to five times as likely for OCD[31].

The rates of autism were even higher: trans people were five to six times as likely to have an autism diagnosis as people who weren't trans[32]. This relationship went the other way as well: people diagnosed with autism were five to six times as likely to be transgender or otherwise gender diverse[33].

Autism itself is a risk factor for other psychiatric diagnoses. A large meta-analysis found that in comparison to the general public, autistic people are more likely to have ADHD, anxiety, depression, bipolar disorder, schizophrenia, obsessive-compulsive disorder, and sleep-wake disorders[34]. In particular, ADHD is the most common co-occurring psychiatric diagnosis in adults with autism[35]. The two are highly linked.

Gender transition itself doesn't seem to be the origin of these higher rates of mental health issues: a 2005 study of the Swedish population found that men who had ever been aroused by crossdressing had about three times the odds of receiving a psychiatric diagnosis in the last year compared to men who hadn't[36]. This suggests that autoheterosexuality itself is associated with higher odds of having mental health issues.

The data is clear: trans people deal with mental health difficulties at much higher rates than the broader population. And since many mental disorders are mostly heritable, we cannot attribute trans people's mental health difficulties to societal conditions alone. The situation is more complicated than that.

TRANSGENDER SUICIDALITY

Have you ever heard the statistic that 41% of trans people[37] have previously attempted suicide?

That study wasn't a fluke: another large transgender survey with similar methodology found basically the same result: 40% reported a prior suicide attempt[38].

Given that only about 5% of Americans report a prior suicide attempt[39], does this mean trans people are eight times as likely to attempt suicide as people who aren't trans?

To explore this question, I will stick to measures of prior suicide attempts. Although this isn't the only way to measure suicidality, I use prior suicide attempts as a metric here because it's what studies of transgenderism often use. In addition, measuring the same type of outcome makes it easier to compare the results of different studies.

Estimates of attempted suicide in trans people tend to vary widely, but all are above the levels in the general population. Studies measuring suicidality in gender-dysphoric people have found widely varying rates of past suicide attempts (9–47%)[40]. Fortunately, studies usually find estimates below 41%.

A study on transgender Virginians found that 25% had previously attempted suicide[41]. Another study found that 28–31% of trans women in the New York metropolitan area had a prior suicide attempt[42]. Two surveys in the UK found that 21–25% of trans people had attempted suicide more than once, and overall, 35% of them had done so at least once[43].

In China, suicidality among trans people is also higher than the general population. At an attempted suicide rate of 16%, Chinese transgender people are about five times as likely as the broader population to have previously attempted suicide[44].

In the overall world population, an estimated 2.7% of people have previously attempted suicide[45], so these trans suicide rates seem absurdly high by comparison.

It isn't only gender minorities who have escalated rates of suicide—nonheterosexuals do too[46]. Among nonheterosexuals, bisexual females are the most likely to have previously attempted suicide[47].

The way researchers find study participants has a huge impact too: multiple meta-analyses of suicidality in homosexuals have found that community samples result in estimates of past suicide attempts that are approximately double those found in population-representative samples (20% versus 10–11%, respectively)[48].

If this difference between community samples and population-representative samples applies to trans people too, it's good news. Many of the transgender studies I just referenced were community samples (including the one that found a 41% rate), so they might be overestimating suicidality.

Altogether, heterosexuals have the lowest rates of suicide attempts among sexuality- and gender-based identity groups. Homosexuals have two to three times the rates of suicide attempts as heterosexuals, and bisexual females have a higher rate yet. Trans people make suicide attempts at 1.5 to two times the rate of homosexuals.

Although sampling biases may contribute to high reported rates of trans suicide attempts such as the famous 41% statistic, it appears that trans people truly do have the highest risk of suicide among all sexual and gender minority groups.

TRANSGENDER SUICIDALITY: MORE THAN GENDER DYSPHORIA

What is responsible for the high rate of suicide attempts among trans people? Is it societal discrimination? Gender dysphoria? Mental disorders?

Yes. All of these play a role.

In general, the more mental disorders an individual has, the more likely they are to have made prior suicide attempts or successfully suicided (see Table 4.2.1)[49]. Trans people are, at root, *people*, so it's likely that the high prevalence of mental disorders among trans people contributes to their high rate of suicide attempts. And since mental disorders are highly heritable, a significant part of this tendency is inborn and independent of society or culture.

As important as genes are, however, society and culture definitely still contribute to transgender suicidality. Not all the potential for suffering is inborn. For example, anxiety and depression contribute to suicidality, yet they're less heritable than many other types of mental disorders.

The availability of transgender medical care also matters to trans people: many studies show that getting such care is associated with better outcomes among trans people[50].

Personality matters too. Research on sexual and gender minorities has shown that these groups have noticeably different rates of past suicide attempts depending on personality traits such as neuroticism, agreeableness, or conscientiousness[51].

Study	Kessler 1999	Nock 2008	Too 2019
Location	United States	Developed countries	Meta-analysis
Criteria	Ever attempted Suicide	Ever attempted Suicide	Suicide
	Odds ratio	Odds ratio	Risk ratio
Female	2.2	1.7	-
Any anxiety disorder	3.2	4.8	4.1
Any mood disorder	12.9	5.9	12.3
Any impulse-control disorder	-	4.2	-
Any substance use disorders	5.8	4.2	4.4
Any personality disorders	-	-	8.1
Any disorders	6.7	6.4	7.5
Exactly 1 disorder	3.8	0.8	-
Exactly 2 disorders	6.1	1.9	-
3 or more disorders	19.7	8.9	-

Table 4.2.1: Mental health disorders drastically increase the odds of attempted and completed suicide.

In addition, trans people who have previously attempted suicide report that gender issues weren't the only contributor to their suicidality: in a UK study, 65% of trans people reported that trans-related reasons played a part in their prior suicide attempts, while 61% said that factors unrelated to transgenderism contributed to their prior suicide attempts[52].

DISCRIMINATION AND MISTREATMENT INCREASES SUICIDALITY

There is a large body of literature suggesting that discrimination harms the well-being of sexual and gender minorities[53].

By pointing out that suicidality in trans people is not purely a function of gender issues, I'm not saying gender issues are irrelevant. They definitely matter. But how others treat trans people matters too.

For instance, a study of MTFs in the New York metro area found that gender-related psychological or physical abuse were both significantly associated with increased suicidality and depression, especially when that abuse happened during adolescence[54].

A study of transgender Massachusetts residents found a similar association between mistreatment and suicidal thoughts: having been on the receiving end of physical violence, sexual violence, or gender-related discrimination was associated with a higher risk of having contemplated suicide in the past[55].

Additionally, study participants who had transitioned or were planning on transitioning had a higher risk of prior suicidal thoughts than nontransitioners. Consistent with the general pattern of higher suicidality in females, FTMs were approximately twice as likely to have prior suicidal thoughts for every single one of these risk factors[56].

When researchers analyzed results from the massive 2015 US Transgender Survey to examine contributing factors to suicidality, they found that the rate of prior suicide attempts differed based on a whole slew of factors and past experiences[57]. Many of these decrease well-being in people in general, but some were transgender specific.

Transgender people with higher income, educational attainment, age, and general health had made fewer past suicide attempts, whereas those with drug use, past arrests, psychological distress, disability, and homelessness had made more past suicide attempts. Sex mattered too: FTMs had more prior suicide attempts than MTFS.

Social rejection also made a big difference. There were higher past suicide attempt rates among trans people who had unsupportive family, classmates, or coworkers, or those who had experienced rejection by their family of origin, intimate partner, child, or religious community.

Trans people who had experienced a professional intervention that attempted to stop them from being trans or change their sexual orientation also had higher odds of past suicide attempts. Those who'd been physically attacked, had unwanted sexual contact, or experienced intimate partner violence of any kind all had a higher chance of past suicide attempts, as did those mistreated by police or denied access to restrooms corresponding to their gender identity.

Of the discrimination trans people experienced that they attributed to being transgender, there were four types of experiences that had the greatest impact: being evicted, experiencing homelessness, being physically attacked, and being fired from a job[58]. Trans people who had experienced none of these negative events in the previous year had only a 5.1% risk of suicide attempt during that time, whereas those who experienced all four types of discrimination had a 51% risk—a tenfold increase[59].

The trend is clear: having less money, being younger, and being socially rejected or mistreated for being trans are all associated with higher odds of prior suicide attempts.

IN SUM

* Transgender people are much more likely to have previously attempted suicide than the general population. Even if using more conservative estimates, transgender Americans appear to have at least five times the odds of prior suicide attempts. Trans people in China also have similarly elevated rates of prior suicide attempts.

* Trans people have much higher rates of mental disorders than the general population. They are more likely to have highly heritable mental disorders like ADHD, autism, and bipolar disorder, as well as moderately heritable mental disorders like anxiety, depression, and OCD. Trans identity aside, prior arousal from crossdressing is itself associated with much higher odds of a recent psychiatric diagnosis.

* Mental disorders are associated with much higher rates of suicidality among the general population, so it's likely that transgender suicidality can be largely attributed to trans people's elevated rates of mental disorders. Since these mental disorders tend to be moderately to highly heritable, a significant proportion of transgender suicidality is probably due to inborn factors independent of societal conditions.

* However, societal conditions matter too. Transgender suicidality is highly linked to social class as well as discrimination for being transgender. The treatment trans people experience certainly influences their mental health outcomes. Genes aren't everything.

AUTISM

AUTISM CONTRIBUTES TO GENDER VARIANCE

Autism studies show that autistic people are more likely to be gender variant or transgender, and transgender studies show that trans people are much more likely to be autistic. The relationship goes both ways.

One study found that autistic people are about 5.5 times as likely to identify as nonbinary[1], showing that autism's relationship with gender variance isn't limited to binary trans identities.

Similarly, a study utilizing parental reports found that both autism and ADHD were associated with higher gender variance in children: kids with either disorder were seven to eight times as likely to have repeatedly expressed the wish to be the other sex[2].

ADHD and autism are both part of my mental makeup, so this overlap with gender variance doesn't surprise me—I have long noticed that autistic-identified people are particularly common in online trans spaces.

After surveying the scientific literature connecting autism to sexuality and gender variance, I noticed three ways that autism appears to contribute to greater gender variance:

* Increased rates of nonheterosexuality
* Increased rates of nonvanilla sexuality (and thus more autoheterosexuality)
* Autistic gender alienation

Rates of nonheterosexuality are significantly higher in autistic people. One study specifically exploring sexual orientation in autistic people found that both sexes were more likely to report homosexual, bisexual, or asexual identities and attractions than non-autists of their sex[3].

Other autism studies have also found this same overall pattern of increased nonheterosexuality[4], with one finding that all the nonheterosexual groups of participants had markedly higher levels of gender dysphoria than the heterosexual group[5].

Nonvanilla sexualities tend to cluster within individuals[6], so someone with one form of nonvanilla sexuality is likely to have another form of it. Since autoheterosexuality is a nonvanilla sexuality and nonvanilla sexualities are more common among autistic people, it's likely that autism is associated with higher rates of autoheterosexuality. This correlation is another way that autism may contribute to gender variance.

Studies looking into the relationship between nonvanilla sexuality and autism have found that autistic males have significantly higher rates of nonvanilla sexuality than typical males[7]. One study that asked autists an open-ended question about their turn-ons found 5% of autistic males reported autogynephilia and 12% reported arousal from crossdressing[8]. They reported these experiences without being asked about them directly, so I suspect these were consistent sexual interests in the people who reported them.

Researchers have also found that autistic traits are associated with higher levels of gender dysphoria[9]. This correlation was noticeably stronger in females, which suggested that autistic traits were more likely to contribute to gender dysphoria in females[10]. Even though autistic females had higher gender dysphoria scores, however, autistic males were more likely to be on cross-sex hormones[11].

Other research examining mental health outcomes found that autism, nonheterosexuality, and gender dysphoria were all associated with a negative impact on a person's well-being: membership in just one of these three groups significantly added to stress, depression, and anxiety, while also lowering well-being[12]. Gender dysphoria had the greatest negative impact of the three, and being in all three groups simultaneously was associated with even worse mental health than being in any one group on its own[13].

AUTISTIC GENDER ALIENATION

A qualitative study that asked autistic and non-autistic participants about their gender feelings and experiences found drastic differences between the two groups[14].

Compared to the non-autistic control group, members of the autistic group were far more likely to say that they felt different from their own sex, that they felt more like the other sex, or that they had struggles understanding their gender identity. They were also much less likely to say their birth sex aligned with their self-conception or fit their gender role.

Some of these autists felt alienated not just from their gender but also from humanity itself. After researchers asked one participant how she fit in with either sex, she said, "It's like asking me if I feel more affinity to girl aliens or boy aliens"[15].

Consequently, autistic people in this study were far more likely to identify as androgynous or nonbinary, state that gender wasn't important to their personal identity, have an undetermined sexual orientation, or say that a romantic partner's companionship mattered more than their gender.

In sum, autists are more likely to feel alienated not only from the gender associated with their sex, but also human gender as a whole. Understandably, autists place less emphasis on gender—a pattern that shows up in their self-identity, sexual orientations, and sexual partner preferences.

AUTISM IS ASSOCIATED WITH NEUROLOGICAL MASCULINIZATION

The empathizing-systemizing theory (E-S theory) of autism holds that, on average, females are better than males at perceiving another person's mental state and responding with an appropriate emotion (empathizing), while males are better at analyzing or constructing rule-based systems (systemizing).

In E-S theory, empathizing and systemizing are two poles of a spectrum on which the sexes tend to differ, and it conceives of autism as a shift in the male-typical direction, toward systemizing[16]. One of the largest psychological differences between the sexes is that females prefer to work with people and males prefer to work with things[17], so E-S theory's prediction about female-male differences in empathizing and systemizing isn't surprising.

A *gigantic* study involving over 600,000 participants demonstrated the same patterns predicted by E-S theory: within autistic and non-autistic groups, females showed more empathizing and males showed more systemizing. Autists of both sexes were higher in systemizing and lower in empathizing than their non-autistic counterparts, and this difference predicted autism far better than any demographic characteristics, including sex[18].

The most obvious sign that testosterone exposure may contribute to autism is that males are much more likely to be autistic. There are, however, several other lines of evidence supporting the idea that testosterone plays a role in the development of autism.

When scientists measured fetal testosterone levels, they found a positive association between fetal testosterone levels and autistic traits[19]. On the other hand, testosterone usage among trans men later in life doesn't seem to correlate with different levels of autistic traits[20], so the timing of testosterone exposure matters.

There is other evidence suggesting autism has a link to testosterone exposure: autistic females are more likely to report testosterone-related health issues such as polycystic ovarian syndrome, hirsutism, unusually painful periods, or a history of severe acne[21].

Female autists are also more likely to be attracted to women or to have been tomboys as children[22], both of which are associated with masculinization. They are also much more likely to be transsexual or have gender dysphoria[23]. Unsurprisingly, autoandrophilia in females is also associated with autistic traits[24].

In addition, congenital adrenal hyperplasia—a disorder of sexual development that leads to elevated testosterone levels—is associated with increased autism traits and nonheterosexuality in females, as well as decreased female gender identity[25].

AUTOHET TRANS PEOPLE HAVE HIGH RATES OF AUTISM

In general, it's estimated that less than 1% of people are autistic, perhaps about 0.6%[26]. Among trans people, though, autism is far more common.

Research conducted by gender clinics has found that trans people with nonhomosexual orientations or late-onset gender dysphoria are more likely to show autistic traits. This pattern implies that autism is particularly associated with autohetero-sexual transgenderism.

A study at a London-based gender clinic found that 7% of FTMS and 5% of MTFS met the threshold for an autism diagnosis[27]. Perhaps not coincidentally, *all* of the transsexuals with marked autistic traits were nonhomosexual[28] and nearly all of them said their gender dysphoria started at or after puberty[29]. In addition, nonhomosexual orientations predicted higher scores of autistic traits[30].

A different study from England found that 30% of FTMS and 5% of MTFS in their sample met the threshold for an autism diagnosis. Nonhomosexual MTFS had significantly higher scores than homosexual MTFS, but this same relationship wasn't found among FTMS[31].

Children and adolescents at gender clinics also seem to have elevated rates of autism. A study from a famous Dutch gender clinic—The Center of Expertise on Gender Dysphoria at the VU University Medical Center Amsterdam[32]—found that 7.8% of children and adolescents referred there had autism[33]. Adolescents were more likely than younger children to be autistic, which suggested that autism was more closely associated with a later onset of dysphoria. Among adolescents themselves, the autistic ones tended to be older[34], and most of them were nonhomosexual[35].

Altogether, these patterns suggest that autism contributes to gender variance in several ways and that it's particularly associated with autoheterosexual transgenderism.

IN SUM

* Trans and nonbinary people are much more likely to be autistic. In turn, autistic people are much more likely to be gender dysphoric or gender variant. This association goes both ways, and it shows up repeatedly across many studies.

* Autistic people are more likely to be nonheterosexual, have nonvanilla sexualities, or feel alienated from their default gender—each of which contributes to gender variance in its own way.

* Autistic gender alienation makes it likely that autists will feel different from their own sex or feel similar to the other sex. They are far more likely to identify as androgynous or nonbinary and may even feel alienated from other humans to a degree that gender itself seems irrelevant. In short, autistic gender alienation contributes to gender issues.

* Autism is associated with neurological masculinization: males are more likely to be autistic, and autistic females are far more likely to report testosterone-related health issues, gender nonconformity in youth, or attraction to women. Furthermore, fetal testosterone levels are positively associated with higher scores on measures of autism later in life.

* Studies from gender clinics show that autistic traits are more common in trans people who have nonhomosexual orientations or whose dysphoria started around puberty. These patterns indicate that autism is particularly associated with autoheterosexual transgenderism.

PART 5

DEMOGRAPHICS OF SEXUALITY AND TRANSGENDERISM

HOW COMMON IS AUTOHETEROSEXUALITY?

TOO COMMON TO LACK A NAME FOR IT

Autoheterosexual and homosexual preferences occur at similar rates, yet there is a huge imbalance in awareness about these two sexual orientations.

Where does this imbalance come from? Why is homosexuality mainstream knowledge while autoheterosexuality is comparatively unknown?

A lot of this imbalance originates in differences between allosexuality and autosexuality. Allosexuality motivates sexual union with other people, which drives an external search for compatible sexual partners.

Gay people need to find each other in order to fulfill their sexual and romantic needs. They often move to cities big enough to support community infrastructure (e.g., gay bars), which helps gay people develop a shared identity and become visible to broader society.

In contrast, autosexuality can exist in isolation, as a closed loop. It doesn't require others.

In the past, autohets typically formed heterosexual partnerships and participated in society as their default-gender selves while keeping their cross-gender selves confined to their homes. However, the recent cultural ascendance of transgenderism has changed the game: it's safer than ever for autohets to express their cross-gender selves in public.

EXACTLY HOW MANY AUTOHETEROSEXUALS ARE THERE?

Depending on how researchers find study participants and ask them questions, they arrive at different estimates of the prevalence of autoheterosexuality.

These estimates tend to be on the higher side when researchers ask "have you ever" questions because even one recalled instance of cross-gender arousal, behavior, or fantasy gets recorded as a "yes". Similarly, questions about sexual fantasies tend to get more "yes" responses than questions about past experience because people don't always act on their fantasies.

Some small studies on college undergrads[1] found autohetero-sexuality or erotic transvestism prevalence rates anywhere from just a few percent all the way up to 15%. A recent online study of more than 4,000 people found that 15% of females and 25% of males reported at least a bit of sexual interest in behaving or dressing like the other sex[2].

We can best interpret double-digit estimates like these as indicators of the number of people who have a touch of cross-gender sexuality or can at least see the appeal. However, the number of people who are definitively into erotic crossdressing or cross-gender fantasy is certainly lower.

Since "transvestite" used to be the technical term for trans people, many researchers thought that the act of crossdressing itself was what mattered. They didn't realize they were witnessing autoheterosexuality and that crossdressing was just one of many ways to symbolically evoke the idea of being the other sex.

As a result, researchers often asked study participants about crossdressing and neglected to ask about crossdreaming (imagining oneself as the other sex). Unfortunately, this approach underestimates autoheterosexuality rates in females because they tend to be less interested in transvestism.

Since prevalence estimates of crossdressing and crossdreaming vary so widely between studies, I've collected some figures from formal studies and presented them in Table 5.0.1 to make them visible at a glance[3].

Only a couple of these studies asked about crossdreaming. Of these, one surveyed a representative sample of the French population and found that 4.9% of females and 3.6% of males often felt as though they were the other sex during sexual fantasies[4]. The other was conducted on an online sample by Justin Lehmiller for his book *Tell Me What You Want*[5]. In Lehmiller's sample, approximately 2% of females and 3% of males often fantasized about physically becoming the other sex[6].

In these two studies, sex differences in crossdreaming prevalence are rather small. But the transvestism prevalence estimates in Table 5.0.1 suggest that sex differences in crossdressing are greater. I calculated weighted averages from these estimates and found that approximately 4–5% of males have been aroused by or are sexually interested in crossdressing, whereas less than 2% of females are into erotic transvestism and less than 1% have experienced past arousal from crossdressing.

This data suggests that females and males differ more with respect to transvestism than they do with respect to cross-gender fantasy itself.

THE CZECH AUTOHET PREVALENCE ESTIMATES

In early 2020, Czech sexual researchers published the biggest study to date on the population prevalence of nonvanilla sexual interests in a representative sample of a country's population[7]. It had over 10,000 participants.

These researchers were thorough—they collected data for five dimensions of sexuality: preference, arousal, behavior, porn use, and fantasy. Since definitions of sexual orientation often

Measured aspect of sexuality	Sexual Interest	Female ♀ N	(%)	Male ♂ N	(%)	Population	Study
Ever crossdressed and become aroused	TV	3898	0.5	2092	4.6	Finnish twins cohort, ages 18–32	Baur et al. (2016)
Ever crossdressed and become aroused	TV	565	3.5	475	6.5	Quebec, ages 18–64, somewhat RS	Joyal and Carpentier (2016)
Ever crossdressed and become aroused	TV	1171	0.4	1279	2.8	Swedish national probability sample, RS	Långström and Zucker (2005)
Experience with crossdressing	TV	1404	3	1329	6	US residents, somewhat RS	Janus and Janus (1993)
Paraphilic interest >6 months, with distress	TV	394	1.8	477	0.8	Students, University of Calabar, Nigeria, non-RS	Abdullahi et al. (2015)
Often fantasize about dressing as other sex	TV	1919	2.5	2043	5	Americans, online survey, non-RS	Lehmiller (2018)
Desire to experience crossdressing	TV	565	5.5	475	7.2	Quebec, ages 18–64, somewhat RS	Joyal and Carpentier (2016)
Often fantasize about physically becoming other sex	Autohet	1919	2	2043	3	Americans, online survey, non-RS	Lehmiller (2018)
Often feel as though of other sex in fantasies	Autohet	1128	4.9	1329	3.6	French national probability sample, RS	Spira et al. (1994)
Ever crossdressed and become aroused	TV	-	-	367	2.7	Men ages 40–79, Berlin, Germany, non-RS	Ahlers et al. (2011)
Transvestism present in favorite sexual fantasy	TV	-	-	214	2.8	Online or residents of Trois-Rivières, Quebec, non-RS	Joyal et al. (2015)

Table 5.0.1: Prevalence estimates of autohet-related eroticism.

TV = transvestism, RS = representative sample.

include the element of preference[8], I will call upon their figures for sexual preference.

These Czech researchers presented the prevalence of transvestism and autoheterosexuality at two different levels of intensity, which I'll categorize as "mild-moderate" and "strong".

Due to the size and quality of this Czech sample and the care researchers took to differentiate among different strengths of sexual interest, I consider these prevalence estimates for autoheterosexuality to be the most reliable, so all further calculations in this book that rely on autohet prevalence estimates will use them.

In Table 5.0.2, I've listed the transvestism and autoheterosexuality prevalence estimates from this study along with ratios inferred from them. These ratios help illuminate how females and males differ with respect to imagining themselves as the other sex (crossdreaming) and its sartorial expression (crossdressing).

	Female ♀		Male ♂		Sex Ratio, F : M	
	Mild-Mod	Strong	Mild-Mod	Strong	Mild-Mod	Strong
Transvestism	2.0%	0.3%	5.4%	1.1%	1 : 2.7	1 : 3.7
Autoheterosexuality	4.9%	0.8%	7.9%	1.7%	1 : 1.6	1 : 2.1
Ratio, TV : Autohet	1 : 2.5	1 : 2.7	1 : 1.5	1 : 1.5	-	-

Table 5.0.2: Prevalence of sexual preference for transvestism and autoheterosexuality in the Czech population, and derived ratios. *Source: Bártová et al 2020.*

In comparison to females, males were more likely to have a sexual preference for crossdressing or crossdreaming. This sex difference was even more apparent when it came to strong preferences, which were even more likely to happen in males.

In both females and males, sexual preferences for crossdreaming were more common than sexual preferences for crossdressing. This is what we should expect to see if sexually motivated crossdressing is ultimately a downstream effect of autoheterosexuality which occurs in a subset of autohets.

Although females were about half as likely to have strong autoheterosexual preferences, this is still far too common to deny that female autoandrophilia exists, or that it plays a major role in FTM transsexualism.

COMPARING AUTOHETEROSEXUAL AND NONHETEROSEXUAL PREVALENCE

In order to estimate the size and composition of the broader etiological population from which almost all transsexuals originate, I'll use the findings of the Czech study[9] in tandem with sexual orientation prevalence estimates from the US[10].

Both of these sources used a five-point scale. In the Czech study, 1 indicated no interest, 2 to 3 was mild to moderate interest, and 4 to 5 was strong interest[11]. From the US sexual orientation prevalence estimates[12], I'll treat "completely heterosexual" as no same-sex attraction, "mostly heterosexual" and "bisexual" as mild to moderate levels of same-sex attraction, and "mostly homosexual" and "completely homosexual" as strong levels of same-sex attraction.

This method isn't perfect and arguably has its flaws. For example, a bisexual person could be strongly attracted to both sexes equally, so this method of interpretation would not capture their degree of same-sex attraction adequately. However, attraction to one sex is usually associated with weaker attraction to the other, so this potential flaw isn't a deal-breaker.

Another limitation is that I'm comparing estimates from one Eastern European country with estimates from all over the United States, a country with more cultural and genetic diversity. European ancestry is quite prevalent in the US, though, so there will still be significant genetic overlap.

Despite these limitations, I'm using these studies because they use large samples of the general population, and they differentiate among five degrees of sexual interest in ways that allow for reasonable comparison between nonheterosexuality and autoheterosexuality.

Within both sexes, there are roughly three autoheterosexuals for every four homosexuals. Males are about twice as likely to be autoheterosexual or homosexual. Females are much more likely to report bisexuality, and males are more likely to report some autoheterosexuality.

Using these prevalence rates and assuming a population that is half female and half male, I've estimated the size of the broader etiological population from which transsexuals originate, as well as the theoretical size limit of the gender-based part of the LGBTQ coalition.

According to the two-type model, transsexuals are either homosexual or autoheterosexual. Assuming that only people who are strongly homosexual or autoheterosexual have enough gender issues to become transsexual, the broader etiological population from which transsexuals originate is approximately 2.9% of the population.

HOW COMMON ARE LGBTQ SEXUALITIES?

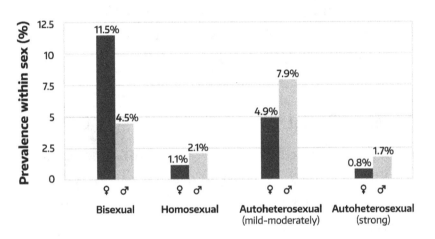

Same-Sex Attraction:
Source: Sexual Orientation, Controversy, and Science (2016)
Authors: J. Michael Bailey, Paul L. Vasey, Lisa M. Diamond, S. Marc Breedlove, Eric Vilain, and Marc Epprecht

Autoheterosexual Preference:
Source: The Prevalence of Paraphilic Interests in the Czech Population: Preference, Arousal, the Use of Pornography, Fantasy, and Behavior (2020)
Authors: Klára Bártová, Renáta Androvičová, Lucie Krejčová, Petr Weiss & Kateřina Klapilová

Figure 5.0.3: Estimated prevalence of nonheterosexuals and autoheterosexuals.

As I pointed out previously, membership within the gender-based part of the LGBTQ coalition depends on two sexual propensities: same-sex sexuality or autoheterosexuality (nonhet or autohet).

After adding up everyone who has even just a bit of same-sex attraction or autoheterosexuality, it seems that the LGBTQ coalition comprises up to about 17% of the population—one in six people. (I say "up to" because this method will double-count autohets with nonheterosexual partner preferences, and not everyone with these orientations considers themselves part of the LGBTQ coalition).

Nonheterosexuals represent just under 10% of the population, and people with any degree of autoheterosexual interest represent 7–8% of the population. The numerical wisdom of appending TQ to LGB is clear: doing so greatly increases the number of people included in the coalition.

AUTOHETEROSEXUALITY AND SAME-SEX ATTRACTION

It is unknown exactly how many homosexuals and bisexuals owe their same-sex attraction to autoheterosexuality instead of conventional same-sex attraction, but it's clear that some do. This is especially clear for bisexuals.

As seen in the preceding section, an estimated 4.5% of males and 11.5% of females in the US report that they are either bisexual or mostly heterosexual[13].

However, bisexuality is way more common in autohets. Among people who admit to even the slightest bit of sexual interest in dressing or behaving as the other sex, an estimated 30% of males[14] and 48% of females[15] identify as bisexual.

Transgender Americans have high rates of bisexuality too. In the 2015 US Transgender Survey, more than half of nonhomosexual trans people reported sexual identities indicative of bisexuality such as "queer", "pansexual", or "bisexual"[16].

What could be causing these high rates of bisexuality?

Meta-attraction is one potential source of this increased bisexuality. Attraction to androgyny is another. Both sexual propensities are common among autoheterosexuals, and both are associated with bisexuality.

Using the method described in this endnote[17], I estimated that among Americans who report bisexual or mostly heterosexual attractions, approximately one-fifth of females and three-fifths of males ultimately do so because of autoheterosexuality. If these estimates are close to the mark, it's quite possible that autoheterosexuality is involved in most cases of male bisexuality.

Relatedly, Israeli researchers found that among people who identified as bisexual or mostly heterosexual, there were positive associations between same-sex attraction and cross-gender sentiments such as feeling like the other sex or wanting to be it[18]. This connection was present in both sexes, but noticeably stronger in males. These bi and mostly het males also reported a greater desire to be the other sex than other groups.

Although autoheterosexuality is more often associated with bisexuality than preferential homosexuality, it occurs in some people with same-sex preferences too. For example, in that same autosexuality study which found high rates of bisexual identity among autoheterosexuals[19], approximately one in six autohet females reported greater attraction to females, and approximately one in twenty-five autohet males reported greater attraction to males.

This finding isn't a fluke. Other researchers have documented similar overlaps between autoheterosexual interest and homosexual preference. For example, autoandrophilia is more common among lesbians than the broader female population[20]. Similarly, studies of trans women have consistently found that a proportion of those who get categorized as homosexual report past experience of autoheterosexual arousal[21].

IN SUM

* Depending on the study, prevalence estimates of autoheterosexuality vary widely. Online surveys commonly produce double-digit estimates, but representative surveys generally indicate that about 3–6% of people have sexual interest in crossdressing or crossdreaming. Females tend to be on the lower end of this range, while males tend to be on the higher end.

* When it comes to strong sexual preferences, there are about three autoheterosexuals for every four homosexuals. Males are approximately twice as likely to be autoheterosexual or homosexual. Females are more likely to be bisexual but less likely to show sexual interest in crossdressing.

* Autoheterosexuality is a significant contributor to bisexuality. Much of this contribution stems from attraction to androgyny and meta-attraction—both are common among autohets and both contribute to

bisexuality. Much of male bisexuality, perhaps most, is ultimately autohet-related. A smaller proportion of female bisexuality is autohet-related.

* In both sexes, some people with homosexual preferences are autoheterosexual. This overlap is more common in females.

ARRIVING AT THE TWO-TYPE MODEL

HOW SCIENTISTS FIGURED IT OUT

Categorizing effeminate males into two types is nothing new.

Centuries before Western scientists began to study homosexuality and transvestism, Islamic legal scholars wrote about effeminate males known as *mukhannathun*, which roughly translates to "effeminate ones" or "ones who resemble women".

These scholars were trying to prescribe social rules rather than understand gender or sexuality, but the two types of mukhannathun they described closely resemble the two types of MTFS we know exist today.

The mukhannathun didn't fit neatly into either gender role, so legal scholars discussed how—and if—they ought to be incorporated into society.

Writing in the eleventh century AD, a scholar named al-Sarakhsi differentiated between two types of mukhannathun when addressing the question of whether they ought to be allowed in a harem, the part of the house where women dwelled. One type of mukhannathun could be permitted entry, but the other:

> "In evil acts is, like other men—indeed, like other sinners—prohibited from women; as for the one whose limbs are languid and whose tongue has a lisp by way of natural constitution, and who has no desire for women and is not *mukhannath* in evil acts, some of our shaykhs would grant such a person license to be with women."[1] [Some Arabic words removed for clarity]

The naturally effeminate type who was not interested in women had permission to enter a harem, but the type that was attracted to women was barred.

A few hundred years later, a scholar named al-Kirmani also wrote about mukhannathun. He defined them as men who imitate women in speech and behavior, and he differentiated between two types of male effeminacy: constitutional and affected[2]. Later writers also distinguished between intentional and unintentional effeminacy, suggesting that this difference was a recurring pattern across generations.

Taken together, these observations suggest that the scholars were aware of two different kinds of effeminate males:

* Those who innately spoke and moved like women, yet had no desire for them
* Those who could be attracted to women and whose feminine behavior seemed intentional

Although there's no way to know for sure whether they were describing the same two types we know of today, the resemblance is obvious.

HIRSCHFELD'S TRANSVESTITE TAXONOMY

Until Magnus Hirschfeld published *Die Transvestiten* in 1910, scientists usually saw male femininity as a sign of homosexuality. But after Hirschfeld conclusively demonstrated that male transvestites were usually attracted to women and driven by a love of female beauty, it was clear that transvestism was distinct from homosexuality.

This finding ultimately led to a new question: *how many types of transvestites are there?*

Hirschfeld classified them into four categories based on sexual orientation—homosexual, heterosexual, and bisexual groups based on attraction to men, women, or both, plus a fourth group that was either asexual or *automonosexual* (attracted to themselves and no one else)[3].

Unfortunately, Hirschfeld's sexual research and political activism for the liberation of sexual minorities encountered changing political tides. In 1920, he was brutally assaulted[4]. In 1933, Nazis ransacked his sexual institute, burned all the books and case notes in a giant bonfire, and likely killed the sexual minorities they found inside.

After Nazis suppressed Hirschfeld's work, decades passed before scientists dove back into the search for a reliable classification system for trans people.

DIFFERENTIATING TRANSSEXUALS FROM HOMOSEXUALS AND TRANSVESTITES

Following Hirschfeld, the next serious attempt at categorizing trans people appeared in Harry Benjamin's *The Transsexual Phenomenon*[5], the first book about transsexualism to reach a wide audience.

Benjamin's taxonomy, the Sex Orientation Scale, placed MTFS on a six-point scale ranging from *pseudo-transvestite* all the way to *true transsexual*. Half the categories described different types of transvestites, and the other half described different types of transsexuals.

His scale was intended to categorize MTFS based on medical necessity, not etiology. Its purpose was to help determine whether they would be good candidates for hormones or vaginoplasty; it didn't categorize based on discrete developmental pathways.

Unfortunately, to qualify as a "true transsexual" on the scale, a patient had to be mostly attracted to men. This contributed to a tradition of gatekeeping MTFS who preferred women—a pattern that continued for decades afterward. In fact, this type of gatekeeping still happens sometimes when clinicians aren't hip to the two-type model.

This gatekeeping incentivized trans women to portray themselves in whatever way would allow them to have the surgeries they wanted. In order to get the medical care that could ease their suffering, they had to fit the transsexual category as described in the academic literature.

ADDRESSING SUFFERING: GENDER DYSPHORIA SYNDROME

In 1974, Norman Fisk introduced the concept of *gender dysphoria syndrome* in an influential paper[6] that shifted the focus toward alleviating suffering rather than deciding if patients were "true transsexuals".

After seeing that patients had strikingly similar stories, Fisk felt that many MTF gender patients had read the scientific literature on transsexualism and portrayed themselves as textbook cases in order to get the surgeries they needed.

Many of those patients were satisfied with the results of the surgeries, so he concluded that it was more pragmatic for clinicians to focus on improving a patient's quality of life rather than trying to determine whether they fit the transsexual mold. He saw that transsexuals were "in full flight from either effeminate homosexuality or transvestitism"[7] and that they sought a trans-sexualism diagnosis for valid reasons.

Treating gender-related suffering directly instead of trying to decide if any given patient was "actually transsexual" was a big deal. This shift in perspective started the push toward a new treatment approach that reduced the strict gatekeeping previously commonplace in transgender medicine.

ARRIVING AT THE TWO TYPES: EFFEMINATE HOMOSEXUALS AND TRANSVESTITES

In the 1970s, researchers turned their attention to understanding the underlying causes of transsexualism. They had known for some time that their transsexual research subjects bore a remarkable similarity to either effeminate gay men or transvestites, but they still weren't sure how many distinct types of transsexualism there were.

John Money proposed one of the first two-type taxonomies in 1970, dividing MTF transsexuals into "transvestitic" and "effeminate-homosexual" types[8].

The homosexual group was gender nonconforming as children, only felt attraction to men, and didn't experience erotic transvestism. By contrast, the transvestitic group wasn't solely attracted to men or very gender nonconforming as children, but they did report a history of cross-gender arousal[9].

Six years later, Peter Bentler proposed a three-type MTF taxonomy that separated transsexuals into homosexual, heterosexual, and asexual groups[10]. Interestingly, *none* of the asexual group had considered themselves homosexual before surgery, but over half had thought of themselves as heterosexual[11].

Bentler sought to understand the developmental pathways that led to different transsexual outcomes, as well as "the inter-relationship that transsexualism has with transvestism and homo-sexuality"[12]. Even though his transsexual taxonomy had three types, he pointed to only two related groups from which they came.

A couple of years later, a pair of Australian researchers—Neil Buhrich and Neil McConaghy—published "Two Clinically Discrete Syndromes of Transsexualism", a paper that provided some preliminary numerical evidence for the two-type model[13].

They divided transsexual participants into those who admitted to past arousal from dressing as women and those who denied it. Those who admitted to prior arousal from crossdressing showed significantly more physical arousal to erotic media with women[14]. They were also more likely to have had sex with women, to be married to one, and to be older[15]. From this pattern, the researchers concluded that MTF transsexuals "can be divided into two clinically discrete groups on the basis of whether or not they have shown fetishistic arousal"[16].

Taken together, these papers and studies show that by the 1970s, sexologists were converging on a two-type model of MTF transsexualism in which one type was associated with gender-nonconforming homosexuality and the other with erotic transvestism. These studies were still too small to be conclusive, but that was about to change.

A gender clinic in Canada was using fancy new computer technology to create a database of responses to questionnaires filled out by patients during the intake process. With the help of this computer database, clinicians at the gender clinic within the Clarke Institute of Psychiatry in Toronto, Canada, were about to play a major role in transgender history.

RESEARCH AT THE CLARKE INSTITUTE OF PSYCHIATRY

Throughout the 1980s, researchers at the Clarke Institute made a concerted effort to find out how many types of MTF transsexualism there were, as well as what distinguished them.

In "Two Types of Cross-Gender Identity"[17], Kurt Freund and others investigated the relationship between gender patients' reports of prior arousal from crossdressing and their reports of cross-gender identity. The researchers divided gender patients based on whether they reported prior arousal from crossdressing as well as their reported strength of cross-gender identity. Those who reported continuously feeling like a woman for at least a year were classified as transsexuals; those who reported a lesser degree of cross-gender identity were classified as transvestites or borderline transsexuals[18].

Almost all nontranssexual subjects were heterosexual and reported sartorial arousal[19]. In general, researchers found that past arousal from crossdressing was associated with heterosexuality rather than homosexuality.

More than 90% of transsexuals who didn't report sartorial arousal were classified as homosexual. However, only about half the transsexuals who admitted to sartorial arousal were classified as homosexual[20]. Even among homosexual-classified transsexuals, those who didn't report sartorial arousal were significantly more attracted to men (and less to women) than those who reported sartorial arousal[21].

The average age of initial contact with the gender clinic varied too. Averaging just under twenty-six years of age, homosexual transsexuals who denied sartorial arousal were the youngest[22]. Transsexuals who reported past sartorial arousal were older: the homosexual group averaged about thirty-two years of age and the heterosexual group about thirty-nine years of age[23]. Overall, youth was associated with homosexuality and no prior crossdressing arousal, while older age was associated with heterosexuality and crossdressing arousal.

This was similar to the patterns found by Australian researchers a few years prior[24]. Based on these findings, the authors concluded that "there are two discrete types of cross-gender identity, one heterosexual, and the other homosexual"[25].

At the end of "Two Types of Cross-Gender Identity", a postscript added that another researcher at the clinic had recently made a similar dataset, and looking at it left the authors with the impression that "the two types are even more distinct"[26]. This other researcher was a newer hire, and he was about to spearhead the MTF taxonomy research at the gender clinic. Before the 1980s were over, he would publish three empirical studies on the subject and ultimately pin down the essential difference between the two types of MTF transsexualism.

His name? Ray Blanchard.

BLANCHARD'S TRANSSEXUALISM RESEARCH

Although the research published by Blanchard's colleagues suggested there were two types of cross-gender identity, Blanchard
himself didn't start from that premise. Instead, he referred back
to Hirschfeld's four-type taxonomy separating transvestites into
homosexual, heterosexual, bisexual, and asexual groups[27].

Blanchard started with these four groups and combined them
when evidence suggested they were ultimately the same type.
The empirical core of Blanchard's taxonomy research consisted
of three studies, all of which shared some methodology[28]:

* The data came from self-administered, multiple choice,
  paper-and-pencil questionnaires
* Patients were asked, "Have you ever felt like a woman?"
  and those who responded, "At all times and for at least
  one year" were categorized as transsexual
* Patients were sorted into four groups (homosexual,
  heterosexual, bisexual, and asexual) using their
  responses to the Modified Androphilia and Modified
  Gynephilia Scales

In his classic typology study, "Typology of Male-to-Female
Transsexualism"[29], Blanchard tallied the number of trans
women in each group who reported prior sartorial arousal, and
he found drastically different rates for homosexual versus nonhomosexual groups.

BLANCHARD FOUND THAT EROTIC CROSSDRESSING IS MUCH MORE COMMON IN NONHOMOSEXUAL MTFs

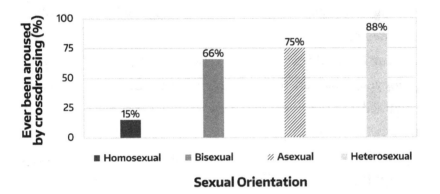

Source: Typology of male-to-female transsexualism (1985)
Author: Ray Blanchard
Note: Sexual orientations are in relation to birth sex

Figure 5.1.1

This difference suggested a shared underlying etiology for all three nonhomosexual groups, but its exact nature wasn't yet clear. Still, it had *something* to do with cross-gender arousal.

In Blanchard's second typology study[30], "Nonhomosexual Gender Dysphoria", he took the sixteen most representative subjects from each of the four sexual orientation groups and compared them with respect to age and childhood gender nonconformity[31].

The homosexual group reported significantly more childhood gender nonconformity than all three nonhomosexual groups, but the nonhomosexual groups weren't significantly different from one another[32].

The homosexual group also presented at the gender clinic at a significantly earlier average age (23.6 years) than the nonhomosexual groups, all of which had an average age in their 30s[33]. This finding that nonhomosexual transsexuals tended to be older matched previous findings[34].

Blanchard's third and final typology study, "The Concept of Autogynephilia and the Typology of Male Gender Dysphoria", solidified the two-type MTF typology by demonstrating there were two legitimate types of transgenderism. When people talk about his MTF typology work, they're often alluding to this study.

In this influential study, Blanchard presented compelling evidence that there were two distinct types of MTF transsexualism, and he also introduced the concept of autogynephilia that tied it all together[35]. He'd solved the typology problem, at least for the foreseeable future.

To create a scale to measure autogynephilia, Blanchard statistically analyzed questionnaire items asking about cross-gender sexual fantasy and sexual interest in other people. He found that they clustered into three main factors[36], which he developed into psychological scales:

* The Core Autogynephilia Scale, which measured past arousal from thoughts of being a woman (core AGP) or having a female body (anatomic AGP)
* The Autogynephilic Interpersonal Fantasy Scale, which measured past arousal from the thought of being admired as a woman by others (interpersonal AGP)

✳ The Alloeroticism Scale, which measured sexual interest in other people (allosexuality)

In combination with scales that measured prior arousal from crossdressing (the Cross-Gender Fetishism Scale) and prior heterosexual experience (the Heterosexual Experience Scale), Blanchard created a coherent explanation regarding the factors that set the different nonhomosexual groups apart and what they had in common.

FEW 'HOMOSEXUAL' MTFs ARE AUTOHETEROSEXUAL, ASEXUAL MTFs AREN'T INTO OTHER PEOPLE, AND BISEXUAL MTFs HAVE META-ATTRACTION TO MEN

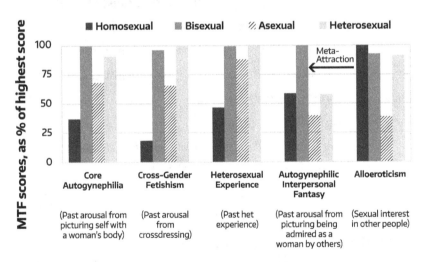

Source: The Concept of Autogynephilia and the Typology of Male Gender Dysphoria (1989)
Author: Ray Blanchard
Note: Sexual orientations are in relation to birth sex

Figure 5.1.2

The nonhomosexual groups (heterosexual, bisexual, and asexual) *all* scored much higher than the homosexual group on measures of Core Autogynephilia, Cross-Gender Fetishism, and Heterosexual Experience, which indicated they were attracted to women and to being a woman far more than the homosexual group[37].

Scores on the Autogynephilic Interpersonal Fantasy Scale showed that the bisexual group was particularly sexually interested in having their feminine persona admired by others[38]. Blanchard proposed that this desire for feminine validation was behind their bisexuality. He referred to this gender-affirming attraction to men as "pseudobisexuality"[39].

The asexual group scored almost as high as the bisexual and heterosexual groups on the Heterosexual Experience Scale, but far lower than all other groups on the Alloeroticism Scale[40]. This result seemed contradictory, so Blanchard checked the clinical charts of some trans women whose questionnaire responses suggested almost complete asexuality, and he noticed that their charts commonly contradicted their questionnaire responses— their testimonies were unreliable[41].

This finding didn't rule out the possibility that some bona fide asexuals existed in the asexual group[42], but it did show that some gender patients weren't being 100% accurate in their self-reports, perhaps because strict medical gatekeeping strongly incentivized patients to say what they thought clinicians wanted to hear.

Overall, Blanchard's three MTF typology studies convincingly demonstrated that all (or virtually all) trans women were either homosexual or autoheterosexual.

These two groups took consistent forms:

* The homosexual group was only attracted to men, feminine from an early age, didn't have a history of cross-gender arousal, and presented at the gender clinic in their mid-twenties on average.

* The autoheterosexual group was attracted to women, both men and women, or neither. They were also less innately feminine, had a history of cross-gender arousal, and first presented at the gender clinic in their thirties on average.

This way of sorting trans women—where homosexual trans women are of homosexual etiology and nonhomosexual trans women are of autogynephilic etiology—is often referred to as *Blanchard's transsexualism typology*.

Blanchard theorized that asexual trans women lacked interest in other people because their autogynephilia overshadowed their allogynephilia to the point that they lacked interest in women[43], and bisexuals were those whose interest in men was a by-product of a desire to have their femininity validated by others[44]. Combining these two theoretical insights, it follows that some autogynephilic people will have homosexual partner preferences because their autogynephilia overshadows their attraction to women while also creating a contextual attraction to men.

Seemingly Accurate, but Controversial

Blanchard's theory neatly synthesized decades of previous research into a coherent picture that finally made sense of MTF transgenderism. Despite its apparent validity, however, many trans women today vehemently oppose this model and critique the underlying research.

They may point out that *not all* the nonhomosexual groups reported a history of cross-gender arousal, and some of the homosexual group reported a history of cross-gender arousal[45]. If Blanchard's taxonomy was accurate, they may argue, shouldn't have 100% of the nonhomosexual subjects reported cross-gender arousal and 0% of the homosexual subjects reported cross-gender arousal?

Furthermore, the personal narratives that many trans women have about themselves, their histories, and their motivations do not match up with their conception of autogynephilia.

It's fair to wonder: if so many trans women disagree with the model, isn't it likely incorrect?

These critiques are worth addressing, and they raise important questions: Can people be wrong about themselves? And can people understand themselves accurately yet still give unreliable testimony?

The answer on both counts is yes—*of course they can*. No one has perfect knowledge of themselves or the world around them.

Trans women are as human as anyone else. Just like other types of people, they will respond to incentives and have aspects of their inner world that they don't want to examine in-depth or share with others.

Just How Reliable Is the Testimony of Gender Patients?

When thinking about Blanchard's empirical research and the reliability of the self-reports he used, it's important to consider the context in which he collected that information.

His study subjects were gender-dysphoric patients at a gender clinic. Many of them had to travel great distances to get there and wanted to be approved for cross-sex hormones or surgeries. They knew the clinic didn't grant permission to everyone who wanted those, so they had a strong incentive to present themselves in a way that would increase their odds of obtaining gender-affirming care.

Blanchard was aware of these incentives, so he conducted two studies to investigate the reliability of their testimonies (and in which ways they skewed, if any).

The first one tested how the normal human tendency to portray oneself in a socially desirable way (social desirability bias) impacted the self-reports given by gender patients[46]. Blanchard found the responses from homosexual gender patients didn't correlate with measures of social desirability bias, except for the question that asked whether they felt like women[47].

By contrast, the responses from heterosexual gender patients[48] correlated with social desirability bias in a way that skewed toward the conventional picture of an MTF transsexual:

* More attraction to men, and less to women
* More feminine gender identity
* Less erotic transvestism

Based on this finding, Blanchard concluded that nonhomo-sexual gender patients tended to portray themselves in a way "that emphasizes traits and behaviors characteristic of 'classic' transsexualism"[49]. Prior researchers had also noted this tendency[50], but now there were numbers to back it up.

In a second study[51] that examined the reliability of testimony from gender patients, Blanchard and his colleagues tested how self-reports of sartorial arousal compared to actual genital blood flow upon hearing spoken narratives of dressing up in women's clothing.

All groups of heterosexual gender patients in that study—*even those who said they'd never been aroused by crossdressing in the past year*—had a stronger genital response to narratives of cross-dressing than to neutral narratives[52]. In addition, groups who reported little to no arousal from crossdressing had the strongest erotic response to the meta-androphilic fantasy of having sex with a man as a woman[53].

Taking people's testimony at face value is likely to result in a flawed picture, so it's important to take all types of evidence into account, not just self-reports. When self-reports are used, it's important to keep in mind the incentives and biases that may affect responses.

REPLICATING THE TWO-TYPE MTF TYPOLOGY

After Blanchard unveiled the concept of autogynephilia and presented a coherent two-type model of MTF transgenderism, typology research came to a standstill. It took more than fifteen years for other scientists to publish large-scale empirical studies that could either replicate or refute his findings.

The next study[54] came out in 2005. It was conducted by Anne Lawrence, an autogynephilic transsexual woman and proponent of Blanchard's theory.

Lawrence sent a survey to transsexual women who received vaginoplasty from the same surgeon[55]. The survey asked about their sexual experiences, sexual attractions, and sexual functioning both before and after getting bottom surgery[56].

Perhaps because the study participants were all able to afford surgery from an expensive private surgeon, the sample skewed heavily toward nonhomosexual MTFs[57]. Based on their reported sexual attractions before surgery, 91% were nonhomosexual[58].

In ways that should be familiar by now, the group that reported a sexual preference for men differed noticeably from the groups that reported attraction to women.

This androphilic group reported higher rates of childhood femininity and first wished to change sex at a younger age. On average, they started living as women fourteen years before the other groups[59]. They were also less likely to report a past of autogynephilic arousal[60].

When Lawrence sorted study participants by sexual orientation, their rates of past autogynephilic arousal closely resembled the rates of crossdressing arousal that Blanchard had found[61]. The vast majority of nonhomosexual MTFs had experienced autogynephilic arousal before, and nearly half of MTFs overall had experienced it hundreds of times or more[62].

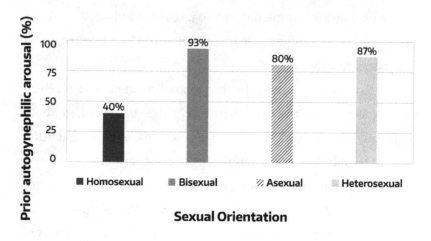

A FAMILIAR PATTERN: NONHOMOSEXUAL MTFs REPORT MORE AUTOGYNEPHILIA

Source: Sexuality Before and After Male-to-Female Sex Reassignment Surgery (2005)
Author: Anne Lawrence
Note: Four of the six "Homosexual" participants who reported past autogynephilic arousal said it happened "Hundreds of times or more". Two had kids and had been married.
Note: Sexual orientations are in relation to birth sex

Figure 5.1.3

Dutch Researchers Replicate the MTF Typology

Around the same time that Lawrence's study came out, so did one from the Dutch gender clinic at the VU University Medical Center in Amsterdam[63]. Researchers investigated whether their gender patients had different rates of transvestic arousal based on their sexual orientation. They categorized patients based solely on self-identification, so their sorting was somewhat flawed, but they nonetheless found the usual types of differences.

On average, the homosexual MTFs recalled more childhood gender nonconformity and applied for surgery about a decade before the nonhomosexual group[64]. They also reported less erotic crossdressing during adolescence (30% of homosexuals versus 54% of nonhomosexuals)[65]. Based on these differences, the researchers agreed that there seemed to be two different types of MTFS[66].

Lawrence noticed that a significant fraction of the homosexual MTF group had been married to women or reported past female sexual partners, so she reached out to the authors to see if those subjects were more likely to report sartorial arousal[67].

After recategorizing participants as nonhomosexual if they were previously married or had previous female sexual partners, the Dutch researchers found that the gap in sartorial arousal rates widened: only 14% of the homosexual group reported arousal from crossdressing during adolescence, whereas 53% of the nonhomosexual group still reported arousal[68].

The Most Convincing Replication

In the mid-to-late 2000s, researchers in New York City were working on a study intended to refute (or replicate) Blanchard's first typology study. This new study used a sample that was three times bigger, more ethnically diverse, and set in the modern day.

It had been more than twenty years since Blanchard's first taxonomy study. The cultural milieu had changed. Trans people were more accepted than before, and gay marriage was about to become the law of the land in America.

If sex and gender were social constructions and unrelated aspects of oneself, *surely* this study would turn up significantly different rates of erotic crossdressing than Blanchard found in his study, right?

RESEARCHERS REPLICATE THE 2-TYPE MTF TYPOLOGY

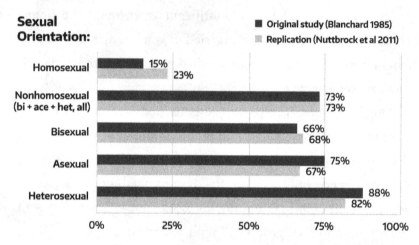

Sexual Orientation:

■ Original study (Blanchard 1985)
▨ Replication (Nuttbrock et al 2011)

Homosexual — 15% / 23%
Nonhomosexual (bi + ace + het, all) — 73% / 73%
Bisexual — 66% / 68%
Asexual — 75% / 67%
Heterosexual — 88% / 82%

0% 25% 50% 75% 100%

Ever experienced arousal from crossdressing

Source: Typology of male-to-female transsexualism (1985)
Author: Ray Blanchard
Source: A Further Assessment of Blanchard's Typology of Homosexual Versus Non-Homosexual or Autogynephilic Gender Dysphoria (2011)
Authors: Nuttbrock, L., Bockting, W., Mason, M., Hwahng, S., Rosenblum, A., Macri, M., & Becker, J.
Note: Sexual orientations are in relation to birth sex

Figure 5.1.4

Nope.

Like Blanchard, these researchers found that 73% of nonhomosexual MTFs reported prior arousal from crossdressing (see Figure 5.1.4). Their homosexual group had a slightly higher rate (23%) than Blanchard's (15%), but it still fit the same overall pattern[69].

Once again, researchers had replicated the results of Blanchard's first typology study.

I consider this replication to be the most important because the researchers were transparent in their opposition to Blanchard's two-type model. They *extensively* downplayed the fact that their study replicated Blanchard's and made it clear to readers that his theory was politically contentious. In fact, the very first sentence of their summary begins, "In a series of important but now highly controversial articles, Blanchard..."[70].

These researchers also brought up a political problem that Blanchard's research posed: his work was essentialist, and it implied a direct link between sexual orientation and gender identity, which directly conflicted with the orthodox stance within the transgender movement that "sex and gender are separate, socially constructed dimensions of personal identity"[71].

They described the book *The Man Who Would Be Queen* as "highly polemic" and said that in author Michael Bailey's framework, "transgenderism was essentially reduced to sexuality"[72].

When discussing their results, they portrayed the association they found between sexual orientation and sartorial arousal as "strong but clearly not deterministic" because the rates of prior sartorial arousal in the homosexual and nonhomosexual groups were 23% and 73%, respectively, rather than 0% and 100%[73]. They framed this prevalence as "at odds with Blanchard's predictions"[74] even though it was fundamentally the same result that Blanchard found.

Despite this misleading framing, the numbers were clear: Blanchard's findings were replicated a generation later, in a larger and more racially diverse cohort, by a study seemingly conducted with the aim of refuting his findings.

Before any of this research, it was already well established that homosexuality existed, that it was associated with gender non-conformity, and that it had occurred throughout human history. Like homosexuality, autoheterosexuality is perennial. It occurs across generations and has been part of the human story for a long time.

Taken together, these studies present strong evidence that when males have an intense, persistent desire to change sex, they are either homosexual or autoheterosexual.

FTM TYPOLOGY

There are some telltale signs that autoheterosexuality is also a driver of FTM transsexualism. Search for "euphoria" or "gender euphoria" in an online FTM forum, and you'll get plenty of results that seem like the autoandrophilic counterpart to male autogynephilia.

It's super easy to find trans men talking about how they experienced gender euphoria after being addressed as a man, peeing while standing, using men's hygiene products, seeing themselves after getting top surgery, or wearing a packer. To respect the privacy of the trans men who wrote these accounts, I'm not going to directly cite any here. Just know they exist and are easy to find.

Unfortunately, there hasn't been much formal research into whether or not trans men are motivated to transition by an attraction to being the other sex. There's barely any research on transmasculine crossdressers either. Historically, researchers have neglected female sexuality in favor of studying male sexuality, and the lack of research on female autoheterosexuality is just one manifestation of this pattern. Still, there are some signs of autoandrophilia in the official literature.

The study from the Dutch gender clinic[75] that partially corroborated Blanchard's results found that four of fifty-two homosexual FTMS and one of twenty-two nonhomosexual FTMS reported prior sartorial arousal during adolescence[76]. Another group of researchers found that seven of twenty-two gay and bisexual trans men (32%) reported prior arousal in response to wearing men's clothing[77]. This rate is less than half that reported by nonhomosexual MTFS in prior studies[78], but it's not a dealbreaker for the autoheterosexuality hypothesis.

As mentioned previously, females are less likely to have sexual interest in crossdressing, so measuring the presence of autoheterosexuality with questions about crossdressing is especially likely to underestimate its true prevalence in females.

It's also not yet known why females report less sartorial arousal:

＊ Is men's clothing less sexually appealing in general?

＊ Is it comparatively easier for people who have a vulva instead of a penis to overlook or otherwise fail to notice the presence of sexual arousal?

* Are females less likely to be fetishistic than males, thus focusing more directly on whole bodies and less on specific body parts or the objects around them?

* In matters of sexuality, do males have a greater fixation on visual form, while females care more about the quality and nature of interpersonal interactions?

These hypotheses are my current best guesses as to why females and males have such different reported rates of sexual interest in dressing as the other sex, but ultimately the contributors to this disparity are still unknown.

An Exploratory FTM Typology Study

There has been at least one study[79] exploring the possibility that gay and bisexual trans men are of a different type than trans men who prefer women. It came out in 2000, so even though its sample size of thirty-eight was good for its time, it's small by contemporary standards.

Researchers asked trans men whom they fantasized about then partitioned those who preferred women into the homosexual group and those who were bisexual or preferred men into the nonhomosexual group.

As with MTFs, the homosexual group was less white and reported more childhood gender nonconformity[80]. They also had more interest in women, especially straight ones. But that's not a surprise: they were assigned to that group based on their preference for women.

By contrast, the nonhomosexual group had a strong preference for masculine sexual partners[81]. More specifically, they were *very* interested in gay men. Although they reported moderate interest in other types of sexual partners, gay men appealed to them most of all[82].

If autoandrophilia drove their desire to transition, we would expect this strong interest in gay men. By partnering with gay men, they can be with their preferred gender and be sure their partner is legitimately attracted to them as men.

In their write-up, researchers suggested that the rarity of strong, persistent nonvanilla sexual interests in females made it unlikely that nonhomosexual FTMS were autoandrophilic[83]. Unfortunately, this assumption has kept some leading researchers from realizing that a generalized two-type model can be applied to both sexes.

Is There a Typology for Trans Men?

Even though the two-type typology for MTFS classifies nonhomosexual MTFS as autogynephilic, it has not yet been established through formal research that FTMS can be sorted in the same way.

One potential issue is that female and male sexual orientation appear to function differently[84]. When exposed to erotic stimuli in the lab, females show less category specificity in their sexual response than males[85]. Female sexual orientation also seems more prone to shifting over time[86].

Furthermore, some preliminary research suggests transgender identification may spread socially within peer groups, especially among females[87]. If further studies account for autoandrophilia and still show a similar pattern, it may be the case that some FTMs are neither homosexual nor autoheterosexual.

However, even if scientists find solid evidence for more than two developmental pathways leading to FTM transgenderism, there is already ample evidence that both homosexuality and autoheterosexuality can motivate females to transition and live as men. The real question is whether there are more than these two types of FTM transgenderism, not whether these two types exist in the first place.

IN SUM

* Centuries ago, Muslim legal scholars differentiated between two types of effeminate males—those who innately spoke and moved like women yet lacked desire for them, and those who were attracted to women and whose feminine behavior seemed intentional. Both resemble the two known MTF types found in contemporary society.

* Magnus Hirschfeld created the term "transvestiten" to describe people who wore clothing of the other sex as valid symbols of inner personality. Based on their sexual partner preferences, he categorized transvestites into four groups: homosexual, heterosexual, bisexual, and asexual.

* When medical technology advanced to the point that it could help trans people fit into society as the other sex, the category of "transsexual" was born. Harry Benjamin created a six-category scale that spanned the transvestite–transsexual spectrum for the purpose of deciding which patients should get access to surgeries. A patient's sexual orientation and the intensity of their desire for surgery were the two main criteria considered. Attraction to women disqualified patients from a "true transsexual" diagnosis.

* Norman Fisk realized that patients were falsely portraying themselves to medical gatekeepers in order to get hormones and surgeries. However, there seemed to be few regrets, so he reconceptualized the gender situation that clinicians were trying to treat as a type of psychological pain he called "gender dysphoria syndrome". This new way of thinking about gender issues began to reduce the sexual-orientation-based gatekeeping that had been standard practice in transgender medicine.

* In the 1970s, researchers began to converge upon a two-type model of MTF transgenderism in which one type was related to effeminate homosexuality and the other to transvestism. In the 1980s, researchers in Canada utilized new computing technology to conduct the first large-scale quantitative studies of transsexualism, and they, too, found evidence for a two-type MTF model.

* After conducting three empirical studies as part of his MTF typology research, Ray Blanchard concluded that homosexual MTFS and nonhomosexual MTFS were of different etiologies. He proposed that nonhomosexual MTFS had an underlying sexuality characterized by arousal at the thought or image of themselves as female, which he called "autogynephilia".

* Later researchers replicated one of Blanchard's key findings: nonhomosexual MTFS are far more likely than homosexual MTFS to report prior arousal from crossdressing. Even researchers who showed overt hostility to Blanchard's typology got results that were nearly identical to Blanchard's. The two-type typology of MTF transgenderism has been replicated several times— empirically, it still stands strong.

* There has been little formal research into whether or not the two-type model applies to trans men. Some trans men report prior arousal from crossdressing, which suggests that some trans men are autoandrophilic. Researchers exploring the possibility of a two-type FTM typology found that androphilic-leaning trans men had less childhood gender nonconformity and were especially attracted to gay men—both of which are expected if androphilic trans men are of autoandrophilic etiology.

CHANGING IDENTITY, CHANGING PREFERENCES

META-ATTRACTION AT WORK

Many transgender people report that their sexual preferences changed after they transitioned gender.

Some trans women who only ever had eyes for women report that men started to become attractive after they transitioned. Some trans men who thought they were only into women say that gay and bisexual men began to draw their attention after transitioning.

For some, their sexual preferences shifted when they adopted a transgender identity or started hormones. For others, it may have started when they socially transitioned or started passing. Depending on the individual, the timing varies.

In order to better understand this phenomenon, the authors of a 2013 paper on sexual orientation in trans men used an internet survey to ask approximately 500 trans men about their attractions before and after transitioning (identification, social transition, or medical transition)[1].

An astounding 40% of these trans men reported shifts in attraction after transitioning. Most shifted toward interest in men. Testosterone usage didn't predict changes to sexual orientation[2], which suggested that hormonal changes weren't behind these shifts.

	Attracted to:		
	Men	Both	Women
Before Transition	13%	33%	54%
After Transition	18%	55%	27%
Attraction Shift	**+5%**	**+22%**	**-27%**

Table 5.2.1: Shifts in attraction before and after FTM transition.
Source: "Measures of Clinical Health among Female-to-Male Transgender Persons as a Function of Sexual Orientation" (Meier et al 2013).

Remember the autoandrophilic FTM developmental trajectory I mentioned previously[3] in which an autoandrophilic trans man may ultimately come out three times?

(1) lesbian/bi woman → (2) trans man → (3) gay/bi trans man

The shifts in sexual preference reported in this study suggest that this identity development sequence is a recurring pattern among autoandrophilic trans men.

REALISTIC RESEARCHERS ADDRESS AUTOHETEROSEXUALITY

A year later, in 2014, another group of researchers published a paper on trans people's sexual orientation changes, but this time they drew from a clinical population[4]. Like previous researchers, they found that reported changes in sexual orientation weren't associated with taking hormones[5]. These changes weren't associated with surgeries, either, or even the age when participants started to feel dysphoria, take hormones, or transition socially[6].

None of these factors seemed to have a significant impact.

To make sense of their findings, these researchers seriously considered the possibility that these changes were related to autoheterosexuality.

They noted how written responses from study subjects suggested autoheterosexuality was behind many of the reported changes in sexual orientation. They also reviewed past studies presenting both qualitative and quantitative evidence for the existence and relevance of autoheterosexuality[7].

These researchers noted that the heterosexual transsexuals they studied were most likely to report a change in sexual orientation, and suggested their true orientation was actually autoheterosexual[8]. They also advised that "researchers should explicitly ask for autogynephilic and autoandrophilic sexual orientation"[9].

Unfortunately, researchers rarely follow this sane and rational advice.

META-ATTRACTION INFLUENCES SEXUALITY SHIFTS

A network of gender professionals in Europe have coordinated their actions in order to research transgenderism and gender variance in larger cohorts across different European countries.

The group they formed, the European Network for the Investigation of Gender Incongruence (ENIGI), carried out a three-year longitudinal study of transgender people. With 902 participants at the start, the study had a massive sample size[10].

As part of this research, participants were asked about 1) their sexual attractions, 2) their sexual fantasies, 3) the sexual identity of their current partner, and 4) which sex role they played in their sexual fantasies. They were asked this same set of questions just before starting hormones, three months later, and then after one, two, and three years[11].

Just like the prior studies, the researchers didn't find any effect of hormones or surgeries on sexual orientation outcomes[12]. At this point, it seems fairly established that hormones or surgeries don't directly cause the sexual orientation changes that trans people commonly report after transitioning.

However, meta-attraction can account for many of these changes. Since autohet meta-attraction can drive a desire to play a cross-gender sex role with a same-sex partner (meta-homosexuality), it's likely that meta-attraction is behind many of the reported changes in sexual orientation.

Between the check-ins at years one and two, trans men and trans women both reported a large increase in sexual fantasies in which they played a sex role associated with their birth sex. If meta-attraction drives the changes to sexual orientation that trans people report, we'd expect them to report fewer sexual fantasies about people of the same sex over this same period.

That's exactly what happened: fantasies about people of the same sex decreased.

META-ATTRACTION DRIVES SHIFTS TO SEXUAL PREFERENCES: 1–2 YEARS INTO TRANSITION, CIS FANTASIES SURGE WHILE FANTASIES ABOUT SAME-SEX PARTNERS DECLINE

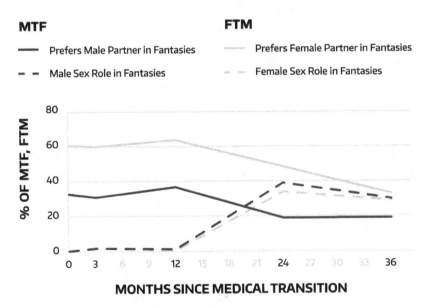

MTF

— Prefers Male Partner in Fantasies

- - Male Sex Role in Fantasies

FTM

Prefers Female Partner in Fantasies

Female Sex Role in Fantasies

Source: Sexual orientation in transgender individuals: results from the longitudinal ENIGI study (2021)
Authors: J. Defreyne, E. Elaut, M. Den Heijer, B. Kreukels, A. D. Fisher and G. T'Sjoen
Note: Researchers found that neither hormone levels or surgeries had a significant association with partner preferences in sexual fantasies, gender role in sexual fantasies, sexual attractions, or sexual identity of current sexual partner.

Figure 5.2.2

This change wasn't limited to fantasies either. These shifts also showed up in reported sexual attractions and even affected their choice of sexual partner (see Table 5.2.3). For both trans women and trans men, measures of same-sex interest declined across the board. It wasn't as large as the decline in cross-gender fantasies, but that's to be expected: only a subset of autoheterosexuals experience meta-homosexuality.

Changes, Year 1 to Year 2	Cis Sex Role in Fantasies	Same Sex Fantasy	Same Sex Attraction	Same Sex Partner
MTF	+38%	-18%	-11%	-17%
FTM	+34%	-16%	-15%	-19%

Table 5.2.3: Shifting identities, attractions, fantasies, and partner choices in the second year of medical gender transition. Data sourced from Defreyne et al., 2021.

Interpreting these research findings with the awareness that autoheterosexuality is the most common cause of transgenderism makes the pattern blatantly obvious, but these researchers didn't even mention autogynephilia or autoandrophilia. And for some strange reason, they presented their findings as a series of truly awful bar charts that obscured the pattern.

The first time I read this study, I saw no clear takeaways. Neither the charts nor the discussion that followed them seemed to indicate any noteworthy patterns. But a few months later, I entered the data into a spreadsheet, plotted it as a line graph, and the pattern jumped out.

It was obvious. As cross-gender sexual fantasies plummeted, so did same-sex fantasies, attractions, and partner choices. Meta-attraction was behind these changes.

It's not as if the researchers were oblivious to the existence and relevance of autoheterosexuality, either: *the very first citation in their paper* pointed to the study I discussed in the previous section in which the authors explored the relevance of autoheterosexuality for several pages and explicitly advised other researchers to ask study subjects about autoandrophilia and autogynephilia[13].

When this ENIGI report came out, it represented the largest study of sexual orientation changes in trans people ever conducted. Its sample size absolutely dwarfed those of all previous similar studies, and it was the product of teamwork between researchers across several countries.

What is the likelihood that this team of transgender health professionals forgot to consider the most common kind of transgenderism when they interpreted and wrote up their findings? Is it likely that none of these researchers noticed this curious pattern of same-sex interest declining in tandem with cross-gender fantasies?

IN SUM

* Trans people commonly report changes to their sexual orientations around the time they undergo gender transition, but empirical studies have repeatedly found

these changes aren't associated with hormones or surgeries. Something else is behind them.

* Research results from the massive ENIGI study suggest that meta-attraction can account for these reported changes in sexual orientation. During the same time period that trans people reported a dramatic drop in sexual fantasies in which they played a cross-gender sex role, there was a corresponding drop in sexual interest toward people of the same sex—a change that showed up in their fantasies, attractions, and partner choices.

WHICH KIND OF TRANS IS THE MOST COMMON?

ESTIMATING THE RELATIVE PREVALENCE OF THE TWO TYPES

Taking into account both sexes and both known transgender etiologies, there are four distinct groups of transgender people. Using data on their reported sexual orientations, it's possible to estimate the relative prevalence of each group with the two-type typology.

Recall that the two-type typology sorts trans people based on their sexual orientation with respect to their birth sex. If they're strictly homosexual, they go into the homosexual category. If they're nonhomosexual (heterosexual, bisexual, or asexual), they go into the autoheterosexual category.

Since some autohets do have same-sex partner preferences, estimates that rely on the two-type typology will underestimate the true prevalence of autoheterosexual transgenderism, but they're a good start.

Before I present etiology prevalence estimates that categorize the transgender community into its four main groups, I want to illustrate some of the fuzziness inherent to this effort to make clear these are estimates, not exact figures.

Many factors affect the sort of data transgender researchers receive. Depending on whom they talk to and the sorts of questions they ask, they get different answers.

MEASURING SEXUAL ORIENTATION: IDENTITIES AND ATTRACTIONS

Depending on how people are asked about their sexual orientation, they give different responses. For instance, the sexual identities they report don't always match their attractions, fantasies, or behavior.

The gender-flipping nature of transition makes things even more confusing. The meaning of identities associated with homosexuality and heterosexuality become ambiguous: if a trans person says they're heterosexual, is that with respect to their gender identity or their sex?

Asking only about sexual identity is probably the worst way to get accurate information on people's sexual orientations—it's also important to ask about their attractions, behavior, or fantasies. Imagination is the only limit when it comes to sexual fantasy, and sexual orientation is commonly defined based on attraction, so it's smart to ask study participants about attractions and fantasies.

Although there are many ways to ask about sexual orientation, most measures get in the same general ballpark. What matters is that it's measured, and getting a few measures is better than just one.

THE IMPACT OF TIME, SPACE, AND CULTURE ON ESTIMATES OF TRANS ETIOLOGY

The way in which transgenderism researchers find their study participants affects the relative proportions of homosexuals and nonhomosexuals in their samples. Internet-based studies[1] tend to find more nonhomosexual trans people than studies from gender clinics[2].

There's also the issue of *timing*: is the study surveying pre- or post-transition trans people? As seen in the prior chapter, the sexual orientations that trans people report often change based on where they are in their gender trajectory.

Timing also matters on a societal level. In recent years, there has been a major shift in the types of people seeking gender-affirming medical care. Adolescent referrals to gender clinics have become female-dominant[3]. People with nonhomosexual orientations are showing up more often too[4].

These changes over the past few decades demonstrate that culture impacts the proportion of trans people who fall into each of the four groups.

For example, race and ethnicity impact the proportion of trans women who belong to either etiology. In the large study of trans women in the New York metropolitan area that replicated

PREVALENCE OF THE TWO TYPES OF TRANS WOMEN VARIES BETWEEN RACIAL/ETHNIC GROUPS

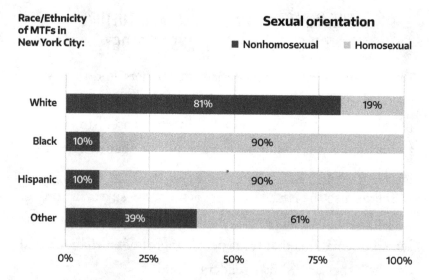

Source: A Further Assessment of Blanchard's Typology of Homosexual Versus Non-Homosexual or Autogynephilic Gender Dysphoria (2011)
Authors: Nuttbrock, L., Bockting, W., Mason, M., Hwahng, S., Rosenblum, A., Macri, M., & Becker, J.
Note: Sexual orientations are in relation to birth sex

Figure 5.3.1

Blanchard's first typology study, researchers found drastic differences based on race and ethnicity: 90% of the Hispanic and black trans women were homosexual[5], but only 19% of the white trans women were homosexual (see Figure 5.3.1).

If these patterns hold for other places in the US, then among Americans, white trans women are usually autoheterosexual, and black or Hispanic trans women are usually homosexual.

I suspect that culture impacts this difference more than genes, because culture strongly influences etiology ratios among trans women. In particular, the degree to which a society is individualistic or collectivistic ("I" versus "we") strongly predicts the proportion of trans women who come from either etiology[6].

Anne Lawrence figured this out. In her model, about three-fourths of nonhomosexual MTF prevalence was predicted by societal individualism[7]. Individualistic countries clearly had the most nonhomosexual MTFs, while collectivistic countries had the least (see Figure 5.3.2)[8].

This difference in societal organization makes a massive impact: it's apparently far more feasible in Western, individualistic countries for autohet MTFs to live as women.

As a freedom-lover, I like what this finding implies: the relative prevalence of autoheterosexual transgenderism is an indirect indicator of how free we are to live in alignment with our strongly held feelings.

When we see autohet trans people where we live, it's a sign that we are free to live in the way that suits us.

CHOOSING YOUR OWN LIFE PATH: WESTERN INDIVIDUALISTIC SOCIETIES HAVE MORE AUTOHETEROSEXUAL TRANSGENDERISM

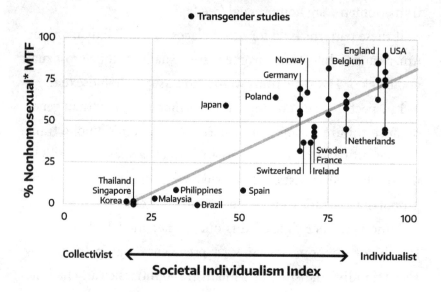

Source of most data: Societal Individualism Predicts Prevalence of Nonhomosexual Orientation in Male-to-Female Transsexualism (2010)
More Evidence that Societal Individualism Predicts Prevalence of Nonhomosexual Orientation in Male-to-Female Transsexualism (2013)
Author: Anne Lawrence
Additional data points: Iantaffi & Bockting 2011; James et al, 2016; Grant et al, 2011; Auer et al, 2014; Wierckx et al, 2014; Jones et al, 2011; Herman et al 2002; Nuttbrock et al, 2011; Hess et al 2020
*Note: In relation to birth sex

Figure 5.3.2

TRANSGENDER AMERICANS ARE USUALLY AUTOHET

Hopefully it's clear by now that estimates of trans people's sexual orientation vary depending on their race or ethnicity, their stage of transition, the degree of individualism in their cultural milieu, and whether their answers have potential consequences for receiving medical care (gender clinic versus online).

There are undoubtedly other factors as well, and there is an inherent fuzziness to figuring out this ratio that we can't fully eliminate. Still, I anticipate some readers will want to know some numbers they can cite as a reasonable statistic when talking about transgenderism.

For that, I'll reference two enormous surveys of Americans: the 2011 National Transgender Discrimination Survey (2011 NTDS)[9] and the 2015 United States Transgender Survey (2015 USTS)[10].

All the trans people who took these surveys were from the US, and a little over 80% of them were white. Except for the 7% of respondents in the 2011 NTDS who filled out their survey in-person[11], everyone took these surveys over the internet.

Almost 80% of those who filled out the 2011 NTDS in-person were not white, while those who took it online were 80% white[12]. This suggests that online surveys will underestimate the true prevalence of trans people who aren't white—and since non-white trans people are more likely to be of homosexual etiology than white trans people, online surveys will likely underestimate the true prevalence of homosexual transgenderism.

These three factors—white race, individualistic culture, and online survey—are all associated with higher estimates of nonhomosexuality and, therefore, higher estimates of autoheterosexuality.

Despite these limitations, I chose these data sources for a few reasons:

* They had massive samples
* They weren't administered in a medical setting, so the trans people taking them knew their answers couldn't be used to withhold medical care
* Dozens of researchers have used these two datasets to publish studies of their own, which implies that many researchers consider them worthwhile

The 2011 NTDS and 2015 USTS asked about sexual orientation in terms of sexual identity as bisexual, queer, asexual, gay/lesbian/same-gender-loving, straight/heterosexual, or other/not listed. The 2015 USTS also had a pansexual category.

In line with contemporary transgender social norms, I interpreted "straight" and "heterosexual" responses in relation to gender identity, which placed them in the homosexual etiology. I sorted "gay/lesbian/same-gender-loving" responses into the nonhomosexual etiology by this same logic.

I interpreted "pansexual" as a synonym for "bisexual" and categorized both as nonhomosexual. Asexuals went into the nonhomosexual category as well.

"Queer" is ambiguous by design and its meaning can be hard to pin down, but it's just another way of saying *nonalloheterosexual.* A previous study showed that almost three-quarters of queer-identified trans men in their sample had nonhomosexual attractions[13], so I sorted queer trans men accordingly. I lacked a comparable reference for sorting the 6–7% of trans women who identified as queer, so I put them all into the nonhomosexual category.

MOST TRANSGENDER AMERICANS ARE AUTOHETEROSEXUAL

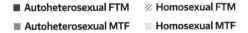

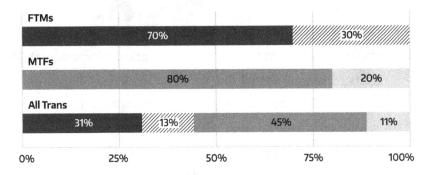

Source: 2-type typology applied to self-reported sexual orientations in 2011 National Transgender Discrimination Survey and 2015 US Transgender Survey
Note: Sexual orientations are in relation to birth sex

Figure 5.3.3

I placed trans people who selected "other/not listed" as their sexual orientation in the nonhomosexual category—I figured if their sexual identity was too unique to pick "heterosexual" or "straight", they were probably nonhomosexual.

Based on this typology-based sorting, autoheterosexuals are by far the most prevalent etiology among transgender Americans. About 70% of trans men and 80% of trans women in America are of autoheterosexual etiology.

Overall, autogynephilic MTFs are the most common type of transgender American. Autoandrophilic FTMs are the second-most common. Homosexual MTFs and FTMs each represent about an eighth of the overall total.

Approximately three-quarters of transgender Americans are of autoheterosexual etiology. The rest are of homosexual etiology.

IN SUM

* The two-type typology sorts trans people into different etiologies based on their sexual orientation. Homosexual trans people are sorted into the homosexual etiology, while nonhomosexual trans people are sorted into the autoheterosexual etiology. Given that there are two known transgender etiologies in each sex, it's possible to sort trans people into four distinct groups based on their reported sexual orientations and thus determine the relative prevalence of each group.

* Study methodologies affect these estimates of etiology ratios. Researchers usually arrive at different estimates for the sexual orientations of trans people based on whether they ask about sexual identities, attractions, behaviors, or fantasies. The way they find trans participants makes a difference too: internet-based studies tend to have a higher ratio of nonhomosexual trans people than gender-clinic-based studies. Whether study participants are pre- or post-transition matters, as does whether or not it's a recent study.

* Culture strongly influences the relative prevalence
  of homosexual and autoheterosexual trans people.
  Homosexual transgenderism is more common
  in collectivistic societies, and autoheterosexual
  transgenderism is more common in individualistic
  societies. Another sign of culture's influence is the
  drastically different etiology prevalence ratios among
  trans women based on their racial or ethnic group.
  Data from New York City suggests that in the US, black
  or Hispanic trans women are usually of homosexual
  etiology, while white trans women are usually of
  autoheterosexual etiology.

* Applying the two-type typology to the largest surveys
  of transgender Americans yields an estimate that
  approximately 70% of trans men and 80% of trans women
  are autoheterosexual. In America, autohet trans people
  are approximately three times as common as homosexual
  trans people.

MORE FEMALES ARE TRANSITIONING

FEMALES ARE CURRENTLY MORE SUSCEPTIBLE TO DEVELOPING GENDER ISSUES

Starting around the years 2005 to 2006, referrals to gender clinics for gender dysphoria began shooting up. Patient demographics have shifted too. Males used to be the majority of referrals, but now females are[1].

At the Dutch gender clinic, homosexual males went from being the largest subgroup to being the smallest (see Figure 5.4.1). Homosexual females became the largest group, and nonhomosexual females went from being virtually nonexistent to being about as prevalent as nonhomosexual males[2].

MALES USED TO TRANSITION MORE OFTEN THAN FEMALES BUT NOW FEMALES TRANSITION MORE OFTEN THAN MALES

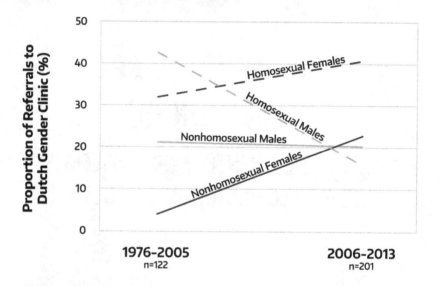

Source: Evidence for an Altered Sex Ratio in Clinic-Referred Adolescents with Gender Dysphoria (2015)
Author: Aitken et al

Figure 5.4.1

Trends in gender identification also suggest that females are currently more susceptible to developing gender issues. Approximately 75–80% of people with suprabinary gender identities (identities beyond female or male) are of the female sex[3]. Most transgender-identified adolescents are female too[4].

Age distributions also reflect the recent surge in transgenderism among females. The 2011 NTDS and 2015 USTS both found that 90% of trans men were younger than forty-five years of age and that people with suprabinary gender identities were similarly young[5].

As seen in Chapter 5.0, females are about half as likely to be either autoheterosexual or homosexual. Since these orientations likely occur at similar rates across generations, these two main causes of transgenderism are unlikely to be the sole contributors to the changing composition of the transgender population. Other factors likely act in tandem with these orientations to create the recent demographic shifts.

SOCIAL MEDIA

Widespread adoption of social media began around the same time that gender clinics started receiving more referrals for gender dysphoria.

Myspace started in 2003. Facebook started in 2004 and introduced the news feed in 2006. Twitter started in 2006, Tumblr in 2007, Instagram in 2010, and Snapchat in 2011. Through these platforms, transgender people could share their stories and advocate for themselves at an unprecedented level. These virtual communities also gave gender-dysphoric people access to information that could help them understand their situation.

Less helpfully, social media also enabled people to compare themselves to the misleadingly positive presentations of their peers' lives. Whitewashed images of happiness and beauty had previously been largely confined to professionally produced media like advertisements, television, and film, but now acquaintances and friends produced them as well, making them seem even more real.

Social media also enabled the spread of a very specific set of postmodern gender ideas which are being inserted into school curriculums, propagated by major nonprofit organizations, and spread by millions of believers through their social media accounts.

RAPID-ONSET GENDER DYSPHORIA (ROGD)

Sexual researchers have proposed that some adolescents and young adults who are claiming to be gender dysphoric or transgender are being influenced to do so by social forces[6]. The technical term for these social forces is "social contagion", which the American Psychological Association defines as "the spread of behaviors, attitudes, and affect through crowds and other types of social aggregates from one member to another"[7].

This type of gender dysphoria supposedly affects females more than males. It has been named *rapid-onset gender dysphoria* (ROGD) because it often appears in adolescents whose parents didn't notice significant gender nonconformity in their younger years. The parents of these adolescents are often surprised to hear of their child's gender dysphoria or transgender identity. Many report that prior to this revelation, their child had increased social media usage or one of their friends came out as trans.

Perhaps not coincidentally, ROGD arises during or after puberty—the same age when autoheterosexual gender dysphoria usually manifests.

Lisa Littman conducted the first study exploring the possibility of ROGD by surveying parents who reported that their child had a sudden onset of gender dysphoria during or after puberty[8]. About 80% of the children were female[9], and a similar proportion of the parents said their child's announcement of being either gender dysphoric or transgender caught them by surprise[10].

Most parents said their children were using social media more often just prior to their announcement of gender dysphoria[11]. After coming out as trans, most of them experienced a boost in popularity within their friend group. An average of 3.5 kids in these friend groups had become gender dysphoric, and in more than a third of friend groups, *a majority* of the friends became transgender-identified[12]. Only 3% of parents reported that their child was the first in their friend circle to come out as trans[13].

Although would-be transgender people tend to befriend each other, and the cultural environment is becoming increasingly friendly to trans people, these rates of transgender identification within friend groups are absurdly high. The influence of social contagion is definitely worth examining.

On the other hand, the subjects' rates of homosexuality and nonhomosexuality were similar to the broader transgender population[14], which is what we'd expect to see if most of these cases of gender dysphoria were ultimately just cases of homosexual or autoheterosexual gender dysphoria.

Littman's study didn't ask parents whether their kids showed any signs of autoheterosexuality, so there's no way to know how many of these adolescents were autoheterosexual. Still, it's important to consider the possibility that many cases of rapid-onset gender dysphoria are actually cases of autohet gender dysphoria. Like ROGD, autohet gender dysphoria usually makes itself known during or after puberty, and the announcement of a transgender identity by autohets often comes as a surprise to their friends and family.

SEX, ETIOLOGY, AND GENDER ISSUES

In order to infer which sex and which etiology contributes more to gender issues, I compared the etiology breakdown within the transgender population to that of the broader etiological population from which they come (the combined homosexual and autoheterosexual population).

To estimate the size of the broader etiological population, I combined American estimates of strong same-sex attraction with Czech estimates of strong autoheterosexuality (those featured in Figure 5.0.3). I assumed a fifty-fifty ratio between females and males. I also assumed the prevalence of homosexuality and autoheterosexuality wouldn't significantly differ between the two countries. Using this method, the broader etiological population made up about 2.9% of the total population.

As expected, the proportion of trans men within the transgender population exceeded the proportion of females in the broader etiological population: being female increased the odds of gender transition. Likewise, the proportion of autoheterosexuals in the transgender population far exceeded their proportion in the broader etiological population, suggesting that autoheterosexuality is a stronger driver of gender transition than homosexuality.

Within the etiological population from which transgender people originate, being either female or autoheterosexual increases the odds of gender transition.

AUTOHETEROSEXUALS ARE MORE LIKELY TO TRANSITION THAN HOMOSEXUALS

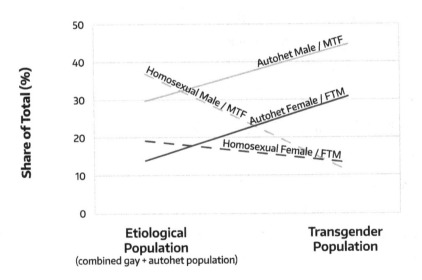

Sources:
Autoheterosexual preference prevalence: The Prevalence of Paraphilic Interests in the Czech Population (Bartova et al 2020);
Homosexual attraction prevalence: Sexual Orientation, Controversy, and Science (Bailey et al 2016);
Transgender etiology prevalence: 2-type typology applied to reported sexual orientations in 2011 NTDS and 2015 USTS
Note: Sexual orientations are in relation to birth sex

Figure 5.4.2

This is especially apparent for people who are both autohet and female: although autohet females are the smallest subgroup within the broader homosexual and autoheterosexual population, autohet FTMs are the second-most common type of transgender person in the US. And data from the 2011 NTDS[15] and 2015 USTS[16] suggest their proportion is increasing. Using the same sorting methodology described in Chapter 5.3, I found that the relative proportion of nonhomosexual FTMs increased 9% between 2008 and 2015.

During this time, the relative proportion of homosexual FTMs stayed constant, nonhomosexual MTFs decreased 4%, and homosexual MTFs decreased 5%. These shifts suggest that more females than males transitioned during this time, and that much of this increase was driven specifically by autohet FTMs.

WHY ARE AUTOHET FTMs BECOMING MORE PREVALENT?

Trans men increasingly understand that their partner preferences don't impact the legitimacy of their trans identity. Androphilic trans men such as Lou Sullivan were behind this change. However, it took a while for this knowledge to percolate throughout the broader FTM population.

For years, influential researchers such as Blanchard and Bailey expressed certainty that homosexual transgenderism existed in both sexes, but they were comparatively doubtful there was a female counterpart to autogynephilic MTF transgenderism[17]. This stance likely kept some autoandrophilic people from realizing they had legitimate gender issues that could be ameliorated through medical transition, thus reducing the number of trans men who sought such treatment.

Another possible contributor to FTM gender transition is related to sex differences in affinity for objects. Females tend to prefer people-centered, relational occupations, whereas males tend to prefer object-centered, technical occupations[18]. This greater male affinity for objects also shows up in sexuality: males are more likely to report transvestism or sexual fetishism (sexual interest in nonliving objects or nongenital body parts)[19].

This sex difference may seem benign at first, but it can have massive consequences for the development and management of gender dysphoria throughout one's life: object-mediated sexuality offers some protection against gender dysphoria.

Object-Mediated Sexuality Reduces Dysphoria

When early sexologists such as Magnus Hirschfeld and Havelock Ellis analyzed cases of autohet transgenderism, they considered those who eschewed crossdressing to be the most intense manifestations of the orientation. Recall that Hirschfeld described these patients as the "congenitally most strongly predisposed"[20], while Ellis said they were "less common but more complete"[21].

Blanchard found that among gender clinic patients with a history of transvestism, autogynephilia and fetishism were significant predictors of whether they had a constant cross-gender identity or wanted to get sexual reassignment surgery[22]. MTFS who admitted to autogynephilia were far more likely to report a cross-gender identity and a desire for surgery. Fetishism had the opposite effect: those who admitted to fetishism were less likely to report a cross-gender identity or a desire for surgery[23]. (This is why the DSM-5 includes the specifiers "with fetishism" and "with autogynephilia" for diagnoses of Transvestic Disorder[24]).

Although transvestism and fetishism are conceptually distinct, both involve the use of objects. Autohets who can derive symbolic worth from clothing or other objects have a tool for attaining cross-gender embodiment that others lack.

However, females tend to show less sexual interest in transvestism or fetishism. Therefore, when comparing autohet females and males whose autoheterosexuality is of similar strength, the autohet females are likely more susceptible to developing strong gender dysphoria.

PSYCHOLOGICAL SEX DIFFERENCES AND OTHER FACTORS

In addition to the previously discussed factors, there are a few more that I suspect work in tandem to increase gender transition and transgender-identification among females:

* Psychological sex differences
* Postmodern gender ideas
* Patriarchy

Females are more likely to be high in neuroticism (tendency to have negative moods)[25]. This means that, *on average*, they are more prone to strong emotional reactions and negative mood states like anxiety, fear, depression, envy, or loneliness.

Females are more susceptible to anxiety disorder and major depressive disorder[26]. They're also more likely to have obsessive compulsive disorder[27], eating disorders[28], or body dysmorphia[29].

In short, females are more prone to negative mood states and more likely to fixate on the state of their body and ruminate about it at length. The ability to compare themselves with peers on social media probably doesn't help matters either.

It also might be the case that some adolescents transition as a coping strategy for dealing with unwanted emotions. This is another one of the hypotheses proposed by Littman for making sense of ROGD[30]. With all the new ideas about gender floating around, it's inevitable that some people will misinterpret their negative mood states as evidence that they are transgender.

Postmodern Gender Memeplex (the New Gender Ideas)

The bundle of new gender ideas that have spread rapidly and become popular in the past few years are likely increasing the number of people who decide to transition.

Some critics of these new gender ideas refer to them as "gender identity ideology"[31]. While the ideas do often take the form of an ideology, I'd rather call the phenomenon the *postmodern gender memeplex*. It's more neutral and descriptive, albeit less catchy.

A memeplex is simply a bundle of ideas or concepts that tend to propagate together as a group. Postmodern thinking entails skepticism toward overarching narratives and the ability to know objective truths, as well as an obsession with the power of language.

One of the foundational ideas within the postmodern gender memeplex is that "gender is a kind of imitation for which there is no original"[32]. Other nonsensical ideas in the postmodern gender memeplex include these:

* Sex isn't binary[33]
* Sex is a label assigned at birth[34]
* "Sex and gender are...separate, socially constructed dimensions of personal identity"[35]

Beliefs like these are emotionally comforting to autoheterosexuals who are wedded to the idea of being the other sex/gender, and it's to these emotional benefits that these ideas likely owe their staying power.

The postmodern gender memeplex expands the importance of gender and shrinks the role of sex (ostensibly to help trans and gender-nonconforming people). Placing greater emphasis on gender and less on sex makes gender transition seem like a more powerful intervention, so this shift in emphasis likely encourages more people to undergo gender transition.

Patriarchy

Another potential contributing factor behind increased rates of FTM gender transition is *patriarchy*, the social system that privileges males over females.

Patriarchy is built into our bodies and psychologies. In many primate species, males fight for social dominance among one another and treat females poorly in order to gain access to their reproductive capacity[36]. This approach represents the optimal mating strategy for many male primates, which is partly why males are bigger and stronger than females.

Some of patriarchy's downsides can be mitigated by thoughtfully changing human culture (this is the work of feminism). However, patriarchy is not a human invention or a mere social construction. Although feminists are still chipping away at patriarchy, it won't fully disappear anytime soon.

In addition to this collective approach to curtailing patriarchy, there is also an individualistic approach to minimizing the downsides of patriarchy—FTM gender transition. By medically transitioning, someone born female can be seen and treated as a man instead of as a woman.

To clarify: I am not arguing that females are transitioning *solely* because of patriarchy, the new gender ideas, or sex-based psychological differences—only that these are potential *contributing factors* that, in combination, may partially account for recently increased rates of FTM gender transition ever since social media and transgenderism became mainstream. I still think that someone who is neither homosexual nor autoheterosexual is unlikely to undergo gender transition.

It also doesn't require a stretch of imagination to conclude that social media has influenced the dramatic rise in FTM gender transition. The surge in transgenderism started around the same time that social media really took off, and online platforms are the primary channel through which the new gender ideas have spread. Social media is a powerful conduit for social contagion—we shouldn't discount its impact on the propensity for gender transition.

IN SUM

* Several lines of evidence indicate a recent surge in transgenderism among females. Most referrals to gender clinics used to be male, but the sex ratio shifted around 2006. Now, female patients are more prevalent at gender clinics. Most transgender-identified adolescents and most people with suprabinary gender identities are female.

* The rise in transgender identification among females happened around the same time that social media really started to pop off (Twitter started in 2006, Tumblr in 2007, and Facebook's news feed was introduced in 2006). This overlap in timing is unlikely to be a coincidence.

* Reports from parents whose children had a sudden onset of gender dysphoria during or after puberty have revealed patterns that suggest transgender identification can spread quickly through friend groups and reach

prevalence rates within those groups that far exceed population norms.

* By comparing the etiological makeup of the transgender population to the broader etiological population from which it derives, it's possible to infer that 1) being female is a stronger contributor to gender issues than being male, and 2) autoheterosexuality is a more powerful driver of gender transition than homosexuality. Unsurprisingly, autoandrophilic FTMs are the fastest-growing segment of the trans population.

* Historical ignorance of nonhomosexual FTM transgenderism may have reduced the amount of nonhomosexual FTMs who sought medical transition (because they couldn't see themselves in the transsexualism literature). Object-mediated sexuality can help reduce gender dysphoria, but females are less likely to have interest in object-mediated sexuality. This leaves autohet females comparatively more susceptible to developing autoheterosexual gender dysphoria.

* Psychological sex differences and patriarchy both contribute to gender issues in females: females are more susceptible to negative mood states and body dysmorphia, and transitioning to live as a man has more social benefits under patriarchy. Postmodern gender ideas contribute to

greater gender transition rates in both sexes. Under the influence of the new gender ideas, adolescents are more likely to think they might be transgender if they don't like their bodies or their sex traits.

PART 6

AUTOHETEROSEXUAL CROSS-GENDER DEVELOPMENT

6 . 0

AUTOHET CROSS-GENDER DEVELOPMENT

CONSTRUCTING THE CROSS-GENDER SELF

Autoheterosexual cross-gender identities form over time through reinforcement.

The original, default gender identity forms by three years of age. Autoheterosexual cross-gender identity grows alongside this default gender identity.

Moving through life as the default gender strengthens the default self. Cross-gender embodiment strengthens the cross-gender self. Both selves grow in parallel.

Initially, the default self tends to be much stronger than the cross-gender self. The stronger their autoheterosexuality, the faster an autoheterosexual's cross-gender side tends to form: the cross-gender wish starts earlier, develops more quickly, and is more likely to become dominant in the end.

For the most strongly predisposed autoheterosexuals, wishing to be the other sex is often one of their earliest memories. Their ability to recall these memories later in life signals their continued significance: these memories stood out as important throughout development and weren't pruned like so many others. They persisted.

Wherever autoheterosexuals are in their gender journey, it's the result of thousands of gender-related thoughts, feelings, behaviors, and experiences—all of which have the power to alter how they think about their place in the world of gender as well as their relationship to it. In a sense, they are always transitioning.

The cross-gender journey starts before they are even aware of it. In the background, their orientation influences how they perceive and evaluate the worth of different forms of gendered embodiment. Well before they've expressed themselves sexually, their orientation is already present, making being the other sex and embodying the traits associated with it seem more appealing.

Gender euphoria raises their mood, while gender dysphoria lowers it. These good and bad feelings are inextricably linked.

Just as the lack of a good feeling feels worse than experiencing that good feeling, the lack of a bad feeling feels better than experiencing that bad feeling. In this way, gender euphoria and gender dysphoria are two sides of the same coin, which is why the authoritatively titled *Gender Dysphoria Bible* proclaims, "anything that can be a source of dysphoria has an equal and opposite euphoria"[1].

Gendered aspects of bodies, clothing, behaviors, social interactions, and ways of thinking all potentially hold symbolic power that signifies to an autoheterosexual how they're embodying gender. The relative significance of these different types of embodiments is specific to each person. It changes over time and varies between individuals.

Initially, more attainable aspects of gender such as clothing and behavior are often enough to satisfy their need for cross-gender embodiment. With repetition, these forms of embodiment may become normal, unremarkable parts of daily life, at which point the less attainable aspects—bodies and social roles—start to hold more significance.

This progression from embodying attainable aspects of gender and later desiring to embody the more elusive aspects may culminate in a longing for gender transition because medical and social transition allow for the highest degree of cross-gender embodiment.

This developmental sequence—which starts with crossdressing or crossdreaming and sometimes progresses to transgenderism or transsexualism—is the historical pattern. It will continue to occur in autoheterosexuals who don't want to begin with social or medical transition.

The ascendance of the transgender movement has also opened other developmental possibilities: hormones are more accessible than ever, new ideas about gender have become culturally wide-spread, and society is more welcoming to gender variance.

In this environment, some autoheterosexuals begin with hormones and only switch to overt cross-gender expression if they start failing to pass as their natal gender. This path is emotionally safer for people who feel highly invested in what others think about them, have paranoid tendencies, or live in areas unfriendly to trans people.

Another increasingly common developmental sequence involves initially coming out as nonbinary, genderqueer, or some other intermediate gender identity. These identities can help autoheterosexuals test the waters by dabbling in cross-gender expression, using nondefault pronouns, and navigating their social environment as a gender-variant person.

After a bit of this experience, autoheterosexuals who have a stronger cross-gender wish may realize that they want to actually *be* the other gender instead of an intermediate one, at which point they may commit to a deeper level of gender transition.

Even though this process starts with occasional reinforcement, it can eventually culminate in a sort of internal revolution within the self system—the cross-gender identity gains control, with the default gender identity subsumed within it:

> "The cross-gender identity seems to grow stronger with practice and with social reinforcements...In unusual cases, the end result is a kind of revolution within the self system. The balance of power shifts in favor of the cross-gender identity..."[2]

Later in life, a transfem named R. L. wrote retrospectively about her experience with this cross-gender development. Although R. L. knew she wanted to be female prior to puberty, her internal feminine self expanded over time until her thoughts, desires, and sentiments reflected the desires of her inner woman:

> "From the age of 8 I have had this desire, which has been continuous, and growing in strength, yet I am not outwardly effeminate, but it is as if the soul of a woman had been born in a male body, and had been engaged in overcoming the physical nature, until now the spirit and mind long for pleasures that are contrary to the physical sex."[3]

It's common for autohets on the transsexual path to form the cross-gender wish before puberty[4]. With the onset of puberty, however, the cross-gender development process picks up speed and intensity.

THE PUBERTY CRISIS

Once libido ramps up after the onset of puberty, the cross-gender drive accelerates.

For many autoheterosexuals, puberty is a time of crisis, confusion, and inner tension. At the same time their bodies are transforming in sex-typical ways, they want to resemble or simply *be* the other sex more than ever.

This desire catches some autoheterosexuals off-guard. They may become confused about why they're thinking about being the other sex and being the people they're attracted to. The perennial "do/be" question asserts itself: "do I want to *do* them, or *be* them?"

Many autohets privately grapple with these feelings and thoughts on their own. Some feel ashamed and inadequate for failing to live up to the societal expectations of their sex. Others dread the ways their body is changing but keep their struggles to themselves, lest they invite rejection or ridicule by revealing their thoughts.

In order to circumvent the existential crisis presented by puberty, contemporary autoheterosexuals increasingly try to circumvent their natal puberty by going on puberty blockers. It's unknown whether this approach is medically wise, but on an emotional level it's certainly understandable.

SOCIETAL REPRESSION SLOWS CROSS-GENDER DEVELOPMENT

Until fairly recently, gender nonconforming people often faced intense social sanctions. Depending on the place and time, auto-heterosexuals expressing their cross-gender side could face the loss of friends, family, and jobs, or be arrested and caged for public crossdressing.

This legal and cultural environment strongly incentivized repression and secrecy.

For autohet males, crossdressing at home was the norm. For those who couldn't pass as the other sex, home was the only place they could be their cross-gender self. In the outside world, they had to look and play the part expected of men. At work, social events, and businesses, they had to present in a way that reinforced their default gender.

When these two modes of existence scarcely overlapped, the two selves sometimes grew in a parallel, nonintegrated way. This could lead to internal tension and psychological instability, so transvestite magazines and newsletters commonly advised their readers to integrate their two sides as one united whole[5].

In this restrictive cultural environment, it took a *long* time for autoheterosexual males to develop a cross-gender identity to the point of adopting a feminine name—a milestone that, on average, they reached after twenty-one years of crossdressing[6].

Today, the outlook isn't so bleak. Things have improved.

A BRAVE NEW GENDER WORLD

Autoheterosexuals growing up today face a completely different cultural environment than their predecessors. The rapid ascent of the transgender movement has drastically reshaped the world that young autohets enter as they grow up.

Trans people have formed vibrant online communities with their own subcultures, as well as a shared language that helps them understand each other. They don't have to feel so isolated anymore.

Now, kids learn about transgenderism in school. The broader population has also been hearing about gender identity and gender dysphoria, so there is widespread understanding that some people feel emotional pain because they're not the other sex.

People have also learned the basics of pronoun usage (e.g., that if they're not sure of someone's pronouns, they should ask).

"They" is also gaining ground as a pronoun. The nonbinary identity has shot up in popularity, which has allowed people to feel they're opting out of the gender binary. Most nonbinary-identified people are female[7].

Barriers to obtaining cross-sex hormones have also been reduced. Hormones are increasingly available on an "informed consent" basis where patients sign a document saying they were informed of potential health risks, and then they walk out with a prescription.

More people are transitioning than ever before. Average transition age has dropped. Puberty blockers are increasingly available to gender-dysphoric children, and some even get gender-affirming surgeries before they are legally adults. Such practices will be curtailed once the lawsuits start rolling in, but still, these possibilities didn't exist before.

The gender game has changed.

À LA CARTE TRANSGENDERISM

As a cultural phenomenon, transgenderism has shifted to a more nebulous place. Countless bitter arguments over who counts as "trans" attest to this ambiguity.

Is legitimate transgenderism determined by identification? Social transition? Medical transition?

There's no clear agreement, and that's okay. The recent increase in gender freedom allows for more possibilities than before.

In the gatekeeping days, trans people had to endure a "real-life test" of living as their desired gender for a year or two before clinics would give them hormones. Now, it's the other way around: they can start with hormones and socially transition later, after physical changes make such transition feasible.

Psychologically, the "hormones first" approach is gentler because it doesn't require social transition, so trans people increasingly take this approach.

For example, some MTFS take hormones while still wearing masculine clothes with the hope that they'll start failing to pass as their birth sex. If they do, they'll start wearing feminine clothes, come out as trans, and adopt a feminine name. Even if they never start passing as the other gender, they may keep taking hormones. Doing so helps them feel better about their body, and by lowering libido, it also lowers their autogynephilic drive.

For these reasons, some MTFS take hormones with no intention of ever coming out. There are even a few autogynephilic people who only get a vaginoplasty because their genital configuration was their biggest gender issue. No hormones. No social transition. Just a vagina.

With these new possibilities, the path forward isn't as obvious. The decision-making process is complicated, and the rise of countless new gender identities doesn't make it any simpler. However, these new options make it more likely that trans people can get where they want to go, on a path of their own design.

THE AUTOHETEROSEXUAL SKINNER BOX

In the last century, scientists found they could change an animal's behavior by administering rewards or punishments after the animal enacted a behavior they wanted to change.

If, after an animal behaved in a certain way, researchers did something the animal liked or took away something it didn't like, those reinforcements would make the behavior happen more often. On the other hand, if researchers did something the animal didn't like or took away something it liked, those punishments would make the behavior happen less often.

This approach to changing behavior through reinforcements and punishments is called *operant conditioning*. The chamber that holds an animal during these experiments is informally known as a "Skinner Box", named after B. F. Skinner, a pioneer in the study of operant conditioning.

Gender-related feelings from autoheterosexuality are themselves innately rewarding or aversive stimuli, so they have the capacity to shape behavior. Gender euphoria is rewarding; gender dysphoria is aversive. These positive and negative mood shifts influence the frequency of the behaviors that preceded them.

Attainment of cross-gender embodiment increases good gender feelings and reduces bad ones, which reinforces the behaviors that lead to cross-gender embodiment. Shortfalls of cross-gender embodiment increase bad gender feelings and reduce good ones, which punishes the behaviors that lead to shortcomings of cross-gender embodiment.

Together, gender euphoria and gender dysphoria tend to make the default gender feel less comfortable and relatable to autoheterosexuals over time. Eventually it may feel aversive, alien, or even actively hostile.

In contrast, the other gender offers sanctuary. This source of comfort and place of inner peace can feel like home, and at a certain point, autoheterosexuals may never want to leave.

SHIFTING GENDER ATTITUDES AND SENTIMENTS

Even if autoheterosexuals don't start out deeply admiring the other sex and holding their own in low regard, thousands of little nudges over years tend to shift their sentiments in that direction.

What starts out as a pleasant thought experiment can eventually develop into dissatisfaction due to the chasm between desire and reality. As Ellis's patient R. M. put it, "I began to think that it would be very nice to be changed into a girl for a time, to see what it was like. Gradually this idea became regret that I had not been born a girl"[8].

These gender attitudes can be present from a young age in those most strongly predisposed to autoheterosexuality. Recalling her childhood self, one transfem confessed, "I would have sacrificed my entire life if only I could have been a girl just for three days"[9].

Hirschfeld absolutely nailed it when he wrote about the gender sentiments of his male transvestites: "Everything about the body that recalls masculinity is perceived with distaste; everything, absolutely everything, that signifies femininity is craved"[10].

This statement is just as true today, and it'll be just as true centuries from now.

Autoheterosexuality tends to make people value attributes of the other sex and devalue those of their own. The other sex rests on a pedestal while their own flawed sex lies in a ditch. They prize, exalt, or glorify the other sex while believing their own is best left unmentioned.

In extreme cases, this dynamic can make existence feel worthless or like a cruel joke. Thankfully, most autoheterosexuals don't reach such extremes. But left unchecked, their gender sentiments are more likely to develop in this direction.

TRANSITION DECISION(S)

Rather than being born already transgender or transsexual, people are born predisposed to developing gender issues because of autoheterosexuality or homosexuality, and they later come to identify as trans or choose to undergo social or medical transition as a way of addressing their gender issues.

Some people are so strongly predisposed to gender issues that transitioning is practically inevitable—they are the ones who became transsexuals in decades past when knowledge of transgenderism was rare and gender nonconformity was heavily stigmatized.

Today, far more people are transitioning than ever. Some people present this rapid rise in transgender identity as evidence of social contagion, but I don't think it's the main story—at least not for adults.

More people are transitioning because there are greater benefits and fewer downsides to transitioning than ever before, and gender transition has become much more widely known and accessible. In effect, more homosexuals and autoheterosexuals are choosing to transition after making rational decisions about how they want to live their lives[11].

But mainstream models of transgenderism fail to account for these two distinct types of transgenderism. This is a problem.

When making highly consequential decisions about whether to undergo gender transition, it helps to have an accurate mental model. Using such a model increases the chances that predictions come true, so *actually* understanding transgenderism can aid autohets in the decision-making process around gender transition.

By having a basic grasp of how autoheterosexual cross-gender development works, autohets have a higher chance of steering themselves toward the outcome they think would serve them best. Through self-awareness regarding their gender sentiments and cross-gender behavioral patterns, they can sense their gender trajectory and act in ways that improve their odds of attaining desired outcomes.

Instead of asking, "Am I trans?" they can ask, "Which aspects of gender transition do I want, and are they worth the trade-offs?".

For autohets, the single most important factor may be the comparative strength of their autosexual and allosexual sides. If their allosexual side is dominant, then transition might not help them overall. If their autosexual side is clearly dominant, however, then transitioning might offer greater rewards than they could get otherwise.

There are plenty of other factors too. Depending on their values, priorities, beliefs, social standing, mental traits, culture, physique, finances, and health, as well as other aspects of their personhood and life circumstances, autoheterosexuals will make different decisions about the best path forward.

With so many moving parts and such high stakes, the gender transition decision-making process is often long and complex. This complexity makes it absolutely imperative to have a robust, accurate mental model.

Better models enable better predictions, and better predictions enable better outcomes. Autoheterosexuals who truly grasp their situation will be best prepared to make the decisions that are right for them.

IN SUM

* Autoheterosexual cross-gender development is an ongoing process influenced by sexuality, cultural milieu, and personal beliefs. Important sexual factors include libido, the comparative strengths of the allosexual and autosexual drives, and which types of gendered embodiment are desired. Personal beliefs affect how autoheterosexuals conceive of their situation, and cultural milieu affects how safe they feel engaging in cross-gender expression.

* The earlier their cross-gender feelings start, the more likely autoheterosexuals are to develop significant gender issues. The onset of puberty increases the desire to be the other sex at the exact same time the body veers in the opposite direction—an incongruence between desire and trajectory that can make puberty a time of great emotional crisis.

* Autoheterosexual operant conditioning shifts autohets across the gender divide over time. Good and bad gender-related feelings gradually condition them to behave and think differently. This series of rewards and punishments often makes autohets feel less welcome in their default gender and more at home in their cross-gender.

* Autoheterosexuality shifts attitudes and sentiments about gender. Autohets often attribute greater significance to traits associated with the other sex and devalue traits associated with their own sex. What begins as occasional thoughts about being the other sex may ultimately develop into intense regret about not being born the other sex.

* Greater awareness and acceptance of transgenderism has made gender transition more widely available and lowered the social costs, so more autoheterosexuals are transitioning to live as another gender. However, many

are doing so without understanding autoheterosexuality. This is a problem: decisions made under false pretenses are more likely to be poor decisions. By better understanding their orientations, autohets can make better decisions regarding gender transition.

"I came across a lot of her prettily trimmed underclothing, and was seized with the desire to put it on. I did so—and from that moment I date what I term my change of sex. I cannot describe to you the pleasure I felt when thus dressing myself for the first time in female garments. It was exquisite, delicious, intoxicating, far and away transcending anything I had before experienced, and when, after some trouble, I was completely attired as a girl, and placed myself in front of the glass, it was a positive revelation...I was both a boy and a girl at once, and since that time I have never been a male pure and simple again, and today I am actually more female than male, in spite of the actual physical facts to the contrary."

—A. T., as quoted in "Eonism" by Havelock Ellis[1]

GENDER EUPHORIA
GOOD GENDER FEELINGS

Gender euphoria is one of the most cherished parts of the autoheterosexual experience.

Gender euphoria is emotionally compelling because it feels like love, and it feels that way because it *is* love—it comes from union with an autoheterosexual's inner cross-gender self.

Increased heart rate is a particularly common physical response to experiencing gender euphoria[2]. Goose bumps, a feeling of warmth, or butterflies in the stomach are common too. Depending on the particular stimulus and individual, as well as the context and intensity, sexual arousal may also be part of the euphoric response[3].

On the milder side, gender euphoria feels similar to the pleasure of holding hands or cuddling with a loved one. On the more intense side, it provides an intoxicating deluge of joy that truly earns the "euphoria" label.

The intensely euphoric feelings tend to be short-lived, but the milder ones can stick around for the long haul[4]. In general, repeated exposure to the same stimulus yields a weaker euphoria response over time.

INITIALLY INTENSE

As A. T.'s testimony at the start of this chapter shows, the first experience of gender euphoria can be so intense that it's downright revelatory.

Looking back on the fledgling stages of his cross-gender exploration, a queer transgender man recounted how dressing in men's clothes brought forth his masculine self and a new high:

> "In the dressing room, I watched myself transform into the handsome devil I secretly believed I could be. I stood in awe of my new, more definitively masculine figure and aesthetic, and experienced a high I'd never felt before."[5]

The "luxuriously happy frame of mind"[6] produced by cross-dressing can dispel "the most pressing fatigue and dullness"[7], leaving behind a residual feeling of wellness that can last into the next day:

"The miraculous effect of feminine clothes still made me tremble [the] next day at my work. Clear, peaceful, and serene the world seemed to me. Intoxicated with happiness, I went gaily to work under the fading stars. With half the expenditure of energy I did the work of three."[8]

This sartorial union with the inner cross-gender spirit helps autohets feel at home in themselves, providing safety, security, and comfort. Although enjoyable, these feelings aren't always easy to interpret. One transsexual woman reported, "When I put on the dress for the first time, after I let myself relax for a few minutes, I started to cry and felt very safe and at peace. I'm not sure what to make of this"[9].

Not only can these intense feelings be hard to interpret, but they can also be hard to put into words.

THE TRANSFORMATIVE POTENTIAL OF UNSPEAKABLE DELIGHT

Sometimes autohet gender euphoria is so powerful that the people experiencing it have trouble conveying the profound depth of their emotions. These ineffable emotions are transformative.

The Hungarian physician had a life-changing gender experience when she "almost died of hashish poisoning" after consuming a high dose of cannabis extract[10]. During this subjectively near-death experience, she saw herself transform into a woman—a change that was hard to put into words: "All at once I saw myself a woman from my toes to my breast; I felt, as before while in the bath, that the genitals had shrunken, the pelvis broadened, the breasts swollen out; a feeling of unspeakable delight came over me"[11].

Upon waking the next day, she had a phantom vulva and phantom breasts, and she felt herself fully changed into a woman. Although she wrote this account three years after that transformative euphoria, her mental and phantom shifts remained as permanent features of her everyday life.

A modern-day transfem who held back on fulfilling her cross-gender aspirations for the sake of her marriage also wrote about unspeakably delightful gender euphoria. After encountering medical issues that required her to be castrated, she was put on a low dose of estrogen. Force-feminized by fate, she was awash in gender euphoria:

"While all this is certainly unfortunate, painful, and potentially life threatening, I am inwardly welcoming these health problems and their treatment...The flood of emotions concerning the limited fulfillment of my great desire is nearly indescribable."[12]

Her situation was potentially life-threatening and painful, but she was thankful for it. Looking like a woman carried such immense spiritual worth to her that the risk of death felt worthwhile. She isn't alone in accepting this risk—even though gender-affirming surgeries carry some risk of death, thousands of autohet transsexuals get them anyway.

The unspeakably blissful joy of gender euphoria beckons to autoheterosexuals, encouraging them to cross the gender divide one meaningful experience at a time.

THE HIGH OF NEW LOVE

For autoheterosexuals, the start of cross-gender exploration can feel like the excited joy of budding love or the "honeymoon period" of a relationship. The polyamorous refer to this feeling as "new relationship energy"[13]. Trans women sometimes call it "pink haze"[14].

Most people know the feeling of being high on newfound love. It's one of the best feelings in the world. Countless songs, stories, and poems have been written about it.

These loving feelings are a product of our evolutionary history. They help us form strong attachments to others lasting several years—long enough to become pregnant, give birth, and wean the resulting child[15]. For this reason, love is one of the most powerful motivating forces in our lives. It's why some people work jobs they loathe for years on end just to support their loved ones—even if it ends up killing them physically, mentally, or spiritually.

Autoheterosexuality directs that same powerful motivating force toward a cross-gender version of oneself. Since gender euphoria feels like love, it's a powerful signifier of meaning and importance that says you're on the right path. It's like that classic R & B song: "(If Loving You Is Wrong) I Don't Want to Be Right"[16].

After hundreds or thousands of these positive mood shifts, attachment to the cross-gender self grows stronger. Eventually, it may feel more real and vital than the default self. Some auto-heterosexuals even come to believe their cross-gender self is the only version of themselves worth living for, and their default self is a veil or mask which obscures their true self.

If they haven't already transitioned, at this point, autohets may decide that becoming what they love via gender transition is the best path forward—that being true to their most deeply held feelings is the best way to live out the rest of their days.

BECOMING WHAT WE LOVE: THE ROMANCE HYPOTHESIS

The simplest way to make sense of gender transition among autoheterosexuals is to think of it as a form of internal marriage to the cross-gendered self.

Few autohet transsexuals would describe their internal experience in this way, but it's a useful metaphor. In a sense, they love the other sex and want to become what they love. This interpretive lens—which frames autoheterosexual gender transition as the result of an internal pair-bond with the cross-gender self—is sometimes called the *romance hypothesis*[17].

Sexual orientations come with the propensity for attachment and the desire to be in union with the object of affection, so *attachment* to embodying the other sex is a logical consequence of attraction to embodying the other sex. *Of course* attraction leads to attachment—it would be strange if it didn't.

The romance hypothesis was originally proposed because there was an aspect of autogynephilic transsexualism that didn't seem to make sense: if autogynephilic gender transition was motivated by sexuality, but feminizing hormone treatment lowered libido, why were so many trans women sticking with gender transition even after hormones decreased their libido?

By focusing on the emotional and sentimental aspects of gender transition, the romance hypothesis offers a deeper understanding than one that portrays autoheterosexuality as a purely erotic phenomenon[18]. It also helps make autohet transgenderism comprehensible to anyone who has fallen in love before.

In her influential essay, "Becoming What We Love"[19], Anne Lawrence makes a convincing case that we can understand autogynephilic trans women as males who "love women and want to become what they love"[20]. Likewise, we can understand autoandrophilic trans men as females who "love men and want to become what they love".

Seven years prior to his gender transition, Lou Sullivan touched on this theme of internal union in his diary. Just before he got his first leather jacket and began to commit more deeply to transvestism, he wrote, "I love to blend female and male—I think of myself as two people finally coming together in peace with each other. Of my other half, I sing, 'Nobody loves me but me adores you!'"[21].

INTERNAL UNION WITH THE CROSS-GENDER SELF

Although some critics[22] contest the idea that autoheterosexuality can create an internal pair-bond with the cross-gender self, observers have noticed this internal union and remarked on it for generations now.

Before Lawrence proposed that autogynephilic gender transition was a matter of "becoming what we love", Blanchard compared the desire that some trans women had for bottom surgery to a long-term marriage in which the eroticism had waned but the desire to stay together remained[23].

Writing in 1970, a decade before Blanchard embarked on his gender research, H. Taylor Buckner described "the transvestic career path"[24]. He saw these inner unions as an "internal marriage"[25] and said they were a "synthetic dyad within the individual"[26]. He also described the male transvestite as an autoerotic individual "who has internalized his dyadic relationship with an autoerotic object"[27] and noted that after a transvestite incorporates the femme persona into their personal identity, "he begins to relate toward himself...as if he were his own wife"[28].

Sixty years before Buckner's observations, Hirschfeld noted that among the transvestites he studied, "the masculine part in the psyche of these people is sexually excited by their feminine side...they feel attracted not only by women outside themselves, but also more so by the women within themselves"[29]. One of Hirschfeld's patients even admitted, "I was my own best friend", when recalling her solitary cross-gender practices[30].

What are the odds that critics of this "internal pair-bond" idea are right? Were reputable observers like Lawrence, Blanchard, and Hirschfeld mistaken when they alluded to internal unions in autohet trans people?

Probably not—it's unlikely that all these experts are wrong. If anything, the strong emotions in the trans community around autoheterosexuality and the two-type model are what we'd expect to see if many trans people truly do have this inner union and are motivated by inner love to protect their self-image from ideas they regard as threats to it.

IN SUM

* Autoheterosexual gender euphoria confers comfort, joy, and other positive feelings in response to perceptions of cross-gender embodiment. At first, it may cause goose bumps, increased heart rate, or the feeling of butterflies in the stomach. Over time, it can develop into a deeper, more companionate love-bond that persists even if overt eroticism has waned.

* The bliss of gender euphoria can be so intense that it's hard to put into words, and this intensity underlies its transformative potential. These warm fuzzy feelings motivate autohets to cross the gender divide.

* Sexual attraction can lead to romantic attachment. Thus, sexual attraction to being the other sex can lead to emotional attachment to being the other sex. This intuitive insight is the basis for the romance hypothesis, an interpretive lens that treats autohet gender transition as an outward expression of an internal marriage to the cross-gender self.

GENDER DYSPHORIA
BAD GENDER FEELINGS

There's a type of pain that the French call *la douleur exquise*. Translated literally, it means "the exquisite pain".

La douleur exquise is the pain of loving someone you know you can't have.

Maybe your love doesn't love you back, or they live on the other side of the world. Maybe you're having an affair and they can only be with you secretly, but you want a full-fledged public relationship. The details may vary, but *la douleur exquise* gnaws at your soul all the same. You want them so badly, but you can't have them.

Writing about her cross-gender wish over a century ago, a transfem elegantly captured the essence of *la douleur exquise* when she wrote, "The lord brought about feelings that I knew would lead to nowhere"[1].

Unmet desires hurt, especially when it comes to love and attachment. This basic human truth helps make sense of the dissatisfaction and distress associated with autoheterosexual gender dysphoria.

Autoheterosexuality is the most common reason that people have an intense yearning to belong to the other sex. Since that desire involves attachment to the cross-gender self, perceived shortcomings of cross-gender embodiment can trigger negative feelings and downward shifts in mood known as gender dysphoria.

In everyday life, so many things can remind someone of their sex, including mirrors, social interactions, or even the sound of their own voice. For the gender dysphoric, any of these reminders can dampen their mood. Those "whose yearnings are wrecked on the hard rock of reality" may find waking life a nightmare, with dreams at night providing only shreds of solace[2].

In practice, gender dysphoria is a broad, nebulous concept. When someone says they have gender dysphoria, there's so much left unexplained. What triggered it? How strong is it? What are they dysphoric about and why?

Gender dysphoria is not a single entity but rather a complex set of feelings, moods, expectations, and self-evaluations associated with gender[3]. The label indicates a person suffers in some way relating to gender, but not much else.

Gender dysphoria shows up in multiple ways in autoheterosexuals and is accompanied by many flavors of suffering. It may present as a persistent, low-grade emotional ache that lowers their happiness set point throughout life. It can make autohets never want to leave the house, lest anyone see them as their default gender. It can even make them feel like their body isn't theirs, or that the whole world is somehow fake.

It can make them wallow in a deep hole of depression, too bummed out to shower, brush their teeth, or eat decent food because taking care of themselves just isn't worth it. It can make existing as their default gender feel hollow and completely devoid of spiritual worth to the point that existing in their body seems like a sick joke played by a malevolent god.

Luckily, negative gender feelings are usually not this extreme. While autohets may feel sad about their gendered traits at some points in their life, many learn to compartmentalize these feelings or at least keep them at an emotional distance.

Some autohets actively manage their gender sentiments by reminding themselves that there are good things about being their default gender and that there are advantages and disadvantages to being either sex. When this works, the rose-tinted perception of the other gender becomes less prominent in their psyche, and the pedestal they've put it on becomes a bit shorter.

Another way that autoheterosexuals have been able to feel better about their gender situation is by drawing meaning from their default gender role through conventional heterosexual relationships, or by becoming parents and raising children. However, this risky approach doesn't always work, and when it doesn't, it can lead to heartbreak and family dissolution. Anyone who wants to try this approach ought to disclose their sexuality to potential partners very early in the relationship, so they can make an informed mating choice.

As bad as gender dysphoria can be, *it is not inevitable that autoheterosexuals will suffer significantly from gender dysphoria.* I emphasize this fact because I've seen quite a few self-aware autogynephilic males in their late teens or early twenties anxiously obsess over the possibility that even though they don't have dysphoria yet, being autogynephilic means it's inevitable that severe, intractable gender dysphoria will strike long after they've missed their chance at passing as the other sex.

That said, there *is* evidence that autohet males have more gender dysphoria than allohet males[4]. Researchers found a very large effect: if a person were randomly selected from each group, there's a 90% chance that the autohet male would have more gender dysphoria than the allohet male. If this difference were expressed in terms of intelligence, it's almost as big as the difference between average intelligence and the cutoff point for mental disability.

It's almost certainly the case that autohet females suffer more gender dysphoria than allohet females too. As discussed in Chapter 5.5, females and autoheterosexuals seem to be at greater risk of developing gender dysphoria than males or homosexuals, so autoandrophilic females are perhaps the most dysphoria-prone etiological subgroup.

AUTOHETEROSEXUALITY AND THE MEDICAL DEFINITION OF GENDER DYSPHORIA

The DSM-5 defines gender dysphoria as "the distress that may accompany the incongruence between one's experienced or expressed gender and one's assigned gender"[5]. The manual provides six criteria[6] for a gender dysphoria diagnosis in adolescents and adults, two of which must be present for six months or more in order to qualify.

The first is a "marked incongruence" between sex traits and gender. This is the clash between body and mind so commonly associated with transsexualism. The other five criteria pertain to specific aspects of this gender incongruence. All map onto particular aspects of autoheterosexuality, which I've listed in brackets:

2. Strong desire to not have the sex traits of one's default gender [anatomic]
3. Strong desire to have the other gender's sex traits [anatomic]
4. Strong desire to be the other gender [core]
5. Strong desire to be treated as the other gender [interpersonal]
6. Strong belief that one feels or thinks as the other gender does [psyche]

Transsexualism is changing the body to more closely resemble the other sex, so it's fitting that the first three directly relate to anatomy, and two of the latter three do so indirectly. Core autoheterosexuality is associated with a desire to have the body of the other sex[7], and looking like the other sex is the best way to get treated as that gender.

The last criterion is associated with psyche autoheterosexuality, the cross-gender consciousness embodiment that makes autohets feel they have the thoughts, feelings, perceptions, and sensations of the other gender, as if they were looking through the other gender's eyes. This beautiful feeling is a strong driver of cross-gender identity and a contributor to mind–body gender incongruence.

Altogether, the aspects of autoheterosexuality associated with these diagnostic criteria lead to a desire to have the body, mind, and social role associated with the other gender—and to simply *be* that gender. Many gender-dysphoric people want to be the other gender to the greatest degree possible. As one of Hirschfeld's patients said, "My yearning is not limited to women's costumes, but also extends itself to an absolute life as a woman, with all primary and secondary phenomena"[8].

Changing the body to more closely resemble the other sex is the most effective and direct way to embody the gender associated with it. Transsexualism is a clear signal to others in everyday life that someone would like to be seen as the gender to which they've shifted. This permanent physical embodiment helps transsexuals socially assimilate into that gender role, feel like their body is their own, and live a life that is true to themselves.

DISSOCIATION: DEPERSONALIZATION/DEREALIZATION (DP/DR)

Although people who aren't autoheterosexual or transgender can experience dissociation, when it shows up in autohet or transgender people, it might be a manifestation of gender dysphoria.

Dissociation can make autohets feel they aren't real or don't have a self. Lou Sullivan experienced this gender-related dissociation and wrote in his diaries about feeling his mind and body coming apart:

> "Went to bed and began crying. I held myself and stroked my skin like I always do and imagining I was a beautiful boy I was sleeping with, and then it began to get too real and I felt my mind and my body separating."[9]

A few years later, his symptoms of dissociation had become steadier and more permanent. Sullivan felt himself an empty husk, devoid of meaning or direction:

> "I'm a walking zombie and I don't even know where I'm walking. It's as tho my whole inner core of who or what I am is totally stripped away. I wonder how much longer I can continue to function, and that's the truth. I feel more and more alienated from myself."[10]

A few years later, he finally began to medically transition. A mere two to three months after starting hormones, he began reintegrating his two sides. He reported, "I'm trying to integrate my identity and my body in my head", and "slowly slowly I feel the fog lifting"[11].

By bringing his body in line with his identity as a man, Sullivan was finally able to *be* in his body and participate in his own life in a way that wasn't possible before. The veil lifted. Life regained its color. He was a man.

For one of Hirschfeld's transfems, the act of dressing as a woman had a similar palliative effect: "When I cast off everything male and put on the outward trappings of a woman…I can perceive almost physically how falseness and violence rushes out of me and disperses like a fog"[12].

In autoheterosexuals and trans people who experience it, this gender-related dissociation can manifest as depersonalization and derealization[13]. People experiencing depersonalization (DP) feel detached from themselves, and those who experience derealization (DR) feel detached from the outside world[14]. In the former, they feel fake, and in the latter, the world feels fake.

DP/DR symptoms can show up as a fog-like emotional flatness or the feeling of being separated by a veil, or watching oneself from the outside as though separate from oneself[15]. When researchers measured DP/DR symptoms in trans people, they had more than the normative comparison group[16]. However, when researchers dropped the question about body ownership, participants' scores decreased by more than half[17], suggesting their diminished sense of physical embodiment was a large part of their dissociation symptoms.

Another study found a similar result: removing the question about body ownership decreased trans people's DP/DR scores by more than 30%, after which their scores of overall dissociation resembled those of the general population (even before getting hormones)[18]. After receiving cross-sex hormones and other medical help, their DP/DR scores dropped by half[19].

Cross-gender embodiment through meta-homosexuality can also help dissipate the fog of dissociation: a study of transgender Virginians found that a majority of MTFS (70%) and FTMS (55%) agreed that they felt more real when having sex with someone of the same sex, but less than a quarter of them said the same of having sex with someone of the other sex[20].

It's common for trans people to feel that their body is not their own. By alleviating gender incongruence, gender-affirming medical treatment and other forms of cross-gender embodiment may help them be at home in their bodies and selves.

GENDER ENVY

For autoheterosexuals, people of the other sex can seem so beautiful that it hurts. This pain, *gender envy*, tends to be proportional to the beauty on display. R. M. explained it best:

"I always envy a woman in proportion to my love and admiration for her. Still, there are many good women, for whom

I feel sincere regard, and even affection, who are not in any way physically attractive to me, and towards whom I feel neither desire nor envy."[21]

It can be hard for autohets to differentiate gender envy from attraction, which is why the familiar do/be dilemma—"do I want to *do* them or *be* them?"—pops up so often.

Due to sexual dimorphism, autoheterosexuals tend to envy the exact opposite physical features from those that nature bestowed upon them. Autohet females often want to be bigger, more muscular, taller, and hairier. Autohet males often want to be smaller, shorter, and more slender, with smoother skin.

Seeing someone of the same sex successfully attain a form of gendered embodiment can also trigger autohet gender envy in people who long to achieve such embodiment themselves. Masculine women and feminine men can spur these feelings, as can transsexuals.

In fact, seeing someone of the same sex succeed at cross-gender embodiment may cause even more powerful feelings of envy simply because it's a powerful reminder of what's possible. There's a tangible sense of "that could be me" that makes this gender envy cut especially deep.

Autoandrophilic Gender Envy

Men's physical features, such as their flat chests, deep voices, Adam's apples, muscles, and body hair, are common sources of gender envy among autoandrophilic people. And yes, they *do* get penis envy[22]. How could they not? Penises are endowed with great symbolic weight for signifying manhood.

The linearity of men's bodies is enviable too. They're likely to envy the flat butts, small hips, and flat chests that men have. Autoandrophilic people also tend to envy men's size. They almost always want to be taller, and it's common for them to want big, veiny hands and big feet.

Some of them desire to pass so thoroughly as a guy that they could have long hair or wear makeup and still be seen as a man. This is appealing not only because it broadens their range of acceptable gender expression, but also because passing as a man while enveloped in signifiers of femininity is an especially powerful validation of their manhood.

Autogynephilic Gender Envy

Autogynephilic people tend to envy the breasts, vulvas, and big hips of women. They envy their feminine faces, long hair, smooth skin, and high voices. Even women's small hands and feet are a source of envy. As R. M. said, "I could not look at a pretty girl without envying her"[23].

And while autogynephilic people may desire certain feminine features, what those features signify is ultimately the most important: womanhood. Women are enviable simply for being women[24].

Autogynephilic people can also envy those same feminine features on males lucky enough to have them[25]. Perhaps because it's so relatable, this envy can be particularly salient.

R. L.'s account is an especially good example of autogyne-philic gender envy. From childhood, she envied women and feminine men alike:

> "When about 8 or 9, I first had the desire to be a girl, and used to envy a little boy, a neighbor, who lived with two sisters and mother, and who was dressed girlishly, which led me to think that I should like to be him and be brought up as a girl."[26]

Later in life, when R. L. went to shows of feminine impersonators, she would envy them and wish she were smaller and more feminine[27]. Bitter with envy, R. L. even looked down on some women, thinking she would make a better woman and that their femaleness was wasted on them: "I look with scorn and disgust, or at least mild criticism, on some females, knowing how much better I could wear their clothes, conduct myself, and give an impression of a real lady"[28].

R. L. envied just about everything concerning women. She envied their smallness, femininity, clothing, and simply the fact that they were women. Over time this envy grew, manifesting in white-knuckled levels of gender dysphoria: "I was getting miserable, and frequently suffering real pain, for the sight of a well-dressed woman would often cause me to clench my nails into my palms, suppress a groan, sometimes a swear escaping my lips"[29].

Her account clearly shows how intense gender envy can be, how easily it can be triggered, and how much it can detract from happiness.

ANATOMIC DYSPHORIA

Autoheterosexuals can feel dysphoric about the size or shape of their bones, muscles, cartilage, and fat deposits. The location, thickness, color, and quantity of their hair can also cause dysphoria. Ultimately, any bodily tissue that signifies gender can influence gender feelings. Due to sexual dimorphism, these gender feelings are often negative.

Primary and secondary sexual characteristics are powerful signifiers of gender laden with symbolic value. It's these traits in particular that autoheterosexuals yearn to change.

Many autohet females would prefer to have a penis, testicles, flat male chest, strong musculature, and thick body hair. They'd also like to have their female reproductive anatomy removed and feminine fat deposits melted away.

Conversely, a lot of autohet males would prefer to have a vulva, breasts, soft facial features, feminine fat deposits, and bountiful hair on their scalp with almost none elsewhere. Many also want their male reproductive anatomy removed and coarse facial features chiseled away.

One type of autoheterosexual wants bigger bones, the other smaller. One wants bigger muscles, the other smaller. So it goes, for any physical trait that varies between males and females.

It's anatomy that juts out, however, that carries the greatest symbolic value, is the hardest to ignore, and is most amenable to surgical interventions. As a result, transsexuals often prioritize removing protrusive anatomy[30].

The contours of their chests are apparent anytime they look down. The type of genitals they have often is too. If being reminded of your sex hurt your mood, yet every time you looked down your protuberances reminded you of your sex, how would you deal with it?

This is the situation that people with severe anatomic gender dysphoria find themselves in. Even when they avoid catching glimpses of themselves, these problematic protuberances can still remind their owners of their presence by jostling as they go about their everyday lives. By getting top or bottom surgery, these unwelcome protuberances can become a thing of the past. By chest binding or tucking, they can be temporarily forgotten. Aside from these interventions, however, these sensations are impossible to escape.

This is why it's so important that trans people with severe anatomic dysphoria have access to quality medical care: so they can look downward or move around in everyday life without feeling like shit.

Autoandrophilic transsexuals often want testosterone or a double mastectomy. Some also decide to surgically remove their ovaries, uterus, or vagina. Some want a penis strongly enough to endure the long, arduous process of phalloplasty.

Autogynephilic transsexuals often want testosterone blockers and estrogen. Surgically, they may also pursue vaginoplasty, orchiectomy (castration), breast augmentation, or facial feminization.

SARTORIAL DYSPHORIA

Autoheterosexuals often feel uncomfortable in the clothing associated with their sex. This sartorial dysphoria can make them feel stifled, oppressed, weighed down, and caged[31]. Crushed under the immense symbolic weight of these alien garments and estranged from themselves, their mood becomes flattened and their zest for life deadened. The sadness creeps in.

"It's as if my entire world turns grey", lamented a transvestite with over fifty years of crossdressing experience[32]. She tried to resist the allure of ladies' garb, but this repression always led to a sour, irritable mood and the inability to glean pleasure from life.

A European transvestite who longed to live and work as a man felt "constrained and in bondage" in women's clothes[33]. Dressed as a man, he traveled to Rio de Janeiro, San Francisco, Yokohama, and Zanzibar. Dressed as a woman, he stayed in Europe.

Elsa B. absolutely *hated* being forced to wear girls' clothing. In it, he felt ridiculous and dejected:

> "To go out dressed in airy skirts and hats with ribbons and lace made me feel like a dressed-up monkey. Following promenades or visits in such clothing, I would be overcome with a deep depression and was glad when I reached home again and could tear the stuff from my body."[34]

A transsexual man reported that after he dreamt about being forced to dress as a girl, he woke up anxious and upset[35]. When dressed as a woman in waking life, he felt that people "saw through" him[36].

Like anatomic dysphoria, sartorial dysphoria can be triggered through touch alone. Women's and men's clothing feels different on the body. They have different materials, cuts, and styles, which make their texture, heft, and tightness different.

Having to wear clothing associated with their default gender very quickly becomes uncomfortable for autoheterosexuals who have developed sartorial dysphoria. Every little sensation is a symbolic reminder of their sex, whereas with cross-gender clothing, every little sensation helps them forget it.

R. L. described this sartorial suffering eloquently. She had multiple "lives" as a woman, but eventually had to detransition for lack of funds. Her sorrow about undressing for the last time was firmly etched in her memory:

> "It was with very great sadness that I undressed for the last time one night…I slipped out into a world that was particularly distasteful to me, my collar choked me, my trousers oppressed me like bandages, my boots felt clumsy, and I missed the clasp of corsets, and the beautiful feel of underwear."[37]

To people who don't experience these feelings, it may seem frivolous or silly that clothing matters so much. But it does. Autoheterosexuals truly do suffer from being coerced into wearing clothing that goes against their nature.

SOCIAL DYSPHORIA

As social animals, how others treat us has a massive effect on how we see ourselves. Being treated as worthy tends to make us feel we are worthy, just as being denigrated tends to make us feel lesser.

It's the same with gender. Being treated as a woman reinforces our sense of being a woman (or feminine), and being treated as a man reinforces our sense of being a man (or masculine). As a result, autoheterosexuals can experience social gender dysphoria from being treated as a member of their sex rather than the gender to which they aspire.

Dysphoria might occur if they're addressed with pronouns corresponding to their sex, put in single-sex groups according to their sex, or hit on because the potential suitor was attracted to their natal sex traits.

Trans men can also feel burned from being emasculated. For instance, one trans man had anxiety attacks associated with having his masculinity doubted[38]. He also took offense if people thought he wasn't a man, whereupon he would drink alcohol and start a fight with the biggest guy in the vicinity in order to prove his masculinity[39].

Similarly, another trans man felt humiliated whenever he was offered children's tickets for streetcars and trains[40]. He also hated when men hit on him, and the one time he tried having sex with a male, he couldn't relax and ended up fighting him[41].

R. L. felt social gender dysphoria too. For her, the pain was rather acute: "the slightest hint or sign by anyone who knows, that they regard me other than as a real woman is like an icy draught, or a sharp pin-prick"[42].

For autoheterosexuals who have a deeper commitment to the cross-gender self, social dysphoria is one of the stronger types of gender pain. It stands to reason, then, that autohets who have gone through gender transition would tend to be particularly sensitive to it.

This is why the transgender movement has put so much effort into raising awareness of pronouns and their importance to trans people. Honoring their deeply felt cross-gender identification with corresponding pronouns helps them suffer less.

BEHAVIORAL DYSPHORIA

In everyday life, there are some activities that males and females tend to do differently, such as tasks around the house, sexual roles, and how they carry their bodies. Therefore, autoheterosexuals may develop a dislike for any activities they associate with their sex. Something as simple as going to the bathroom in a particular type of gendered restroom can trigger feelings of behavioral dysphoria. One trans guy simply couldn't bear to go to the women's toilet[43], and he also felt "sick" when he was forced to behave in a feminine way[44]. Another trans man, stuck at home "being a thorough woman doing domestic work", couldn't stand it anymore and left home once again to be a sailor[45].

Behavioral dysphoria also affects sexual interactions. Some trans men who prefer to be with women insist on being the active partner and may even have trouble being touched in return. One such trans man described being touched during sex as "nauseating", and when the doctor asked him about the passive sexual role he froze up, unable to speak for several minutes[46].

After detransitioning due to financial limitations, R. L. complained, "instead of my own dainty movements and mental happiness as a woman, I had to act as a man to my great displeasure"[47].

PHYSIOLOGIC DYSPHORIA

Sex-specific physiologic functions such as menstruation, penile erections, and ejaculation carry great symbolic weight. When puberty makes these bodily functions apparent, some autoheterosexuals despair because they're turning into the adult form of the sex they don't want to be.

For autoandrophilic people, the arrival of menstruation can be especially alarming. One trans man described the despair, disgust, and sheer horror he felt when he started menstruating:

"It was embarrassing. It was humiliating. It was deplorable in my mind. It was just the most disgusting thing I could think of. I thought I would rather be dead than have to go through this every month. It was like sheer torture."[48]

In addition to dismay at the features they *do* have, autohets may also grieve the bodily functions they lack. Autoandrophilic people can lament that they don't have penile erections or the ability to ejaculate semen, while autogynephilic people may feel a sad longing for monthly hormonal cycles or the ability to become pregnant.

One transfem who greatly envied her wife's pregnancy and delivery was crestfallen when she was unable to lactate herself: "With what delight…would I have suckled the child, and how sad I was when I once put on the screaming child to my breast and could give it nothing"[49].

Another transfem who envied her wife's pregnancy had physiologic dysphoria so strong that it seemed like the most intense suffering she'd ever felt: "Unnatural as it may appear, when our son was born, the thought that I could not go through the experience myself, or even be with my wife at the time caused me the most acute suffering I ever felt in my life, and I did not get over it for many months"[50].

DEPRESSION AND ANXIETY

In autoheterosexuals, shortcomings of cross-gender embodiment can lead to irritability or melancholy. Unable to express the version of themselves they want to be, autohets may end up "depressed, isolated, and withdrawn"[51].

Would-be transsexuals frustrated in their quest for cross-sex hormones or surgeries may grow despondent, falling into a deep pit of despair. If thwarted by a medical establishment that isn't open to helping them, they can feel that life is hopeless and they have no future.

Transvestites who don't fulfill their drive to dress as the other sex may become sullen and irritable. Their skies go gray. Life loses its luster. Inside, the tension of unmet need gnaws at them.

The wives of transvestites know this all too well. They've shared that when their spouses stopped crossdressing, they became "tense, frustrated, moody, unhappy, or angry"[52]. One said her spouse "felt like a caged lion with no escape"[53].

This existential funk can make autoheterosexuals neglect body maintenance. If their default-gendered self becomes unrelatable, they may struggle to see the point of taking care of themselves. A trans man subjected to this self-alienation by female puberty noted how his basic grooming fell to the wayside:

> "Around puberty, I started to feel like, disconnected from my body...I just wore really baggy clothing and I stopped doing a lot of self-care. I stopped, you know like, brushing my hair, and I just stopped grooming basically. I think I just stopped caring for myself because I didn't know how to."[54]

Another transmasc, one who felt stressed out by the prospect of medical inspection of his genitals, showed up at the hospital hungover and covered in excoriations from endlessly picking at his skin—both signs of anxiety[55].

Even back in the '70s, sexologists recognized that FTMs usually had a history of severe depression. Upon examination, most were depressed to some extent, and almost one in five had made suicide attempts[56].

EGO-DYSTONIC AROUSAL:
BEING UPSET ABOUT WHAT TURNS YOU ON

For many autoheterosexual males, their first forays into wearing women's clothing involve donning femme clothing intending to look like a female and growing erect in response. This unlady-like reaction can be deeply upsetting. Shame comes to the fore. What started as a seemingly innocent desire to look like a girl ends in disappointment or regret.

For some, the cycle of contemplating being the other gender, becoming aroused, and getting upset about that arousal happens repeatedly. One autogynephilic transsexual explained it well:

> "Like many of the other respondents, I too have always had these feelings of arousal at the mere thought of being female. And it always pissed me off! I hated it that putting on a dress, or wearing other feminine attire, or even just fantasizing about being a normal woman would elicit such an un-female response, both physically and mentally. I wanted so badly for the things I was doing to simply feel 'normal.'"[57]

This also happened to transfems back in the day. One whose account was published in 1928 shared, "When first I began to dress as a woman, I was offended by the fact that it induced erection; this irritated me greatly"[58]. Another transfem reported how, as a child, she started to tie her sister's corset around her waist and got her first erection. Startled and unsure of what it meant, she took off the corset and was left deeply dissatisfied with the experience[59].

When arousal conflicts with one's idealized self-image, it is called *ego-dystonic arousal.*

Thanks to scientific advances, the boner-killing powers of feminizing hormone treatment allow autogynephilic transsexuals to enjoy the pleasures of feminine embodiment without their bodies reminding them that their cross-gender inclination is ultimately sexual in origin.

Autogynephilic males who are comfortable living as their default gender but who wear women's clothes as part of their sexual arousal process also experience ego-dystonic arousal. With post-nut clarity comes shame, as they find themselves wrapped in clothing that upsets their image of themselves as masculine men. Back in the hiding spot it goes (at least until next time). For autogynephilic males who want to be men, this type of ego-dystonic arousal is common.

A study of Swedish men found that only 47% of men who'd been aroused by crossdressing considered that arousal acceptable to their sense of self[60]. By contrast, only 3% of men who hadn't been aroused by crossdressing considered the idea of becoming aroused from crossdressing acceptable for themselves[61]. These figures suggest that autohet males are usually ashamed and upset about sartorial arousal at first, and this shame is particularly hard to shake off—only about half had become okay with it.

Interestingly, autoheterosexual ego-dystonic arousal seems far less common in females. One possible contributing factor to this difference is that penile erections are overt signs of arousal that are hard to ignore. Stereotypes of horny males and demure females could also play a role in generating this disparity: if being horny is seen as a guy thing, some autoandrophilic people might feel that arousal from masculine embodiment affirms their masculinity.

SHAME

Autoheterosexuals commonly feel some amount of shame about their cross-gender inclinations. This is likely because of its sexual origins, but they may also feel shame about coming up short in terms of societal expectations for people of their sex.

For some autoheterosexuals, the shame runs deep. *Super deep.*

One of the most illustrative examples of this intense shame comes from a transsexual woman whose mother found a noose she'd been using for the purpose of hanging herself by her genitals. Rather than admit to her gender issues, she allowed her mother to think she was suicidal because that seemed less shameful[62].

Another transsexual woman reported, "I think some of us just never let go of that shame. Of course it's about sex!"[63].

Autoheterosexual shame can make someone repress their cross-gender inclinations in childhood[64] or keep it so secret that they don't tell anyone until they're middle-aged or older[65]. Even if they desperately want to share that part of themselves with friends, they might still remain silent due to shame[66].

This shame also has a huge impact on transgender politics,

because it underlies much of the over-the-top hostility toward the concept of autogynephilia in the transgender community.

The Sex-Positive Approach to Transcending Shame

In 2000, Anne Lawrence made a second attempt to introduce the concept of autogynephilia to the trans community through the *Transgender Tapestry* magazine[67]. The following issue contained many responses from trans women[68]. Virtually all of them stood opposed to the theory. Their responses primarily focused on its implications: concerns about personal identity, discrimination protections, or access to medical treatment.

But one response stood out for its willingness to seriously consider the possibility that the autogynephilia theory might be true. In her piece, "Autogynephilia: What If It's All True?", transgender activist and scholar Jessica Xavier sniffed out the unsavory emotion underlying the trans community's hostility to the idea of autogynephilia: *shame.* She wrote, "I find the harsh condemnation of autogynephilia to be more telling than the theory itself...Behind all the nay-saying, I sense something rotten here—the stench of shame"[69].

Rather than run from a possibility that deeply frightened so many of her peers, she faced the potential reality of auto-gynephilia head-on and modeled a sex-positive approach that renounced shame:

"We need not dumb down our gender or sexual diversity in order to please others. We need not fear our own sacred sex; we should, rather, fear a sexphobic culture that persecutes us for daring to practice it. If it is substantiated by additional research, we need not be ashamed of autogynephilia, but of shame itself."[70]

Unfortunately, the transgender community as a whole was unwilling to seriously consider the possibility that most of them had a type of cross-gender inclination that was ultimately sexual in nature. They turned away from this sex-positive approach and allowed shame to fester.

Over two decades later, the sex-positivity movement has grown. Societal attitudes toward sexuality have loosened. The idea that sexuality is not intrinsically shameful has gained ground. Things have changed.

It's okay to talk about autoheterosexuality. In fact, talking about what makes us feel shame with accepting, open-minded people can be an especially fast way to leave shame behind.

It doesn't have to be a big deal.

REPRESSION

Countless autoheterosexuals have initially repressed their cross-gender inclinations. Faced with feelings and a sexuality that conflicted with their default identity, they tried to push it down and bury it. Some have undoubtedly succeeded, but it's not known how often they succeed, for how long, or at what cost.

I repressed too. But once I learned about autogynephilia, I immediately changed my approach. I realized I couldn't reason my way out of feelings that were ultimately caused by a sexual orientation. After easing my prohibitions on cross-gender expression, I began to see the psychic toll of repression.

Autohet repression requires more than blocking off obviously cross-gendered thoughts, feelings, and behaviors. To contain the cross-gender self, even thoughts *adjacent* to the obviously cross-gendered ones must be kept in check.

This barrier doesn't magically maintain itself either. It requires vigilance. To repress, behaviors and thoughts must be actively monitored to ensure they don't veer too close to The Forbidden Place.

Caged by excessive inhibition, the range of emotional and creative expression narrows. Melancholy and irritability set in. The sense of inauthenticity grows. Pressure builds. Eventually, something has to give.

As Hirschfeld noted, complete repression comes at a severe psychic cost:

> "Undoubtedly many transvestites have great difficulty in bearing the temporary or permanent repression of the impulse to emphasize their femininity. Repression has a crushing and finally crippling effect on their pleasure in creative work and their abilities, and frequently it creates a great inner unrest, accompanied by a feeling of listlessness, anxiety, and deep spiritual depression. These effects can grow until they culminate in suicide."[71]

The testimony of transvestites, transsexuals, and their loved ones speaks to the pain of repressing such an important part of themselves. The wives of crossdressers report that abstaining from dressing sours their spouses' moods and makes them anxious, irritable, and tense[72].

One transfem spoke to the melancholy brought on by abstaining from dressing:

"When I stop, and I often have tried to give it up, it's as if my entire world turns grey. The joy and happiness that I usually get from many activities is reduced. The peaks of satisfaction and pleasure are gone."[73]

Another transfem reported similar feelings, even to the point that food didn't taste good anymore[74].

An autohet FTM reported similar pain, including difficulty eating. When verbalizing his intent to repress his masculinity, he told his doctor, "It must be God's will that I shall be a girl, and it might be a sin not to do His will" and said he would get a job as a domestic servant[75]. During the ten weeks of repression when he dressed as a girl, he felt ill, nauseated, and unreal—and even lost about twenty pounds.

Repressing clearly wasn't a good idea, so he started being manly again. He drank, swore like a sailor, and picked up chicks to show off his masculinity, and quickly regained the lost weight[76].

Attempts to repress their cross-gender aspirations can even make some autoheterosexuals feel suicidal: "Four times this year,

I have decided that...I simply must remain male. And all four times, I became seriously suicidal within a week"[77], reported one autogynephilic trans woman.

Autoheterosexual repression has some consistent patterns. Purging and renewed commitment to heterosexuality are especially common repression strategies. Strategies such as drug abuse, doubling down on the default gender role, and being too busy to have idle time have showed up as well.

Repressing through Purging

A carnival was coming up, and a transfem looked forward to finally getting a chance to dress as a lady in public for the first time. She saved up for months to buy an outfit. But afterward, she wasn't completely satisfied with it. Seized with the impulse to burn it, cloth became smoke and ash[78].

She had purged her feminine possessions. But it didn't last long: "Then my fancy for feminine clothes abated, but after an interval it revived with greater intensity and persistence. I then bought good, well-fitting clothes...including everything a woman has"[79].

Some autohets purge when they don't like how their cross-gender inclinations reflect on their sense of self. This behavior is driven by feelings of shame, guilt, and disgust[80].

Countless transfems have gone through binge-and-purge cycles just like this one. For a time, it seems to work. The urge is gone, seemingly for good. But that state usually doesn't last. Instead, the desire comes back even stronger, and before long, they've bought more clothes than they purged in the first place.

This pattern of behavior quickly gets expensive.

If you're autoheterosexual and thinking of purging your cross-gender possessions, consider leaving them with a trusted friend for safekeeping. Chances are, you'll want them back later.

Repressing through Alloheterosexuality

Countless autoheterosexuals have tried to repress through heterosexual hookups or relationships. Whether enacted through promiscuity or serious commitment, this approach may work for a few months or a few years, but it's usually not a lasting solution.

As the new relationship energy fades, the nagging feeling that something's missing grows: "Like a pendulum...my transsexual desires increased as the novelty of the sexual relationship diminished"[81]. This period of conventional heterosexual expression can give way to even greater gender dysphoria than what came before[82].

One transfem married with the hope that her sexual relationship with her wife would subdue her inner feelings of womanliness. This plan backfired: her wife got pregnant, which caused a burning envy in her[83]. In a similar situation, another transfem lamented: "I had thought love and marriage would make an end of my longing to adopt woman's dress. They did not"[84].

Plenty of autoheterosexuals have married and had kids, yet the cross-gender urge remained. Some kept their gender issues secret until death, while others disclosed their feelings. Some met their needs with occasional crossdressing, while others transitioned gender.

Romantic relationships rarely survive gender transition intact, and even lesser forms of cross-gender commitment often cause relationships to unravel. Autohets are usually in heterosexual relationships, so their cross-gender expression is often incompatible with their partner's sexual orientation.

It's important for autoheterosexuals to disclose their cross-gender sexuality to their partners—the earlier in the relationship, the better. Hiding something that significant from potential partners and spouses is unfair to them. If something could be a deal breaker, it's important for them to know.

CRISIS OF MEANING

Some autoheterosexuals consider living as their default gender to be absolutely devoid of spiritual worth, so they may question the value in continuing to exist if they can't live as the gender they want.

This is a dangerous frame of mind to be in.

Losing a sense of purpose or hope in life can lead to rapid declines in mental state[85]. Drowning in suffering and without a positive vision of the future, people can lose their hold on life and begin to fade away.

Since our sexualities have so much potential to confer meaning in our lives, the inability to express them can render life meaningless, even to the point of suicide.

Hirschfeld saw this dynamic play out plenty of times. In fact, it was the suicide of a young homosexual man that precipitated Hirschfeld's switch from general medical practice to sexology[86].

He knew that homosexuals and transvestites alike were vulnerable to suffering from unexpressed sexuality to a degree that could culminate in suicide: "Sexually abnormal persons who are forced into a lifestyle that stands opposed to their nature often thereby fall into depressed mental states that at times even lead to suicide"[87].

Lou Sullivan reached this point of existential crisis. A little over a year before he finally started testosterone, he languished in deep despair. His life had no meaning:

"Sitting in my apt, crying because I feel so goddamn empty inside. My whole goddamn life is a waste of time—just trying to think up things to do to waste time until I die. Nothing means a goddamn thing."[88]

When every fiber of their being screams out that they ought to be the other sex, yet they feel confined to a body utterly lacking in gendered worth, autoheterosexuals may even feel their predicament is a "trick that nature had played" or an "injustice done…by nature"[89].

To right this cosmic injustice, an autogynephilic child routinely sought the help of God. She had only one wish—to become a girl: "I prayed to God every night…to put right the mistake that was made in me and to transform me into a girl"[90].

Obstructed in their desire to be the other gender, autoheterosexuals may feel they are in a perpetual state of exile[91]. In this state, it can be hard to keep a grip on life.

Eventually, some let go.

SUICIDALITY

In 1903, a thirty-two-year-old transvestite checked into a hotel[92]. The following day, she dressed in the privacy of her room and donned a white wedding dress, complete with a veil. Atop her head, she placed a garland of myrtle.

Later, she laid down in bed, pointed a gun at her chest, and shot a hole through her heart. In the note left by her side, she asked to be buried in her wedding dress.

Six years later, in 1909, Michael Semeniuk came down with a fever[93]. His neighbors grew worried about him and called a doctor. When the doctor came, Michael refused to be physically examined, so the doctor left without making a diagnosis.

Michael's corpse was found the next day. Unwilling to live through the discovery of his sex, he had poisoned himself that night.

The pain of being unable to live as their cross-gender selves can drive autoheterosexuals to kill themselves. The constant desire for something unattainable leads to madness, the frustrations accruing over the years until it all feels hopeless. As Richard T. described:

"Because not one of my wishes was realized I became restless, angry. Especially lately this condition has assumed forms bordering on madness. Even the strongest will is powerless against such a natural force. I have often wished for death as the only solution."[94]

The crisis of meaning underlying gender-based suicidality can be so intense that it takes on spiritual importance. This might be why the Hungarian physician attributed her continued existence to her religious practice: "I have nothing to thank but positive religion; without it I should have long ago committed suicide"[95].

Back in those days, even the inability to wear dresses could bring on suicidality. One of Hirschfeld's patients longed to wear dresses, but the culture of her time prohibited it. She despaired over her condition. The inability to wear dresses rendered life meaningless:

> "If I ever came to the definitive decision that I would never get my wish to wear dresses, I would finally throw my life away, because it would be absolutely worthless to me…Life is completely loathsome to me without dresses!"[96]

Being able to wear a dress was a matter of continued existence for her. In modern times, the advent of medical transition has shifted the goalposts, so autoheterosexuals today can feel a similar despair over the inability to get hormones or surgeries.

IN SUM

* Just as autoheterosexuals can feel good about having bodies, behaviors, clothes, and social roles that they associate with the other sex, they can also feel bad about perceived shortcomings in those same domains.

These bad gender-related feelings are known as gender dysphoria. This gender pain is the outcome of a gender-related conflict between desire and reality. Such feelings can be especially excruciating because they are as significant as those caused by conventional love.

* The medical profession codifies gender dysphoria as distress associated with gender incongruence. The diagnostic criteria for gender dysphoria in the DSM-5 map onto aspects of autoheterosexuality that pertain to the desire to have the body, mind, and social role associated with the other sex. Autohet transsexuals change their bodies in order to grow more at peace with themselves and to help others see them as the gender to which they aspire.

* Autoheterosexuality drives autohets to think of themselves as the other sex, and in the process, it can generate a dissociative alienation from their bodies or the world around them (depersonalization or derealization). Gender-affirming sexual interactions and hormones can help alleviate dissociation by helping trans people feel at home in their bodies.

* For autoheterosexuals, people of the other sex can be so beautiful it hurts. Due to sexual dimorphism, autohets often lack the same traits they admire in others, so it is

common for them to envy people of the other sex. They may also envy people of their sex who possess attributes associated with the other sex.

* An unmet desire for cross-gender expression can make autoheterosexuals feel tense and irritable. The inability to feel peaks of pleasure can flatten their mood and leave them depressed. This existential funk can leave them unable to take pride in their physical appearance and uninterested in taking care of themselves.

* Some autogynephilic people become upset when crossdressing or thinking about being female brings upon arousal. The reason they become upset depends on which self-image this arousal affects. It may conflict with their cross-gender self because it makes them feel unwomanly, or it may conflict with their self-image as masculine men.

* Autogynephilic people commonly feel shame about their sexuality. This unaddressed shame underlies much of the excessive hostility toward the concept of autogynephilia within the transgender community.

* Faced with feelings of shame and a sexual propensity that conflicts with their idealized self-image, some autoheterosexuals try various methods of repressing their

cross-gender proclivity. Engaging in cycles of binging and purging their cross-gender possessions is common, as is repressing through heterosexual relationships. They can also repress by making a concerted effort to adhere to the gender role associated with their sex.

* Since sexuality has so much potential to bring meaning to our lives, some autoheterosexuals consider living as their default gender to be absolutely devoid of spiritual worth. They may question the value of continuing to exist if they can't live as the gender they want. The crisis of meaning brought on by this perpetual inner heartbreak can result in suicide.

WHICH COMES FIRST: SEXUALITY OR IDENTITY?

THE CHICKEN-OR-EGG QUESTION AT THE HEART OF THE CONTROVERSY

Many trans people acknowledge that prior to transitioning they experienced arousal in association with cross-gender embodiment. Often, this response happened while crossdressing or crossdreaming[1].

It is not really disputed that many trans people have experienced cross-gender arousal or cross-gender fantasy at some point in their lives. If anything, it's the norm. The dispute is over what it means.

People who disagree with the two-type MTF typology generally make one of the following arguments:

1. Females can also experience arousal at the thought of being a woman[2]
2. For would-be transsexuals, fantasies about being the other gender are a coping mechanism for dealing with the incongruence between their gender identity and their physical sex[3]

The first argument is beside the point, and the second switches cause and effect.

AUTOGYNEPHILIA IN FEMALES (FEMALE AUTOHOMOSEXUALITY)

If females experience arousal at the thought of being a woman, it would represent *autohomosexuality* (attraction to being one's sex), not autoheterosexuality.

Given that some autohomosexual males experience masculinity dysphoria[4], female autohomosexuality could similarly lead to femininity dysphoria (distress over not being feminine enough).

But autogynephilia in females would not drive gender transition—if anything, it would reduce the urge to transition because it would elevate the worth of femininity. Thus, female autogynephilia is tangential to the question of why some males transition to live as women.

In line with the leading theory[5] of where autosexual orientations come from, we would also expect female autohomosexuality to be present in just a subset of same-sex attracted females. Thus, it wouldn't be prevalent enough to be considered typical female sexuality.

Research has shown that some females answer affirmatively to questions intended to measure the presence of autogynephilia[6]. However, most of these studies used measurement scales that differed from Blanchard's, so it's hard to know how to interpret them in relation to his research.

Fortunately, Michael Bailey and Kevin Hsu administered Blanchard's Core Autogynephilia Scale to four groups of autogynephilic males, four groups of typical males, and two groups of females to explore if females were autogynephilic[7]. They found that *all* groups of autogynephilic males scored far higher on the Core Autogynephilia Scale than *any* of the groups of females or typical males. In comparison, the groups of females and typical males all had far lower scores. It wasn't even close.

At this point, it seems fairly settled that even if some females are autogynephilic, it's nowhere near common enough to be considered typical female sexuality. And besides, whether or not some females are autogynephilic is irrelevant to gender transition: autohomosexuality doesn't drive gender transition, autoheterosexuality does.

AUTOGYNEPHILIA AS A WAY OF COPING
WITH GENDER INCONGRUENCE

If fantasies of being the other gender are just a way of coping with gender incongruence, why are these fantasies far less common among homosexual males who undergo gender transition?

If fantasies of being the other gender are just a way of coping with gender incongruence, what does this imply about the males who have fantasized about being female yet haven't transitioned or stated a trans identity? Do these nontrans males actually have a cross-gender identity? Should they be thought of as would-be transsexuals?

Do males identify as heterosexual because they are attracted to females or because they identify as straight? Are males attracted to males because they identify as gay?

Which comes first: our sexual attractions or our sexual identities?

I think the answer is obvious: attractions come first. People notice who they are sexually drawn to and tend to adopt a corresponding sexual identity. Identities don't cause the attractions. Rather, they're a downstream effect of sexual attraction patterns.

If sexual identities caused our attraction patterns, we could simply change our sexual identity and our attractions would change accordingly. But conversion therapies intended to change sexual orientation don't work[8], so identities are clearly not where sexual attractions originate.

A similar line of thought applies to autoheterosexual attraction and cross-gender identity in trans people who experience both.

Which comes first: cross-gender identity or an enduring pattern of sexual attraction to being the other sex?

Doesn't it make more sense that here, too, people experience attractions that shape their identities, rather than the other way around?

If someone experiences autoheterosexual attraction for years before transitioning to live as the other sex, should we retroactively interpret that cross-gender attraction as a sign of cross-gender identity and thus as a way of coping with gender incongruence? If so, does this reasoning also apply to autoheterosexuals who don't transition to or identify as another gender?

Sexual orientations are enduring patterns of sexual attraction that exist regardless of how we feel about them, even if they offend our sense of self. Our sexual identities may change, but changes to sexual orientation are unlikely.

Most people are heterosexual, didn't choose to be that way, and couldn't become same-sex attracted even if they tried. Although they can change their sexual identity if they want to, their attraction patterns are unlikely to budge.

If someone experiences sexual attraction to being the other sex for years on end, isn't that attraction likely driven by a sexual orientation? And even if their cross-gender identity becomes strong and continuous at some point in their lives, isn't that identity most likely a downstream effect of the cross-gender attractions that preceded it?

These beliefs—that cross-gender attractions, fantasies, and arousal are merely ways of coping with gender incongruence, and that gender identity comes first—have obvious emotional appeal to autohets with cross-gender identities. But these beliefs don't make sense chronologically, and there's insufficient evidence for them.

EVIDENCE FAVORS THE "AUTOHETEROSEXUALITY FIRST" NARRATIVE

Core gender identity usually solidifies by three years of age, but many trans people only come to realize they are transgender after puberty, or even in their twenties or thirties—long after autoheterosexuality is already at work in those who have it.

A lot of trans people say they first wanted to be the other sex and felt gender dysphoria in childhood, long before puberty. Some regard this as evidence that their cross-gender desires weren't sexual in origin.

But people commonly report special longings or attachments during childhood that were congruent with their later-revealed sexual orientations[9]. These early attractions sometimes reach the point of eroticism, too, which also happens with autoheterosexuality.

Sartorial arousal has been documented in males under age three[10], and autogynephilic trans women have retrospectively reported that they had autogynephilic arousal as early as four to six years of age[11].

In autoheterosexuals, their orientations are already present long before their cross-gender identities become their dominant gender identities. Autoheterosexuality comes first, and cross-gender identity is a later development in some autohets.

Orientation precedes identity.

IN SUM

∗ Arguments against the legitimacy of the concept of autogynephilia and its relevance to transgenderism generally focus on two lines of argument: 1) females experience autogynephilia and, therefore, autogynephilia is just typical female sexuality, and 2) fantasies about being another gender are manifestations of cross-gender identity in would-be transsexuals. The first argument is beside the point, and the second switches cause and effect.

∗ Default gender identity usually forms by three years of age, but it's particularly common for trans people to start having gender issues around the time of puberty. Many only come out as transgender in their twenties, thirties, or even later. Autoheterosexuality and its associated cross-gender development process best explain this pattern.

PART 7

AUTOSEXUALITY BEYOND GENDER

AUTOSEXUAL ORIENTATIONS
ATTRACTIONS TO BEING

Heterosexuality isn't the only sexual orientation that can be turned inside out.

It happens with age-based or race-based attractions too. Even attractions to nonhuman entities such as dragons and wolves can be inverted, resulting in a sexual desire to be a dragon or wolf.

What do all these different autosexual orientations have in common?

Each one is theorized to be an *erotic target identity inversion* (ETII).

When it comes to ETIIs, the particular erotic target may vary in gender, race, body integrity, age, or species (i.e., between men, women, amputees, youth, wolves, etc.), but the *direction* of the attraction is the same: inverted toward the self.

Erotic target identity inversions are self-attractions (autophilias), so the names for these orientations take the form of "auto-X-philia", where X is the erotic target being embodied. For example, an inverted attraction to men is auto*andro*philia, and an inverted attraction to animals is auto*zoo*philia.

All of these autosexual orientations have the potential to shift someone's identity closer to that of their erotic target. Just as autoheterosexuality can lead a person to identify as another gender, autosexual attraction to being an amputee can motivate someone to identify as an amputee.

Any of these autosexual orientations can cause shifts toward mentally or physically feeling like the erotic target. During mental shifts, autosexuals feel they are having thoughts, feelings, perceptions, or sensations corresponding to their erotic target. During phantom shifts, autosexuals feel the presence of phantom anatomy corresponding to their erotic target.

People with autosexual orientations often want to embody the same traits they admire in the entities they're attracted to. Different types of entities vary with respect to their physical form, bodily functions, mind, behavior, dress, or social role. Thus, people with autosexual orientations can have sexual or romantic interests that fall within one or more of the following embodiment categories:

* *Anatomic autosexuality*—having the physical traits of an erotic target
* *Physiologic autosexuality*—having the bodily functions of an erotic target
* *Behavioral autosexuality*—behaving as an erotic target
* *Sartorial autosexuality*—wearing clothing or other body adornments associated with an erotic target
* *Interpersonal autosexuality*—being socially treated as an erotic target
* *Psyche autosexuality*—having the consciousness of an erotic target

Regardless of which type of autosexual orientation someone has, emotional suffering sometimes accompanies it. As cross-identity strengthens through reinforcement, autosexuals can feel dissatisfaction and unhappiness from the mismatch between their idealized self-image and their physical form.

The specific type of autosexual dysphoria depends on the type of entity that they want to embody. For example, if someone experiences negative emotions because of their unmet wish to be a dragon or a wolf, they have *species dysphoria*.

Autosexual dysphoria can be described even more specifically based on the specific aspects of the erotic target that an autosexual person wants to embody. For example, if someone is dysphoric because of their unmet wish to have fur, paws, and a tail, they have *anatomic species dysphoria*.

X is an 'Erotic Target'

It's what someone is into. It's their 'type'.

Traditionally, X is about gender/sex.

But attraction can be along other dimensions too:

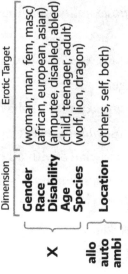

Dimension	Erotic Target
Gender	(woman, man, fem, masc)
Race	(african, european, asian)
Disability	(amputee, disabled, abled)
Age	(child, teenager, adult)
Species	(wolf, lion, dragon)
Location	(others, self, both)

X

allo
auto
ambi

ALLO-X-PHILIA
'other' 'love'

'Love of others as X'
'Love of X'

attraction to
X in others

AUTO-X-PHILIA
'self'

'Love of self as X'

attraction to
X in oneself

**Naming Sexual Orientations:
the 'Where' and 'What' of Love**

Erotic Target	Sexual Dimension	Autosexual Interest	Short-Term Embodiment	Long-Term Embodiment	Identity, Subculture
Men	Sex / Gender	Autoandrophilia	Crossdressing, crossdreaming, temporarily assuming role of man	**Medical Transition:** hormones, surgeries; **Social Transition:** name change, dressing, pronouns, stated identity	Transgender: trans man, transmasc, nonbinary, etc.; fujoshi, some lesbians
Women	Sex / Gender	Autogynephilia	Crossdressing, crossdreaming, temporarily assuming role of woman	**Medical Transition:** hormones, surgeries, permanent hair removal; **Social Transition:** name change, dressing, pronouns, stated identity	Transgender: trans woman, transfem, nonbinary, etc.; sissies, some gay men
People of a Particular Race	Race	Autophylophilia	Dressing, behaving, or imagining oneself as a particular race	**Medical Transition:** surgeries, skin lightening/darkening; **Social Transition:** name change, living as identified race, stated identity	Transracial / transrace / trace
Amputees	Body Integrity / Disability	Autoacrotomophilia	Pretending (bending legs, using crutches, etc.)	Amputation: legs, arms, hands, feet, fingers, toes	Transabled, pretenders, and wannabees
Children	Sexual Maturity / Age	Autopedophilia	Pedovestism, ageplay, age regression, diapers	**Medical Transition:** permanent hair removal, hormones, surgeries; **Social Transition:** full-time diapers or age regression, stated identity	Transage, adult babies, littles
Anthropomorphic Animals	Species	Autoanthrozoophilia	Fursuiting, yiffing, pet play, pet regression, zoovestism (tail, ears, fur, collar, etc.)	**Body Modifications:** piercings, tattoos, implants, teeth filing, etc.; **Social Transition:** name change, full-time zoovestism, stated identity	Transspecies, furry, furry fandom, pet regressors, animal roleplayers
Animals	Species	Autozoophilia	Animal roleplay, pet regression, zoovestism (tail, ears, fur, collar, etc.)	**Body Modifications:** piercings, tattoos, implants, teeth filing, etc.; **Social Transition:** name change, full-time zoovestism, stated identity	Transspecies, therians, otherkin, pet regressors, animal roleplayers

Autosexuals who are dysphoric about their embodiment may wonder if they would be better off living as their erotic target, or if they should get surgeries or body modifications to more fully embody it. But before getting surgeries or making other permanent changes, autosexuals usually embody their erotic target temporarily through clothing or other body adornments, behavior, roleplay, or mental shifts. This temporary embodiment brings comfort, arousal, or a sense of identity and is an important part of the cross-identity development process.

There are particular details unique to each type of autosexual orientation and each individual who has one, but this is the general form that autosexual orientations take.

In brief, this is the *autosexual theory of trans identity*: for each attraction to, there exists a corresponding attraction *to being*, and for each attraction to being, there exists a corresponding type of trans identity—each with its own flavor of embodiment subtypes, euphoria/dysphoria, and shifts.

VARIATIONS IN EROTIC TARGET LOCATION

Most people are attracted to other people: the *location* of their attraction is on *others*—they're *allo*sexual.

When the location of attraction ends up elsewhere, however, it's theorized to be a form of *erotic target location error* (ETLE). It's called this because it's a variation in "where" instead of "what"[1]. The type of erotic target is the same (woman, man, amputee, etc.), but the location is different (self versus others)[2].

The "error" part of the name comes from the evolutionary logic that alloheterosexuality is the optimal orientation for sexual reproduction, so other types of orientations can be considered errors of sexual development to some degree.

As originally envisioned[3], the ETLE concept supposedly accounts for sexual fetishism, transvestism, and autoheterosexuality. Ray Blanchard developed the theory after he found that many gender-dysphoric patients who had been aroused by imagining themselves as the other sex had also been aroused by dressing as the other sex or by certain materials or garments[4].

In this etiological theory, when an erotic target location gets placed on clothing or textiles rather than the body beneath them, it can result in sexual fetishism (attraction to nonliving objects such as clothing, shoes, or materials). When attraction to a clothed person of the other sex gets placed on the self, it results in transvestism. And when attraction to bodies of the other sex gets placed on the self, it leads to autoheterosexuality[5].

Although it's a promising explanation for the origin of autosexual orientations, these orientations clearly exist whether or not the ETLE theory ends up holding true. ETLE is simply the current leading theoretical explanation for what causes them.

WHY HAVE CHAPTERS ON OTHER AUTOSEXUAL ORIENTATIONS?

Learning about other autosexual orientations creates a deeper, more nuanced picture of autosexuality, but that's not the primary reason why I've included these autosexuality chapters. They're here to strengthen the case for autoheterosexuality and its relevance to transgenderism.

There are plenty of essays[6], videos[7], and blog posts[8] claiming that autoheterosexuality and the two-type model are not just incorrect but are also harmful, pathologizing, and transphobic. These critiques are *very* popular among those of my kind who reject the sexuality-based explanation for their situation. Explaining all the little details about how these critiques are mistaken would bore the shit out of too many readers, so I will bypass these critiques instead of addressing them directly.

I've composed chapters on other autosexual orientations and their corresponding trans identities that are based on disability (7.1), age (7.2), species (7.3–7.5), and race (7.6). Acknowledging that even one of these forms of trans identity exists makes the existence of autoheterosexuality and autohet transgenderism seem not only possible, but *inevitable*.

For example, consider the case of draconic identity.

When asked, people who identify as dragons are likely to report sexual interest in dragons as well as sexual interest in being a dragon. Is a dragon identity best explained by saying everyone has a species identity and people who identify as human are cis-species, but sometimes for unknown (and definitely nonsexual) reasons, people end up with a transspecies identity? Or does it make more sense to recognize that autosexual attraction to being a dragon can drive the development of a dragon identity?

I think the latter scenario makes sense not just for draconic identities, but for autosexual trans identities in general. My hope is that readers will see it similarly.

If you're reading this book strictly to learn about autoheterosexuality and aren't interested in learning about other types of autosexual trans identity, you may want to skip ahead to Part 8.

Each autosexual orientation has some language specific to it, and the subcultures associated with each orientation have developed their own way of speaking about their experiences, so you also might want to skip ahead if you've already hit your quota of new vocabulary.

But I hope you'll decide not to skip these chapters. Understanding how autosexuality manifests in other types of attractions will give you a deeper understanding of autoheterosexuality than you can get just by learning about autoheterosexuality itself.

IN SUM

* Autosexual orientations are attractions to being a particular type of entity. Autosexuals are usually allosexually attracted to the same types of entities they wish to embody.

* Erotic target location error (ETLE) theory proposes that location is an aspect of sexual orientation and that autosexual orientations come about when the location

is one's own body rather than the bodies of others. It's a difference in "where", not "what". Autosexual orientations are like allosexual orientations except for their inverted directionality, so they are formally known as *erotic target identity inversions* (ETIIs).

* Autosexual orientations compel people to attain particular forms of embodiment, and they foster attachments to that embodiment over time, thus strengthening feelings of cross-identity. Autosexuals can feel dysphoria in response to perceived shortcomings of cross-embodiment and euphoria in response to perceived attainment of cross-embodiment. The specific types of euphoria, dysphoria, and cross-identity that an autosexual person experiences depend on which dimensions of attraction are part of their autosexuality and which aspects of their erotic target they wish to embody.

* Many autosexuals temporarily embody their erotic target through body adornments, behavior, fantasies, roleplay, or shifts. Some may take drugs, have surgeries, or get body modifications to permanently attain a higher degree of cross-embodiment and more fully become what they love.

TRANSABLED

BEING DISABLED

Although it's uncommon, there are people who have perfectly functional limbs yet want to get them amputated.

This desire comes from *autoacrotomophilia*, a sexual interest in being an amputee.

Autoacrotomophilia is what happens when *acrotomophilia*, a sexual attraction to amputees[1], gets inverted toward the self. This autosexual interest has traditionally been called *apotemno-philia*[2], but that name obscures its autosexual nature, so I'll be calling it "autoacrotomophilia" instead.

Within the amputee admirer subculture, acrotomophilic people are *devotees* and autoacrotomophilic people are *wannabes*.

Most people who are attracted to amputees have also fantasized about being an amputee[3]. This association goes the other way too: most people who want an amputation are sexually attracted to amputees[4].

In order to achieve their desired embodiment, autoacrotomophilic people commonly bend their legs or arms while imagining that their knees or elbows are amputation stumps. This act is called *pretending*. It's analogous to the temporary cross-gender embodiment attained by autohets through crossdressing.

When embodying their amputee selves, autoacrotomophilic people may experience *body integrity euphoria*: positive mood shifts associated with perceptions of disabled embodiment.

Similarly, when perceiving shortcomings of disabled embodiment, they may experience negative mood shifts known as *body integrity dysphoria*. Over time, body integrity dysphoria can develop into enduring dissatisfaction and unhappiness with having fully functional limbs.

People with body integrity dysphoria commonly identify as *transabled*. There are other manifestations of transabled identity based on paralysis, blindness, or other forms of disability[5], but the most common kind of transableism involves a desire for limb amputation.

A study that interviewed fifty-two people with an intense, long-term desire for limb amputation found that most of them first felt that desire by eight years of age[6]. A majority first became aware of their autoacrotomophilia after seeing an amputee, and among those who remembered their first exposure to an amputee, most wanted to get amputated in the exact same location.

The most common primary reason they gave for seeking a limb amputation was to restore their identity as an amputee[7]. The most common secondary reason was either sexual arousal or a sense of well-being[8]. Ultimately, all three reasons were important to them[9]. These same three motivations of identity, sexuality, and well-being are also central motivators for transsexuals.

Many participants in this study also showed signs of gender issues. The group of people who had wished to be the other sex, felt that their body was the wrong sex, or been aroused by cross-dressing was fully *half* the size of the nonhomosexual group as a whole[10]. That's a *far* higher rate than in the general nonhomosexual population—an overlap that aligns with the idea that autoacrotomophilia and autoheterosexuality share a common cause.

All of the autoacrotomophilic people who had their limbs amputated at the preferred location were happy with their decisions. Their testimonies, which touched on themes of identity, sexuality, and well-being, strongly resembled how transsexuals talk about their decisions to undergo sex reassignment surgeries.

One reported, "it finally put me at peace...I no longer have that constant, gnawing frustration". Another said, "The only regret is that I did not have it earlier; since I had it done 5 years ago, I've felt the best I've ever felt"[11].

Other studies on autoacrotomophilia and body integrity dysphoria have found similar results:

* Onset almost always occurs at a young age, between early childhood and early adolescence[12]
* Most autoacrotomophilic people are sexually attracted to amputees, to pretending to be one, and to imagining themselves as one[13]
* The most common reasons given for desiring amputation involve feeling whole or complete, increasing well-being, or attaining sexual satisfaction[14]
* Those who undergo amputation report afterward that it helped them[15]

Like autoheterosexuality, autoacrotomophilia drives a sexual desire to resemble the object of attraction in both appearance and behavior. The testimony of post-op autoacrotomophilic people also accords with the sexual explanation for their condition.

For instance, one amputee said, "There is an aesthetic sexual complex, in addition I find the kind of walking very erotic"[16]. Another derived satisfaction from dealing with the same day-to-day obstacles that other amputees experience: "I have enjoyed working to find ways to overcome these minor difficulties"[17].

After getting surgery, autoacrotomophilic amputees commonly reported feeling euphoric, happy, ecstatic, relieved, or joyful. "I was as happy as I'd ever been and I was really horny, too!" reported one such amputee[18]. Another shared, "I do not regret my choice to get an amputation at all…I love waking up and seeing my stump there. My stump is still very erotic"[19].

Becoming an amputee brought their bodies in line with their idealized self-image, bringing a lightness and ease to everyday life not felt previously. They had a newfound ease in relating to others, and chronic stress dissipated. The most common regret was simply that they hadn't done it earlier[20].

BODY INTEGRITY DISORDER AS A NEUROLOGICAL DISORDER

Some researchers of body integrity disorder have moved away from focusing on sexuality and instead emphasize neurology[21].

Researchers who favor a neurological explanation have shown a preference for the term *xenomelia* over previous terms like *body integrity identity disorder* and *apotemnophilia*[22]. They might point to research indicating reduced activity or structural differences in the right parietal lobe[23] or differences in skin conductance below the desired amputation point[24].

This research may ultimately help us understand the brain structures responsible for creating mental representations of our own bodies, but these differences in brain structure are unlikely to be the ultimate cause of the body integrity incongruence that autoacrotomophilic people experience.

A sexual interest in being an amputee is rare in the general population, but it's the norm among people who seek amputation. This is a strong signal that sexuality drives body integrity dysphoria. The alternative, desexualized explanation overlooks the obvious role that sexuality plays here.

Autoacrotomophilic people commonly report that their desire for amputation increases when they see amputees or when they are lonely[25]. If the desire to truncate limbs comes from sexuality, this response makes complete sense: seeing amputees reminds autoacrotomophilic people of what they long to be, and loneliness is a sign that their sexual needs are unmet.

On the other hand, it's not clear why loneliness would affect the desire for limb amputation if flawed mental self-representations from dysfunctional brain structures are the ultimate cause of body integrity dysphoria.

IN SUM

* Autoacrotomophilia is a sexual attraction to being an amputee. It is the autosexual version of acrotomophilia, a sexual attraction to amputees. It's common for acrotomophilic people to have both the allosexual and autosexual sides of this attraction.

* In order to temporarily embody that which they love, autoacrotomophilic people commonly simulate disability by using prosthetics, bending their limbs, or imagining themselves as amputees. Those who desire permanent embodiment may seek limb amputation.

* Autoacrotomophilia can make someone experience good or bad feelings about the perceived intactness of

their body. These feelings of body integrity euphoria and dysphoria shift how they think of themselves over time, and eventually some of them come to identify as amputees. Autoacrotomophilic transableism is the most common form of transableism, but other forms based on paralysis or blindness also exist.

* Autoacrotomophilic transableism fits the autosexual pattern. It starts manifesting in childhood or early adolescence. It's associated with sexual interest in amputees and sexual interest in being one. Those who desire amputation commonly give reasons such as increasing well-being, expressing their sexuality, or feeling whole or complete. After amputation, they feel more at peace with themselves and their sexuality.

DISCLAIMER

I enjoyed researching and writing almost all the chapters in this book. The transage chapter, however, was not one of them.

I expect that many readers will be grossed out or otherwise turned off by this chapter. Readers who encountered sexual abuse as a child might want to skip it entirely, as might those with sensitive temperaments or rich imaginations.

You have been warned.

With that said, I have a request: please don't harass or otherwise mistreat people simply for showing signs of autopedophilia.

If the autosexual theory of trans identity is correct, many individuals in the subcultures discussed in this chapter are sexually attracted to children. However, it's essential to distinguish between *attractions* and *actions*. Sexual attractions themselves are morally neutral. On the other hand, molesting a child is obviously immoral.

Autosexual orientations are directed toward oneself, however, so acting on autopedophilic urges is not innately harmful. Adults who roleplay or dress as children in the privacy of their homes without real children present are not harming children by doing so.

TRANSAGE
BEING A MINOR

There are people whose chronological age suggests they are adults but who internally feel as if they never finished growing up. Inside, they may feel that they have the mind of a child even as their physical body continues its forward march through time.

A common cause of this feeling is *autopedophilia*, a sexual attraction to being a child.

Autopedophilia can drive an interest in achieving youthful embodiment through clothing, behavior, and interpersonal interactions. For example, autopedophilic people may enjoy dressing as children, wearing diapers, and roleplaying with people who play the role of *caregiver.*

Stimuli that make autopedophilic people feel youthful can cause comfort, relaxation, or arousal. These positive feelings from attaining youthful embodiment are known as *age euphoria*. In contrast, negative feelings about their degree of youthful embodiment are called *age dysphoria*.

As autopedophilic people age, the gap between their chronological age and mental age inevitably grows. Their bodies continue to age and mature, but mentally they feel as if they never developed past a certain age.

The age that autopedophilic people feel themselves to be is a major aspect of their *cross-age identity*. The strength, consistency, and age of this identity varies among individuals. Some feel like a child intermittently; others feel like a child all the time. Some feel like they're two years old; others feel like they're eight.

CHRONOPHILIAS: AGE-BASED SEXUAL ATTRACTIONS

Chronophilias ("chrono" means "time") are age-based attractions[1]. Although age is measured in time, sexual attraction in the dimension of age actually pertains to a particular stage of sexual development—age is merely a proxy.

Age-based sexual attractions are differentiated based on whether someone is attracted to infants/toddlers (*nepiophilia*), prepubescent children (*pedophilia*), early pubescent children (*hebephilia*), late pubescent children (*ephebophilia*), young adults (*teleiophilia*), middle-aged adults (*mesophilia*), or seniors (*gerontophilia*).

Differentiating between attraction to infants/toddlers and other prepubescent children is relevant for research. In this chapter, however, I don't want to split hairs about which prepubertal age someone is attracted to being, so "autopedophilia" will generally be used as an umbrella term for attraction to being any prepubertal or peripubertal age.

AGE REGRESSION: ADULT BABIES AND LITTLES

Some people pretend to be younger than their chronological age through a practice known as *age regression*. These age regressors commonly wear diapers and kids' clothes or roleplay with a partner to foster a headspace reminiscent of youth.

Age regressors tend to take on different identity labels based on the age range they enjoy regressing to. I've listed them here, with the corresponding chronophilia term in brackets:

* *Adult baby* (roughly ages zero to four) [autonepiophilia]
* *Little* (roughly ages four to ten) [autopedophilia]
* *Middle* (roughly ages ten to thirteen) [autohebephilia]
* *Teen* (roughly ages thirteen to seventeen) [autoephebophilia]

In order to regress in age, they may dress as children, put on cartoons, or play with children's toys. Being surrounded by stuffed toys, eating tiny snacks, drinking from sippy cups, sitting on the ground, or coloring with crayons can also help cultivate the headspace they seek.

Some dedicated age regressors even create a special room in their house decorated to suit the age they long to embody. For example, those who like to embody infancy may create a nursery room complete with a crib, toys, and any other baby items that signify babyhood.

Adult babies often like to roleplay as a child while another person, a "daddy" or "mommy", takes on the role of caregiver. Common activities involve bottle-feeding, diaper changing, and being put to bed in a crib.

People who get sexual or emotional satisfaction from wearing diapers are known as *diaper lovers* (DL), while those who focus on the roleplaying and identity aspects of being an infant are *adult babies* (AB)[2].

Together, diaper lovers and adult babies are part of a broader subculture known as *Adult Baby/Diaper Lover* (ABDL). Aside from ABDLs, the other popular sexual subculture that centers ageplay is generally referred to as *Daddy Dom/little girl* (DDlg).

Both of these sexual subcultures foster a sexual dynamic in which one person embodies an adult with a high degree of personal agency—a *caregiver*—while the other person embodies a dependent child, who plays the role of little. Together, the dynamic between caregivers and littles is known as *caregiver/little* (CGL). In this chapter, I'll use "little" in a broad sense that includes any age regressor, regardless of which juvenile age they aspire to.

Roleplaying with a caregiver helps littles shift into a childlike headspace known as *littlespace*. Littles frequently report that littlespace is a calming, enjoyable, and carefree escape from the everyday responsibilities of adult life.

For instance, one well-known adult baby remarked that the feelings elicited by wearing diapers are "like a constant hug from mom"[3]. For him, roleplaying as a baby helps him feel "calm, safe, protected and loved"[4]. Another prominent adult baby has proposed that for ABDLs, diapers evoke feelings of comfort, vulnerability, littleness, safety, and arousal[5].

For many littles, these good feelings and the littlespace mindset are the whole point of being a little. The feelings are an integral part of their emotional world, and littlespace provides an inner sanctuary from the emotional strife of everyday life.

CONGRUENCE BETWEEN EXTERNAL AND INTERNAL ATTRACTIONS

In 2016, Kevin Hsu and Michael Bailey published a study of erotic target identity inversions in pedophilic males that found about half of them were at least somewhat aroused by the fantasy of being a child. A fifth of these pedophilic men were so autopedophilic that they maxed out the eleven-point scale that Hsu and Bailey used[6].

Among the autopedophilic participants, the type of child they wanted to embody often matched the type of child they found most attractive. If they liked boys, they would imagine themselves as a boy. If they liked girls, they'd usually imagine themselves as a girl[7].

A similar pattern emerged with respect to age. When the internal and external attractions matched on both gender and age range, they were more strongly correlated than mismatches of age or gender[8]—a pattern that held for all age ranges.

Overall, this tendency for both gender and age to match between internal and external attractions supports the idea that autopedophilia is an erotic target identity inversion.

I've included a version of Hsu and Bailey's correlation matrix here so that you can see it for yourself (see Figure 7.2.1). I expect that many readers will have little experience interpreting correlation matrices, so correlations of magnitude $r=0.15$ or higher are highlighted to make the patterns more visible.

Other evidence suggesting that autopedophilia is an erotic target identity inversion comes from an ABDL community survey of more than 1,500 ABDLs which found that identities associated with other types of autosexual trans identity were common. About 20% of participants identified as a "sissybaby", an identity that combines transfeminine and transage together. About 15% identified either as a "babyfur" or "puppy", both of which combine transspecies and transage identities into one label[9].

That same survey also found another indicator that age regression is associated with attraction to youth. When participants were asked about issues within the ABDL community, the most common answer was "pedos"[10].

IDENTITY OR SEXUALITY?

Similar to other subcultures associated with autosexual orientations, some ABDLs prioritize the sexual side, while others focus on the identity aspects. Most ABDLs have interest in both.

CORRELATIONS: INTERNAL AND EXTERNAL ATTRACTIONS TO MINORS TEND TO MATCH IN BOTH GENDER AND AGE

AUTOSEXUAL AROUSAL BY THE THOUGHT, IDEA, OR FANTASY OF BEING A:

Boldface when autosexual target = allosexual target

	Female, aged:					Male, aged:				
ALLOSEXUAL ATTRACTION TO:	≥17	15-16	11-14	4-10	≤3	≤3	4-10	11-14	15-16	≥17
Females, aged: ≥17	**0.46**	0.46	0.30	0.09	-0.03	-0.06	-0.17	-0.17	0.04	0.13
15-16	0.44	**0.60**	0.52	0.23	0.04	-0.08	-0.25	-0.22	0.02	0.12
11-14	0.32	0.53	**0.64**	0.45	0.13	-0.08	-0.25	-0.34	-0.11	0.01
4-10	0.20	0.32	0.54	**0.70**	0.35	0.11	0.01	-0.31	-0.16	-0.01
≤3	0.14	0.09	0.18	0.32	**0.60**	0.30	0.05	-0.16	-0.10	0.08
Males, aged: ≤3	0.08	-0.03	-0.01	0.09	0.32	**0.63**	0.37	0.14	0.05	0.08
4-10	-0.11	-0.25	-0.25	-0.17	0.07	0.30	**0.59**	0.41	0.10	-0.01
11-14	-0.19	-0.35	-0.45	-0.49	-0.19	0.00	0.26	**0.56**	0.30	0.02
15-16	-0.06	-0.12	-0.26	-0.32	-0.16	-0.04	0.09	0.37	**0.48**	0.19
≥17	0.14	0.02	-0.14	-0.22	-0.09	-0.04	0.05	0.18	0.42	**0.31**

N=233

Source: Autopedophilia: Erotic-Target Identity Inversions in Men Sexually Attracted to Children (2016)
Authors: Kevin J. Hsu and J. Michael Bailey

Figure 7.2.1

Kevin Hsu surveyed male ABDLs and found that more than 90% reported some degree of sexual motivation in wearing diapers, in using them, or in simply being an ABDL[11]. A smaller proportion, 69%, said that roleplaying as a baby was sexually motivated to some degree[12].

It's plausible that the lower reported rate of sexual arousal from roleplaying as a baby came from the natural human tendency to portray themselves in a flattering light, but it might just be that many adult babies think sexuality detracts from their youthful personas. One adult baby explained, "The AB parts of us are separate from such [an] adult activity as sex. It's done that way to keep our kid side as pure and innocent as possible"[13].

ABDLs interested in the baby identity tend to enjoy being treated like a baby, which is associated with sexual interest in baby objects like clothing, toys, bibs, and pacifiers—but not necessarily with diapers themselves[14]. In contrast, ABDLs who prioritize sexual excitement as part of their ABDL practices are more likely to be sexually aroused by wearing diapers or using non-ABDL sex toys[15].

Although these subgroups prioritize different aspects of ABDL behavior, they both have a high affinity for wearing diapers. The vast majority of ABDLs report that the feel, sound, and smell of diapers is important to them[16].

They tend to find diapers sexually stimulating—and they use them often. They commonly enjoy *wetting* them, and, to a lesser extent, enjoy *messing* them too[17]. For many ABDLs, wetting their diaper is a powerful source of comfort: "The feeling of release and the feeling of comfort of a warm, wet diaper is really something that is very special to me", reported one ABDL[18].

ABDLs also appreciate the convenience of wearing a diaper[19]. While wearing a diaper, they don't have to interrupt what they're doing to go to the bathroom. They can simply *go*.

ABDLs ultimately have a combination of sexual, emotional, and identity-based motivations for the things they do[20]. All these aspects contribute to ABDL behavior, with no single aspect as the sole motivation.

AGE DYSPHORIA

As littles grow older than the age they want to embody, so does the gap between their physical bodies and their ideal forms. This incongruence between desire and reality can lead to unhappiness and dissatisfaction known as *age dysphoria*[21].

Male littles may wish that the hair on their bodies or face would vanish. Female littles may wish that their breasts were smaller or nonexistent. Ultimately, *any* signs of puberty can detract from the illusion of being prepubescent.

Age-dysphoric littles dread the forward march of time. Wrinkles, rough skin, vanishing "baby fat", skin blemishes, lost scalp hair, and thick body hair all conflict with the idea of being a kid.

Above all, many littles long to be smaller than they are. Kids are small, so feeling small enhances the feeling of being one. No wonder the "little" identity is so popular: it directly alludes to the littleness that many littles want to embody.

In response to age dysphoria, some might consider medical interventions to make them look younger or wonder if they'd be better off existing as the youthful age to which they aspire.

Hsu and Bailey's study of autopedophilic males found that 11% had considered hormones or surgery to alter their appearance, and 58% had pondered whether they'd be better off as children[22]. Hsu's survey of ABDLs found similar figures: about 11% had considered medical procedures to look more like a baby, and 38% had considered the possibility that they'd be better off as a baby[23]. In addition, both responses were associated with slightly higher odds of reporting sexual arousal by the fantasy of being a baby[24].

TRANSAGE IDENTITY

Through imagination and roleplay, some adult babies and littles can build a childlike identity within themselves whose age doesn't correspond to their physical age[25]. At first this identity is mild, partially formed, and subservient to the adult identity. It can subtly shift someone's behavior while the adult identity is in charge, but overall, it remains latent and under their control.

Over time, this childlike identity grows in strength and complexity as cross-age experiences accumulate. If someone develops this inner child to a sufficient degree, they may even start to feel they really *are* that age.

Psychologists have described this situation as "age identity disorder"[26], but the people they're describing are unlikely to think of it as a disorder. To them, it's simply their identity. According to ABDL writer Michael Bent, adult babies "put the baby identity on top of the adult identity and seek to assign primacy of identity to the baby"[27].

If age regressors see themselves as a child only some of the time, or if the age they choose to embody fluctuates often, they might think of themselves as *agefluid*. If their sense of being a child is consistent or fairly permanent, they might identify as *transage*.

For a select few, their cross-age embodiment can become a permanent lifestyle[28]. If their age regression drive is particularly strong and they have caretakers who can permanently facilitate their age regression, they may live full-time as a child or baby.

CONNECTIONS AMONG AGEPLAYERS, ABDL, AND AUTOPEDOPHILIA

People who enjoy ageplay or ABDL aren't necessarily autopedophilic. For example, they may be motivated by erotic power exchange, masochism, diaper fetishism, or other sexual interests.

Adults have much more agency and power than children, which makes ageplay a potential avenue for erotic play involving the element of power exchange. When roleplaying as a child, an ageplayer implicitly hands over power to the person in the adult role. This power exchange can be intrinsically erotic on its own, outside of autopedophilic motivations.

Masochism—deriving sexual pleasure from receiving pain or humiliation—might also be behind some instances of ageplay.

Many adults would find it degrading to be forced into diapers or otherwise infantilized. Urinating or defecating oneself, or being punished for having an "accident", would be even more degrading.

There are also people who simply get pleasure, comfort, or arousal from wearing diapers and don't have any interest in imagining themselves as a child or in roleplaying as one. They may simply have a fetish for wearing diapers that is unrelated to symbolizing youthful embodiment.

I feel that it's important to mention these other potential explanations for ageplay or diaper-wearing so that readers don't get the impression that *all* ageplayers are ultimately motivated by autopedophilia. Although autopedophilia is a promising explanation for the behavior of ageplayers who are particularly dedicated to embodying youth, autopedophilia research is in its infancy, and there's still a lot we don't know about it.

MICHAEL JACKSON: THE BOY WHO NEVER GREW UP

For a time, Michael Jackson lived at the Neverland Ranch—an estate he named after the mythical island in the story of Peter Pan, the boy who never grew up.

Jackson's estate had amusement park rides, a train, and a zoo. It also had countless statues and paintings of little cherub boys. One especially striking painting showed Jackson surrounded by little white-skinned cherubs who doted on him by offering flowers or putting them in his hair[29].

All of these features of Jackson's estate appear in *Living with Michael Jackson*, a documentary about Jackson's life that focuses on his love of childhood and children as one of its central themes[30]. In the film, a television journalist named Martin Bashir interviews Jackson several times over a period of months. Bashir felt uneasy about Jackson's love of children and presses him on the issue several times:

> *Bashir*: The inspiration for Neverland: Peter Pan. Why is Peter Pan a figure of such interest and inspiration to you?
>
> *Jackson*: Because Peter Pan, to me, uh, represents something that's very special in my heart. You know, he represents youth, childhood, never growing up, magic, flying, everything I think that children and wonderment and magic...what it's all about, and to me I just have never ever grown out of loving that or thinking that it's very special...
>
> *Bashir*: Do you identify with him?
>
> *Jackson*: Totally.
>
> *Bashir*: You don't want to grow up?
>
> *Jackson*: No, I am Peter Pan.
>
> *Bashir*: No you're not, you're Michael Jackson.
>
> *Jackson*: I am Peter Pan in my heart.

At another point in the documentary, Jackson sits alongside and holds hands with a twelve-year-old named Gavin. Bashir found it strange that a man in his forties was so closely connected to kids, so he asks Jackson about his motivations for spending so much time with boys[31]. Gavin quickly interjects that Jackson was actually four. Jackson agrees and goes on to extol the virtues of children and childhood:

> *Bashir*: But Michael, you're a forty-four-year-old man now.
> What do you get out of this? What do you get out of this?
> *Gavin*: He ain't forty-four, he's four!
> *Jackson*: Yeah, I'm four...I think what they get from me,
> I get from them. I've said it many times: my greatest
> inspiration comes from kids. Every song I write, every
> dance I do, all the poetry I write, is all inspired from that
> level of innocence. That consciousness of purity. And
> children have that. I see God in the face of children. And
> um, man, I just love being around that all the time.[32]

If Jackson's testimony accurately represented his beliefs, then he had a transage identity and identified as Peter Pan.

Some men who came forward saying that Jackson molested them were around the ages of twelve to thirteen when those incidents allegedly happened[33]. It's likely that Jackson was most attracted to boys in early puberty, making him a homosexual hebephile.

His identification as Peter Pan suggests that he had a transage identity that matched his apparent sexual preferences, so he was likely autohebephilic (attracted to being a child in early puberty)[34].

Autohebephilia is the most straightforward explanation for Jackson's intentionally high voice that began after puberty, the countless facial surgeries that demasculinized his face, the Neverland Ranch, and his habit of spending much of his free time in the company of children.

Michael Jackson's Medical Transracialism

Jackson surrounded himself with art and statues depicting white people. In the paintings he commissioned, the children were almost all white[35]. He was usually white in them too. The men who have come forward with allegations of childhood sex abuse also have skin on the lighter side.

If Jackson had autosexual preferences that matched his apparent allosexual preferences, he was attracted to the thought or image of himself as a light-skinned boy, which means his idealized self-image probably had light skin too.

It's unknown if Jackson privately thought of himself as white in a racial sense. However, he was born with skin that easily got him racially classified as black, and he died with skin that was paler than the vast majority of people who get racially classified as white. Few humans are whiter than late-stage Michael Jackson.

In addition, numerous cosmetic surgeries shifted his facial morphology toward a more European look. His nose became narrow and his lips thin.

If Michael Jackson was autosexually attracted to being a white boy, it could account for not only his extensive facial surgeries and medical transracialism, but also countless other details surrounding his life in a straightforward, logically consistent way that provides new insight into the late pop star's life.

IN SUM

* Autopedophilia is sexual attraction to being a child. It drives a desire for youthful embodiment which is often enacted through diapers, clothes, behaviors, or roleplay. Those who embody a more youthful age by mentally shifting into littlespace are known as age regressors. These age regressors commonly refer to themselves as "littles", and many are a part of the adult baby/diaper lover (ABDL) community.

* Among age regressors, the idea that their youthful embodiment has anything to do with sexual attraction to children can be an affront to their identity because pedophilia is the most stigmatized sexuality. It also conflicts with their idea of sexual purity in children. Some age regressors keep their child selves separate from their sexual selves in order to maintain the innocence of their child persona.

* Autopedophilic people are most likely to have autosexual interest in being the same gender and age group they are allosexually attracted to. The presence of pedophilia is a commonly reported issue among participants in the ABDL community, which is to be expected if ABDL is a manifestation of autopedophilia. Atypically high rates

of other forms of trans identity in the ABDL community suggest that a shared cause underlies these different forms of trans identity.

* Age regressors have a combination of sexual, emotional, and identity-based motivations for their behaviors. At first, their child identity is mild. Through mental shifts and roleplaying over time, their child identity grows stronger. They are likely to feel that their body grew up, but their mind stayed a child, and they may experience age dysphoria from the incongruence between their chronological age and subjective mental age.

* Michael Jackson's behavior and statements indicated that he was attracted to embodying youth through his behavior, social role, and state of consciousness. He intentionally spoke with a high voice, surrounded himself with children, and identified as Peter Pan. These age-related behaviors suggest that his idealized self-image was that of a boy on the cusp of puberty or in the early part of it.

FURRIES

BEING AN ANTHROPOMORPHIC ANIMAL

Humans aren't the only beings with four limbs, a torso, and a face with two eyes, a nose, and a mouth. Canines and felines have those features too. So do mythical creatures such as dragons, faeries, and angels.

Perhaps because of these fundamental similarities, people have the capacity to find those animals and mythical creatures sexually attractive. When those animals and mythical creatures have *anthropomorphic* (human-like) characteristics, people are even more likely to find them attractive.

And, of course, a subset of people who are attracted to various nonhuman entities are also attracted to the idea of being one. People like this tend to fall into one or more of these three groups:

* *Furry fandom*—a community of people who share an interest in depictions of animals that have human-like physical or mental characteristics; members of this group and the animals they depict are known as *furries* or *furs*

* *Therians*—people who feel a deep, integral spiritual or psychological connection to a nonhuman animal, often to the point of identifying as that animal

* *Otherkin*—people who identify as not entirely human, often as mythical or imaginary species (i.e., dragons, angels, fairies, elves, Pokémon, etc.)

People in these groups often have a sexual interest in nonhuman creatures. Some even identify as nonhuman. Those who do are *alterhuman*.

Alterhuman is an umbrella term for nonhuman identification that encompasses anyone who experiences "an internal identity that is beyond the scope of what is traditionally considered 'being human'"[1]. People who identify as wolves, tigers, dragons, angels, vampires, or elves are all alterhuman.

Many of these forms of identity are examples of *cross-species identity*—a form of trans identity more commonly known as *transspecies identity*.

People with transspecies identities can experience positive mood shifts (*species euphoria*) in response to stimuli that evoke a sense of cross-species embodiment. In turn, they can experience negative mood shifts (*species dysphoria*) in response to perceived shortcomings of animal embodiment.

These shifts in mood may occur in tandem with mental shifts that evoke a sense of having animal consciousness, or phantom shifts that create the sensation of phantom body parts such as paws, wings, or a tail. Both mental shifts and phantom shifts strengthen transspecies identity.

Although furries, therians, and otherkin are distinct groups, they have overlapping membership. Approximately 20% of furries identify as therian[2] and roughly 5% identify as otherkin[3].

Of these groups, furries are the largest and most well-known. Furry sexuality has also been studied more intensely than therian sexuality or otherkin sexuality, so let's start there.

YIFFING: FURRY SEXUALITY

Have you heard of "yiff", "yiffy", or "yiffing"? If so, you know that *yiff* is a cute, versatile euphemism for sex that is popular among furries.

"Yiff" can describe sex between furs or pornography of it. As a verb, "yiff" means "to have sex" or "to mate"[4]. Furries may also call someone "yiffy"[5] as a euphemism for "sexy".

Although "yiff" has nonsexual uses, it's primarily used to allude to sexuality. The ubiquity of "yiff" in the furry community suggests that furry-themed sexuality is common among furries. Data from furry surveys does too.

Most people in the furry fandom have sexual interest in furry content[6]. It's estimated that about 95% of male furries and almost 80% of female furries look at furry-themed pornography[7].

Furries are also far more likely to be gay or bisexual than non-furries. One survey found that 30% of male furries and roughly 10% of female furries were mostly or fully homosexual[8]. In fact, nonheterosexuality is so common among furries that one study of male furries had participants who were more likely to be gay than straight[9].

Furries are also somewhat likely to report attraction to animals or stuffed animals. One survey of furries found that 17% of them were *zoophilic* (sexually attracted to animals) and 7% of them were *plushophilic* (sexually attracted to stuffed animals)[10].

Furries are a marginalized sexual minority[11], and they often feel that coming out as furry is analogous to disclosing their sexual orientation[12]. But being part of the furry fandom isn't just about sex—it's also about escape, entertainment, community, and a sense of belonging[13].

FURRY EMBODIMENT AS A FORM OF AUTOSEXUALITY

In order to better understand male furry sexuality, sexologists Kevin Hsu and Michael Bailey surveyed 334 of them about their furry sexual interests[14].

Hsu and Bailey proposed the name "anthropomorphozoophilia" for a sexual attraction to anthropomorphic animals, and described a sexual attraction to being one as "autoanthropomor-phozoophilia"[15]. Both of these words are rather long, so I'll shorten them to "anthrozoophilia" and "autoanthrozoophilia" instead.

If someone is sexually attracted to anthropomorphic animals, they're *anthrozoophilic*, and if they're sexually attracted to being one, they're *autoanthrozoophilic*.

A majority of the furries that Hsu and Bailey studied were strongly sexually attracted to anthropomorphic animals as well as the fantasy of being one—approximately 99% were at least a little anthrozoophilic, and more than 90% were at least somewhat autoanthrozoophilic[16].

As expected, the gendered component of their anthrozoophilia showed correspondence between internal and external attractions. Furries exclusively interested in female furs tended to be more aroused by imagining themselves as a female fur, and *all* of the furries exclusively interested in male furs were more aroused by imagining themselves as male furs than female furs[17].

In terms of species, their attractions showed a similar correspondence between autosexual and allosexual attractions. For *all* thirteen species examined in the study, allosexual attraction to a species of anthropomorphic animal was most strongly correlated with autosexual arousal by the fantasy of being that exact same species.

Hsu and Bailey revealed this congruence between internal and external attractions with a magnificent thirteen-by-thirteen correlation matrix that elegantly demonstrates the relevance of the erotic target identity inversion framework for understanding autosexuality. In this matrix, the next-strongest correlations happened when the different species were similar. Being attracted to felines was associated with being attracted to other types of felines. Attractions to canines showed the same pattern.

I'm a huge fan of Hsu and Bailey's furry correlation matrix. I've included a version of it here so that you can see it in its full glory (see Figure 7.3.1). As with the correlation chart in the prior chapter, correlations of magnitude $r=0.15$ or higher are shaded so that you can better discern the patterns within it.

Altogether, Hsu and Bailey's findings strongly support the idea that autoanthrozoophilia is a form of autosexuality, and anthrozoophilia is its allosexual counterpart.

Later, a group of researchers aligned with the furry fandom conducted a study of furries to see how their results compared to Hsu and Bailey's[18]—at 1,113 responses, their sample was several times larger.

Again, the vast majority of furries said they had sexual attraction to furry media, and most reported moderate to strong amounts of attraction[19]. Most also reported sexual arousal by the fantasy of being an anthropomorphic animal, showing that anthrozoophilia and autoanthrozoophilia are both common in male furries[20].

FURSONAS: FURRY IDENTITY

Through meeting like-minded people and developing an anthropomorphic animal representation of themselves—a *fursona*[21]—

CORRELATIONS BETWEEN ALLOSEXUAL AND AUTOSEXUAL INTERESTS IN ANTHROPOMORPHIC ANIMALS

Boldface when autosexual target = allosexual target

AUTOSEXUAL AROUSAL BY FANTASY OF BEING A:

ALLOSEXUAL ATTRACTION TO:	Fox	Wolf	Dog	Lion	Tiger	Cat	Rabbit	Mouse	Raccoon	Horse	Bear	Eagle	Dragon
Foxes	**0.67**	0.45	0.38	0.08	0.11	0.15	0.10	0	0.20	0.09	0	-0.10	0.02
Wolves	0.45	**0.62**	0.47	0.16	0.23	0.13	0	-0.12	0.11	0.10	0.07	0.01	0.09
Dogs	0.40	0.41	**0.60**	0.02	0.06	0.10	0.04	-0.02	0.12	0.13	0.07	-0.09	-0.06
Lions	0.05	0.14	0.08	**0.62**	0.48	0.27	0.14	0	0.11	0.19	0.24	0.12	0.08
Tigers	0.11	0.22	0.15	0.52	**0.65**	0.31	0.18	0.06	0.13	0.14	0.23	0.13	0.07
Cats	0.15	0.08	0.06	0.28	0.30	**0.65**	0.30	0.24	0.22	0.04	0.10	0.02	-0.03
Rabbits	0.13	0.01	0.01	0.16	0.16	0.29	**0.65**	0.45	0.34	0.17	0.15	0.04	-0.09
Mice	0.05	-0.09	-0.03	0.01	0.04	0.14	0.46	**0.70**	0.34	0.13	0.15	0.10	-0.01
Raccoons	0.29	0.16	0.15	0.19	0.15	0.24	0.39	0.40	**0.69**	0.15	0.26	0.12	0.06
Horses	0.04	0.06	0.10	0.24	0.16	-0.03	0.19	0.10	0.08	**0.69**	0.27	0.16	0.18
Bears	0.02	0.11	0.14	0.26	0.24	0.12	0.18	0.17	0.19	0.19	**0.63**	0.18	0.17
Eagles	-0.12	-0.02	-0.09	0.12	0.12	0.04	0.04	0.12	0.07	0.19	0.23	**0.73**	0.32
Dragons	-0.05	0.01	-0.05	0.08	0.02	-0.07	-0.05	0	0.04	0.18	0.18	0.31	**0.74**

N=309

Source: The "Furry" Phenomenon: Characterizing Sexual Orientation, Sexual Motivation, and Erotic Target Identity Inversions in Male Furries
Authors: Kevin J. Hsu and J. Michael Bailey

Figure 7.3.1

furries can explore their identity and express themselves in a supportive, welcoming community.

When picking a species for their fursona, furries are most likely to pick a canine such as a wolf, fox, or dog. Feline species such as lions, tigers, and cats are the second-most popular. Dragons come in third[22].

Furries are far more likely than the general population to consider themselves not fully human or to say they would become completely nonhuman if they could[23]. The frequency and intensity of furry roleplaying is inversely associated with human embodiment[24], which suggests that when furries yiff as their fursonas, it contributes to feelings of nonhumanity.

CROSS-SPECIES IDENTITY AND HUMAN EMBODIMENT

To investigate the relationship between someone's nonhuman identity and their sense of human embodiment, scientists tested how a sample of furries responded to the rubber hand illusion[25]. In this experiment, the participant sits with one hand resting on a table while a rubber hand rests where their other hand would if it were on the table. A cloth draped over their shoulder and the base of the rubber hand allows them to more easily imagine that the hand on the table is connected to them.

The real hand and rubber hand are both stroked in the same spots at the same time with a rubber brush. Once the illusion begins, the person sees the rubber hand as part of their own body and may feel as if they could move it if they wanted to.

They might also proprioceptively sense that their unused hand has shifted closer to the rubber hand's location. This phenomenon is known as "proprioceptive drift". The bigger this shift is, the more they feel a sense of ownership over the rubber hand[26].

Autosexual orientations create attractions to particular states of embodiment. Furries and therians tend to imagine their animal sides with paws, hooves, or wings, not hands.

The dysphoria from shortcomings in the desired type of embodiment can show up as dissociation or alienation from one's own body, so the rubber hand illusion's ability to alter a person's sense of embodiment could let scientists indirectly detect the loss of embodiment associated with species dysphoria and cross-species identity. By testing furries with the rubber hand illusion and using data from a similar study as a control group, scientists were able to measure if being a furry impacted their sense of human embodiment.

It did.

Furries responded less to the rubber hand illusion than the non-furry comparison sample, suggesting that they identified less with the hand. They reported less embodiment and were less likely to feel as if they had lost their hand or that it had disconnected from their nervous system[27].

Furries also experienced less proprioceptive drift than non-furries. This drift was significantly associated with their roleplaying habits[28]. The more frequently and intensely they roleplayed as anthropomorphic animals, the less their real hand felt shifted toward the rubber one, which indicated a lesser degree of human embodiment[29].

Less proprioceptive shift was associated with more negative sentiments toward humanity and a stronger mismatch between their identities and bodies[30]. The therian subgroup of furries felt an even greater incongruence between their bodies and identities and also viewed humanity even more negatively than non-therian furries.

Together, these results suggest furry roleplaying contributes to a reduced sense of ownership over one's human body, which itself is associated with negative sentiments toward humanity as well as a greater mismatch between one's body and identity.

IN SUM

* Furries are fans of anthropomorphic animals. Many furries create and develop fursonas representing their anthropomorphic animal selves. Canine, feline, and draconic fursonas are the most common.

* Furries commonly wear body adornments such as animal ears or a tail as a way of representing their furry side. The more affluent among them may even own fursuits. It's common for them to roleplay with each other as their fursonas, either in-person or online. Most furries are nonheterosexual.

* Furries usually have sexual interest in both anthropomorphic animals and the idea of being one.

Among male furries, sexual interest in a particular species of anthropomorphic animal is strongly correlated with autosexual interest in being that same species of anthropomorphic animal.

* Furry roleplaying is associated with a weaker sense of human embodiment, which itself is associated with negative sentiments toward humanity and greater species incongruence between one's body and identity.

THERIANS
BEING AN ANIMAL

When someone has a deep integral or personal belief that they're a nonhuman animal, it's called *therianthropy* ("theri-" means "wild animal")[1]. People who experience this are *therianthropes*, or *therians* for short[2].

Therians often believe their connection to their inner animal side—their *therioside*—is spiritual or psychological in nature[3]. They're also likely to believe that they were born with a connection to their animal species, that they share traits with it, or that they were that species in a past life[4]. Their animal identification may coexist with their human identity or replace it entirely[5].

A therian's transspecies identity may be accompanied by mental suffering because of perceived differences between their ideal self and physical self[6]. This species dysphoria can manifest as pain, discomfort, or dissatisfaction in response to this mismatch between their animal identity and their human body[7]. Species dysphoria also manifests as emotional detachment from their human form[8]. Some therians have even reported that suppressing their therian side has previously led to severe depression or suicidal thoughts[9].

For therians, species dysphoria can be a powerful confirmation of their cross-species identity[10]. One therian said their dysphoria was "the single biggest reason I don't think it's all just a delusion"[11]. Another saw themselves as "a wolf born into the wrong body"[12].

By contrast, species euphoria strengthens cross-species identity by creating emotionally significant, memorable experiences. For example, when one therian heard a wolf howling just outside their tent during a childhood camping trip, they "broke out into goosebumps" and felt extremely happy and excited for days afterward[13].

This infatuation with wolves is common among therians. In fact, the nonhuman species to which they identify—their *theriotype*—is more likely to be a wolf than any other species[14].

As with furry fursonas, canine species are the most popular theriotypes, followed next by feline species[15]. And if mythical creatures such as dragons count as valid theriotypes, they are the third-most common[16].

Pet ownership trends also follow this pattern. In the US, surveys consistently find that dogs are the most popular pet, followed by cats[17]. Depending on the state, approximately 40–70% of American households have pets[18]. One 1997 therian survey, however, found that 96% of respondents had childhood pets[19].

Since it seems so common for therians to have had childhood pets, and their theriotypes seem congruent with broader pet-ownership trends, perhaps childhood exposure to animals influences a would-be therian's development and alters their eventual theriotype.

SHIFTING

In their minds, therians hold a conception of the appearance, behavior, and consciousness of their identified species. If they perceive that their embodiment matches up with this conception, they shift toward feeling more like their theriotype.

This shift toward an animal mind state is a *therioshift*, but therians usually just call it a *shift*. As a community, they've coined many terms to describe the various types of shifts they experience. These are some of the more common ones:

* *Mental shift*—a change in mindset toward being more animallike and less humanlike, adopting a more animalistic outlook or more animalistic feelings or perceptions[20]

* *Phantom shift*—a distinct sense of having phantom animal anatomy as part of one's body (i.e., a tail, ears, muzzle, paws, fur, four legs, scales, fins, or wings)[21]

* *Perception/sensory shift*—a change in sensory perception toward being more animallike (i.e., more attentive smell or hearing)

* *Cameo shift*—a therioshift toward feeling like a different species of animal than one's known theriotype(s)

* *Dream shift*—being partly or fully an animal within a dream

Mental shifts and phantom shifts are the most common types of shifts among therians[22]. The vast majority of therians have experienced both mental and phantom shifts (see Table 7.4.1).

Therian mental shifts involve embodying the consciousness of a nonhuman animal species. Most types of shifts that have been named involve changes to mental states and are thus ultimately subvariants of mental shifts.

During a mental shift, it's common for therians to behave in a way that more closely resembles their idea of how their animal species behaves. For instance, a wolf therian might walk on all fours, howl, or get the urge to chase someone down as if they were prey.

During a phantom shift, therians experience the sensation of having nonhuman body parts as part of their body. These are usually the same features that their theriotype has, so these can help therians figure out their theriotype or that they're even therian in the first place[23]. Therians are usually a species with tails, ears, and paws, so these are some of the most common features for therians to experience during phantom shifts (see Table 7.4.1).

Shifting Frequency	Mental	Phantom	Past Phantom Anatomy	
Constant	19%	23%	Tail	70%
Daily	24%	20%	Ears	69%
Every Couple Days	20%	16%	Muzzle/Snout/Teeth	61%
Few Times a Month	16%	17%	Paws/Hooves	49%
Few Times a Year	9%	8%	Fur/Mane	37%
Rarely	6.5%	7.9%	Legs	26%
Only Once	2.4%	1.7%	Wings	24%
Never	3.4%	7.6%	Other	20%

Table 7.4.1: Mental and phantom shifting frequency, and previously experienced phantom anatomy.
Source: "Therian Census" (White Wolf 2013). (N=291).

Shifting isn't limited to charismatic megafauna such as wolves, jaguars, and dragons either. An earwig therian can experience it too:

"When it told me via trances, dreams, mirror-talks, and other rather terrifying (at the time) means, that it was moving into my consciousness, I was scared. I thought I was going absolutely insane. I fought it tooth and nail, and yet I could feel that armour plating begin coming up, snapping into place, in daily life...but my inner voice would keep going: 'you are strong, you have discovered a part of you that was hidden away for (family, society, self)'s sake. Now, you can be twice as strong, for though you are small, you are fast, you have self-defence.'"[24]

Unintentional shifts like this can feel more like instincts, thereby strengthening a therian's cross-species identity[25]. These unconsciously induced shifts are known as "involuntary shifts", whereas consciously induced shifts are "voluntary shifts".

As therians learn what triggers their shifts, they can gain more control over when and where they shift. By embodying their theriotype through voluntarily shifting at appropriate times and places, therians can reduce their feelings of species dysphoria[26].

In order to trigger a shift, therians may choose to meditate, surround themselves with nature, behave like their species, or interact with objects associated with their species[27]. For example, one former therian reported that donning a full wolf skin "invariably brings on a strong mental shift"[28]. However, some therians can shift without needing any specific rituals or environments to induce it[29].

Perhaps because so many therians identify as wolves, some of them report that a full moon can increase their shifting ability, cause emotional changes, or increase their sex drive[30]. One therian referred to this species euphoria as a "moon buzz" and noted that it paradoxically caused a restless, manic energy in some therians yet brought calmness to others[31].

Some therians don't shift in a binary fashion between human and animal. Instead, they exist on a spectrum between animal and human, fluidly wavering between the two[32].

Transspecies identity can also be a permanent state of being. Online surveys of therians have found that about one in five report a "constant" mental shift, and slightly more report a "constant" phantom shift (see Table 7.4.1)[33].

If the frequency of shifting that therians report is typical among people with autosexual trans identities, then the vast majority of autohet transgender people also experience shifts, with most doing so at least a couple times a week.

Different types of shifts are likely to have different impacts on feelings and identity. Phantom shifts create the sensation of phantom anatomy and thus can contribute to anatomic dysphoria. Similarly, mental shifts can make someone feel they have the consciousness of a particular type of entity, a sensation that is likely behind the internal sense of identity reported by people with various forms of trans identity.

When I first encountered the concept of shifting, it was a eureka moment for me. I saw it as a conceptual breakthrough that could help autosexuals interpret and speak about their cross-identity experiences more effectively. By creating and developing the concept of shifting, the therian community has made a great contribution to the broader autosexual population.

ZOOPHILIA—SEXUAL ATTRACTION TO ANIMALS

If therianthropy is caused by an erotic target identity inversion, then we should expect therians to report sexual attraction to animals (*zoophilia*) as well as sexual attraction to being an animal (*autozoophilia*).

As expected, therians are sexually attracted to animals at uncommonly high rates. In community surveys[34], about a third of therians admit they are attracted to animals[35], and a higher proportion don't deny being attracted to animals (see Table 7.4.2).

Sexuality Measure	Affirmative (%)	Any amount/ Not "no" (%)	N	Therian Survey
Any sexual attraction to furries	62	-	559	Therianthropy Community Survey #1
Attracted to animals	12	32	107	What kind of therian are you?
Attracted to animals with human brain	27	61	109	What kind of therian are you?
Attracted to theriotype	30	56	108	What kind of therian are you?
Any sexual attraction to animals	37	-	559	Therianthropy Community Survey #1
Sexual/romantic attraction to theriotype	37	-	216	Therianthropy and Gender Experience

Table 7.4.2: Therians' reported attraction to animals.

Studies of other populations find much lower rates of zoophilia. A Quebec-based study of sexual fantasies found that 2–3% of people had previously fantasized about having sex with an animal[36], and a study of male college students found that 5.3% of them had previously fantasized about animals during sexual intercourse[37]. Similarly, a representative survey of the Czech population found that 4% of males and 2% of females reported at least some zoophilic preference[38].

The proportion of therians who admit to zoophilic attractions far surpasses that of more general populations. Even if not all therians are willing to report sexual attraction to animals, enough do that it's reasonable to infer that an enduring pattern of attraction to animals plays a role in their cross-species identity.

This sexual-orientation-based explanation for therianthropy also makes sense of some of therianthropy's other aspects:

* Many therians report knowing of their animal nature their whole life, or at least since childhood
* Therians are likely to believe that therianthropy (or the capacity to develop it) is an inborn trait[39]
* They commonly discover their animal nature "around the ages 10–16 or whenever puberty starts"[40]
* Emulating animals leads to "special comfort and feelings of naturalness"[41]

These are the same sorts of beliefs and feelings reported by people with other autosexual orientations. The developmental timelines are also similar, as are the catalyzing effects of puberty.

Another curious similarity is that therians are more likely to have autism or mental health issues. One study comparing therians to non-therians found that therians were about six times as likely to show high levels of autistic traits and three to four times as likely to have been previously diagnosed with a mental health issue[42]. These elevated rates of autism and mental health diagnoses closely resemble those found among transgender people (see Chapters 4.2 and 4.3).

Data on zoophilia and autozoophilia from Hsu and Bailey's study of male furries also supports the idea that autozoophilia is an erotic target identity inversion. The correlation they found between zoophilia and autozoophilia (r=0.48) was about as strong as the one they found between gynephilia and autogynephilia (r=0.44)[43].

In the course of writing this chapter, I didn't find any formal research on therians that estimated how many of them are sexually attracted to being an animal. The results from therian and otherkin community surveys shown in the next chapter, however, suggest that it's common for therians to be their theriotype in their sexual fantasies or enjoy being treated as their theriotype in sexual contexts.

IN SUM

* Therians are people who feel a deep psychological or spiritual connection to a real, nonhuman animal species. Many of them identify as that species of animal.

* Therians can feel pain, discomfort, or dissatisfaction in response to the mismatch between their nonhuman animal identity and their human body. This species dysphoria can make them feel detached or alienated from

their human form and may serve as confirmation that they are truly therian.

* Therians created the concept of shifting to describe their experiences of cross-embodiment. The most common types of shifts are mental shifts and phantom shifts. For therians, mental shifts create a sense of having animalistic consciousness, and phantom shifts create a sense of having phantom anatomy such as fur, four legs, or a tail. These shifts, which usually correspond to their theriotype, help reduce species dysphoria by conferring a sense of animalistic embodiment.

* Many therians report knowing of their animal nature for all or most of their life, and they are likely to believe being therian is an inborn trait. They experience species euphoria by emulating animals, and they commonly discover their animal nature around the onset of puberty. They are also sexually attracted to animals at uncommonly high rates. Taken together, these traits and developmental patterns suggest that therianthropy is linked to autosexuality.

OTHERKIN

BEING A NONHUMAN ENTITY

Like other pubescent teenagers before them, Rumor was awakening to their inner dragon-like nature:[1]

> "My awakening sucked. It was a slow and painful process. At least, it was for the first few years...I couldn't shake my sense of identification with dragons, though it made no sense to me. I felt like I was a dragon on some level."[2]

Confused and seeking to understand their new feelings, Rumor found others on the internet who were dragons too. Learning that others felt the same way was a revelation, but they initially ran from their dragon identity and suppressed their draconic nature—a "masochistic approach" they later came to regret[3].

After exploring and accepting their identity, they were primarily left with "a sort of quiet sense of wonder". Like countless otherkin who came before them, they had become aware of the parts of themselves that weren't fully human. They had *awakened*.

Otherkin are a subculture of people who identify as not entirely human. They have a deep integral belief that they are a nonhuman entity in mind, spirit, energy, or some other nonphysical manner.

Otherkin have traditionally been fictional or mythological creatures such as dragons, elves, faeries, or vampires. The nonhuman entity that an otherkin identifies as is their *kintype*.

Therians also fall under the otherkin umbrella and can be thought of as otherkin whose kintypes are real, nonhuman animals.

Otherkin who identify as mythological creatures such as dragons, elves, and faeries are *mythkin*, those who identify as characters from fictional media are *fictionkin*, and those who identify as objects such as cars, dolls, or furniture are *objectkin*.

All these different identities are beyond the scope of what is traditionally considered human, so they are all forms of alterhuman identity.

Like therians, the dysphoria that some otherkin experience pertains to the incongruence between their nonhuman identity and their physical human body, so some otherkin are also susceptible to species dysphoria[4]—a sensation that's been described as "feeling displaced in a human body when you feel you should be in an entirely different one"[5]. Otherkin may also feel out of place or feel a homesick longing to return "home"[6].

KINTYPE EMBODIMENT: KINSHIFTING, BODY ADORNMENTS, AND BODY MODIFICATIONS

When otherkin shift, they call it *kinshifting*. It's fundamentally the same phenomenon as therioshifting, so otherkin also use the language around shifting that was pioneered by therians[7].

During a kinshift, otherkin feel more like their kintype in body or mind.

When otherkin undergo a mental shift, they feel more like their kintype mentally. During this experience, they may behave more like their kintype or feel that their sensory perception is similar to their kintype (i.e., a sensory shift).

When in a phantom shift, otherkin can feel the presence of phantom body parts corresponding to their kintype. If they are a dragon, they may feel wings, scales, or a tail. If they are a demon, they may feel horns on their head. However, some otherkin experience combinations of phantom anatomy that don't neatly fit with any singular kintype.

To induce shifts, otherkin may adorn their bodies with costumes, jewelry, makeup, or specially themed garments that remind them of their kintypes[8]. This *species transvestism* is like crossdressing, but for species instead of gender.

In the Nonhumanity & Body Modification/Decoration Survey[9], a survey of otherkin that explored nonhuman embodiment through body modifications and adornments, otherkin were most likely to say they decorated or modified their body for self-expression or aesthetics. Among those who engaged in body decoration, 67% said that relieving dysphoria was a motivator. Only 13% said the same for sexual gratification[10].

When asked to explain their motivations, most spoke about species dysphoria or self-expression. But some spoke to the sexual side of their use of body adornments for cross-species embodiment[11]:

"It makes me feel good, in charge of my sexuality and brings forth my feelings of nonhumanism."

"Everything from 'just plain fun' to sex things to achieving feelings of bodily comfort/euphoria. Many of these things overlap."

"Some of it is for pet play, which itself is something I'm into because of my animal identity."

Even though these reports are primarily about species rather than gender, it's uncanny how similar they are to testimonials from autohet trans people. Translated into the language of gender, that last quote would instead read, "Some of it is for gender play, which itself is something I'm into because of my gender identity".

I've seen this type of statement made by plenty of trans women who believe their sexual interest in female embodiment is an outgrowth of their gender identity or gender dysphoria rather than the other way around. If autosexuality underlies otherkin identity and most cases of transgenderism, this overlap in thought patterns is not only unsurprising, *it's to be expected.*

Perhaps this is why an FTM respondent to that same survey said nonhuman-related body decorations and chest binding cause similar feelings:

> "It greatly eases my dysphoria. Wearing non-human related body decoration as an otherkin gives me a feeling similar to binding my chest as a trans person. It helps me to feel more comfortable in my existence and can even feel therapeutic at times."[12]

Like autohet transsexuals, many otherkin want to permanently modify their body to more fully embody their idealized self-image. In the body modifications survey, many respondents already had conventional body mods such as piercings or tattoos, and those who had not yet gotten body mods usually wanted to get them.

Otherkin also showed interest in unconventional body mods such as getting their tongue split, ears shaped, or teeth sharpened. Subdermal implants and genital modifications were also on their radar. Among otherkin who wanted to get body mods, 75% said it was related to their nonhumanity, and 60% thought that future body mods would help relieve their dysphoria[13].

Otherkin who had already gotten body mods usually said it was done out of self-expression or for aesthetics. Some said they did it for spiritual reasons or to relieve dysphoria. A few said it was for sexual gratification.

Overall, these otherkin wanted body mods for the same reasons as other kinds of autosexuals—to feel at home in their body, to feel whole, or to alleviate dysphoria:

> "To relieve dysphoria regarding having breasts and nipples as an avian."

> "I chose to get body modifications related to my nonhumanity as an attempt to minimize discomfort in the body I am forced to occupy."

> "Just like wearing gear, my body modifications give me a sense of wholeness."

As with autohet transsexuals, otherkin speak of feeling alienated from their body because of mind–body incongruencies and report feeling better after modifying their bodies to suit their identities.

FICTIONKIN AND OBJECTKIN

Within the otherkin community, there are no hard and fast rules about which kintypes are "valid". For instance, otherkin are fairly split about whether people who identify as characters from TV shows, cartoons, or movies have "valid" kintypes[14].

On the other hand, they're seemingly more unified regarding the legitimacy of objectkin: five out of seven respondents to one otherkin community survey said they wouldn't accept inanimate objects as kintypes[15]. In response to this invalidation, an objectkin may defend their identity with their belief in animism (the idea that plants, objects, and natural phenomena have souls) and argue that their identities are just as real and valid as other kintypes[16].

Objectkin are uncommon. Aside from the therian subset of otherkin, most otherkin identify as mythical creatures or as members of mythical humanoid races. But given that people can be sexually attracted to objects (*objectophilic*), it stands to reason that some of them will be sexually attracted to the idea of being particular objects (autoobjectophilic), and therefore a few will even come to identify as those objects.

IDENTITY: DEGREE, AGENCY, AND COPING

In considering nonhuman identity, both the strength of that identity and whether it was consciously chosen are important factors. Although otherkin identify *as* nonhuman beings and this identity is often regarded as involuntary, not all alterhumans have this degree of identity or see their identity as involuntary.

To give voice to their experiences, alterhumans created identity labels that vary depending on the strength of nonhuman identity, whether it was chosen freely, and whether it stemmed from a desire to cope with emotional suffering:

* Strength of stated identity—identifying *as* or identifying *with*?
* Degree of agency—was the identity taken on voluntarily or involuntarily?
* Emotional context—is the identity a means of coping with suffering?

When an alterhuman individual identifies *with* a nonhuman being, they are *other-hearted*[17]. Similar to how someone who identifies *as* a dragon is "dragonkin", someone who identifies with dragons is "dragon-hearted".

Other-hearted individuals identify *with* a nonhuman being, not *as* that being[18]. Although this connection to a type of nonhuman being doesn't quite reach the level of believing that one *is* that type of being, it's still a strong connection.

The distinction is similar to the difference between "kin"—which describes someone's relatives—and "kith", which describes someone's familiar friends and acquaintances. Therefore, other-hearted individuals are also called "otherkith", and the species they identify with is their "kithtype". For example, someone who identifies with vampires can be described as "vampire-hearted" or "vampirekith".

People who consciously choose a nonhuman identity are called "otherlinks" or "otherlinkers", and their "linktype" is the type of entity they've consciously chosen to identify as[19]. The voluntary nature of an otherlink identity differentiates them from otherkin, whose nonhuman identity is considered involuntary.

Since alterhumans have developed this language to tell apart voluntary and involuntary identities, the amount of agency involved in the development of nonhuman identity seems to be a crucial consideration for them.

Whether a person chose the identity or adopted it as a coping mechanism matters too. "Copinglinks" are alterhumans who have consciously chosen to identify as or with a nonhuman entity or fictional human identity as a coping mechanism[20]. But for some reason, the "copinglink" label wasn't too popular among the people it described, so a broader "otherlink" category was created to accommodate voluntary nonhuman identities in a way that didn't seem to portray them as less valid or important.

There's no way to objectively know if a particular alterhuman individual is actually an otherkin, otherkith, or otherlink. As with matters of gender identity, they have to be taken at their word—sometimes quite literally: it might be a word you've never heard before.

XENOGENDERS

Alterhuman identities are beyond the scope of what is traditionally seen as human, so many otherkin have trouble relating to human notions of gender. As a result, otherkin often have a type of nonbinary gender identity called *xenogender*. The prefix "xeno" comes from the ancient Greek word "xénos", meaning "alien".

Xenogenders can't be contained by human conceptions of gender and instead relate to animals, plants, objects, or other concepts not traditionally associated with human gender[21].

Faerie otherkin may describe their gender as "faegender", and dragonkin may describe their gender as "dragongender". Because kintype influences these xenogenders, they are a type of "kingender".

Otherkin have also created labels for the gendered nature of their animal identities such as "buckgender", a gender that encompasses masculine animal energy, and "doegender", a gender that encompasses feminine animal energy.

When it comes to xenogenders, it seems there's no limit to the possibilities. In fact, the limitlessness of xenogenders calls into question whether they truly count as gender identities.

Xenogenders Are Genders If Gender Is "Who You Are"

The idea that gender identity is simply "who you are" is fairly common in the gender-variant community. Even large nonprofit organizations like Stonewall UK sometimes describe gender identity as "who you are"[22]. Given such broad conceptions of gender identity, it was inevitable that xenogenders would arise and that people would promote them as legitimate gender identities.

After all, who can say that an autohet person's internal sense of being the other gender counts as a gender identity, but an otherkin's internal sense of being their kintype doesn't?

Otherkin often see themselves as their kintype during sexual fantasies and also like being treated as such in sexual situations. This preference suggests that otherkin have an autosexual attraction to being their kintype, and thus can also have an internal sense of being their kintype akin to how autoheterosexuals can have an internal sense of being the other sex.

If gender identity is as broad as "who you are", then xenogenders are gender identities just as the cross-gender identities of autoheterosexuals are gender identities.

But if the concept of gender were limited to human femaleness and maleness, then xenogenders wouldn't count as gender identities. They would still be a type of identity, but "gender" wouldn't be the right word to describe them.

OTHERKIN AND HUMAN GENDER VARIANCE

Nonhuman identity and transgender identity coincide too often for their co-occurrence to be a fluke.

An estimated 0.6% of US adults[23] and 1.8% of US high school students[24] identify as transgender. A recent Gallup survey found that among Americans, 1.2% of millennials and 1.8% of zoomers identified as transgender[25]. Overall, it seems that fewer than 2% of Americans identify as transgender.

Otherkin, though, are far more likely to identify as transgender. Otherkin community surveys[26] indicate that about a third of otherkin identify as transgender (see Table 7.5.1), and an even higher proportion have a suprabinary gender identity (see Table 7.5.2).

As seen in Table 7.5.1, community surveys of otherkin from 2013 to 2021 suggest that in recent years, *the proportion of otherkin who identified as transgender increased by approximately 3% per year*—a rate of change that itself exceeds the total proportion of transgender Americans, which is likely under 2%.

TG identity (%)	Year	N	Survey Name
8	2013	112	Werelist Poll of 2013
12	2015	67	KIN survey
27	2020	219	Therianthropy and Gender Experience
29	2021	113	What kind of therian are you?
34	2021	156	Alterhumanity and sexuality

Table 7.5.1: Transgender identity rates in therians and otherkin.

Survey Name	Female %	Male %	Other %	Year	N
2012 Therian Census	37	33	30	2012	134
2013 Therian Census	44	34	23	2013	291
Werelist Poll of 2013	50	33	18	2013	112
KIN survey	36	46	18	2015	67
Otherkin Survey	42	35	23	2018	48
What kind of therian are you?	31	31	38	2021	113
Alterhumanity and sexuality	22	29	49	2021	156

Table 7.5.2: Prevalence of female, male, and suprabinary gender identities in therians and otherkin.

Relatedly, the gender of a therian's animal side is more likely to match their human gender than their human sex.

In 2020, a prominent internet therian named PinkDolphin surveyed the therian community about their therianthropic and gender experiences[27]. In his survey titled "Therianthropy and Gender Experience", PinkDolphin found that the gender of a therian's theriotype was more likely to match their human gender than their human sex: only 32% of therians said their theriotype's gender didn't match their human gender identity, whereas a solid 53% of respondents had theriotypes whose genders didn't match the sex of their human body[28].

Additionally, about a third said they experienced human gender dysphoria because of their theriotype's sex traits[29]. It seems that for some transgender therians, their different dysphorias feel similar. Their personal accounts also suggest that their animal identities can inform their human gender identities, and vice versa.

In this and the following section, I will draw upon written responses from community surveys to support my assertion that autosexuality is the primary cause of transspecies identity. Most responses shown here are unaltered, but I sometimes made small changes to spelling or grammar for clarity.

One therian felt that transgenderism and therianthropy were linked and remarked how their respective dysphorias felt similar:

"I experience gender dysphoria, and I think gender- and species-dysphoria feel very similar. Because of that, I think transness and therianthropy are very similar, and I don't personally have much issue with the term 'trans-species'."[30]

A stallion therian reported that his gender identity and animal identity mutually reinforced each other:

"My gender identity influences my therianthropy and vice versa. My therianthropy doesn't have a separate gender from my gender. I am transgender because I am a man in a female body as I am a therianthrope because I am a horse in a human body. So naturally they come together to make me see myself as a 'stallion.'"[31]

For an FTM therian of unspecified theriotype, the maleness of his animal side helped him realize he was transgender:

"Interestingly, I viewed myself as the male version of my theriotype before I fully came to terms with me being FtM transgender...In a way, my nonhuman identity helped me 'ease' into accepting myself as male."[32]

One otherkin reported that their human-like kintypes impacted their human gender identity more than their theriotypes:

"My human/humanoid fictotypes generally affect my gender identity more than my theriotype does because their experiences with gender are human experiences that relate more directly to my own human experience, while non human animals have a very different experience of gender than humans do."[33]

In another survey of otherkin[34], one respondent described how his gender feelings and species feelings were entwined, making it hard to separate the two. He identified as buckgender, an identity that encompasses nonhuman feelings of masculinity:

"My gender identity and my otherkin identity are deeply intertwined and I find it impossible to compartmentalise and separate my identity feelings into categories of 'gender' and 'species'. My gender, buckgender, is meant to represent the way that I parse/process gender from a non-human perspective."[35]

Understandably, otherkin with identities that aren't carbon-based can have particular difficulty relating to human gender. Some robotkin have reported that their attractions to machines were connected to their intense dysphorias or that their gender identity was best described as "robot":

"A majority of my identity is mechanical. I have attractions to machines and have extreme dysphoria (species and gender) relating to this at times."[36]

"I put 'robot' as my gender on this survey because it is truly how I feel. The level of disconnect to humanity I feel absolutely influences my gender, and describing it in human terms is incredibly hard."[37]

Sexual attractions to machines are pretty rare: it would be quite a coincidence if robotkin were attracted to machines, but sexuality was unrelated to their mechanical identity.

OTHERKIN SEXUALITY:
"ANYTHING SEXUAL MAKES ME SHIFTY AF"

In 2020, the Alterhumanity and Sexuality Survey[38] asked 156 otherkin about their sexuality and got responses that usually indicated the presence of autosexuality: most respondents affirmed they've been their kintype in sexual fantasies or that they enjoy being treated as their kintype by their sexual partners (see Table 7.5.3).

Their allosexuality showed similar patterns: most said they were sexually attracted to their kintypes or that they consume porn of their kintypes.

Even fictionkin (people who identify as characters from fictional media) showed a similar pattern. A majority of fictionkin fantasized about being their fictotype or admitted to consuming pornography related to their fictotype.

This attraction to kintypes is arguably the norm. One therian reported, "I'm zoo for my type...This is *normal* for all therians. If they deny it they are either lying, or it affects them so little, it doesn't matter/register"[39].

When fantasizing, otherkin often imagine they are their kintypes. One dragonkin found this quite arousing, reporting that "the idea of transforming into my kintype is very arousing to me, and of course as a dragon I like the idea of having sex with my own kind"[40].

For one otherkin, a primal headspace was seemingly a prerequisite for them to get turned on: "sex only seems interesting if I'm in a werewolfy or more animal state of mind", reported one werewolfkin[41].

Measure of Sexuality	Affirmative (%)	Any Amount/ Not "No" (%)	N
Consume furry porn	56	78	155
Consume porn of kintype	51	69	156
Find kintype attractive (nonhuman kintype)	54	73	153
Enjoy being sexually/romantically treated as kintype	74	94	128*
Is kintype in sexual fantasies	57	75	154
Fantasize about being fictionkin-type	61	74	61
Consume porn about/from fictionkin-type source	49	66	61

Table 7.5.3: Prevalence of allosexual and autosexual interests in kintypes among otherkin and therians.
*Write-ins excluded; Affirmative = sometimes/somewhat or higher.
Source: Alterhumanity and Sexuality Survey (Lopori 2021).

A dragonkin noted the connection between their dragon side and their sexuality when they disclosed, "when I really start to get in the mood, my dragon side starts to come out more and my sex drive goes from 0 to 10 real quick"[42].

They weren't the only otherkin who shifted while aroused: most respondents said they'd shifted during sex or masturbation before[43]. As one of them noted, sexuality usually brought on shifts: "Phantom sensations everywhere, mental shift, sensory shifts. Anything sexual makes me shifty AF"[44].

Like human-based manifestations of autosexuality, signs of alterhumanity can be present before puberty, and puberty makes its sexual nature apparent. One horsekin reported, "I was a horse before puberty and when I had my wet dream it was about a mare"[45].

Some otherkin have difficulty with conventional sexual expression because they aren't sexually attracted to humans enough to pursue or sustain a relationship with one. If that other human is otherkin, though, it helps: one otherkin reported, "I have very little attraction towards humans, and feel more attraction to people whose identities are more similar to mine, i.e. kin folks, and furries"[46].

Even if their conventional sexuality is intact enough to be attracted to humans, otherkin might feel too much incongruence between their nonhuman identity and their human body to find a sexual way of being that works for them:

"My struggle to connect with my body definitely changes how comfortable I am receiving sexual acts. I think it changes my level of attraction to others as well. I also really struggle to perceive/understand gender, which makes it difficult to define my attraction based on that."[47]

Like furries, otherkin have elevated rates of nonheterosexual orientations. In fact, they're more likely to claim a sexual identity indicating attraction to multiple genders (i.e., bisexual, queer, or pansexual) than they are to say they're heterosexual[48].

When people are sexually attracted to being another species, the knowledge that it's mating season can strongly affect their libido. One deerkin reported peak libido during deer rutting season:

"My sex drive often feels a bit more primal in a sense. I notice this a lot in the kind of kinks that I express as well, such as vore. I also get *mega* horny around deer rutting season."[49]

This deerkin wasn't the only one whose primal side lent itself to an interest in *vore* (a sexual interest in being eaten alive, or in eating a creature or person alive). Most respondents to the Alterhumanity and Sexuality survey reported kinks like this which are difficult or impossible to enact in reality[50].

Among otherkin who reported such kinks, 20% were into vore, and 28% were into *transformation* (sexual interest in transforming into something else)[51]. In her write-up, the survey creator remarked, "It is of no surprise that transformation is so popular; we all like to imagine turning into our kintypes whether in a kinky way or not"[52].

Altogether, these survey results support the idea that otherkin experience cross-species identity and species dysphoria because of autosexual attraction to being their kintypes. Thus, their internal cross-embodiment experiences are just as emotionally significant as those experienced by people with other forms of autosexuality.

IN SUM

* Otherkin are a subculture of people who identify as not entirely human. They have a deep integral belief they are a nonhuman entity in mind, spirit, energy, or another nonphysical manner. The type of nonhuman entity an otherkin identifies as is their kintype. Otherkin may have mythical kintypes such as dragons or demons, fictional kintypes based on fictional characters, or even object kintypes such as dolls or cars. Therians are the subset of otherkin who identify as real, nonhuman animals.

* Otherkin embody their kintypes through mental shifts and phantom shifts. During these shifts, they may feel they have the mind state of their kintype or sense the presence of phantom anatomy corresponding to their kintype. These shifts may be voluntary or involuntary, temporary or permanent. The degree to which an otherkin shifts varies between individuals, as do the types of shifts they have.

* To facilitate nonhuman embodiment, some otherkin adorn their bodies with costumes, jewelry, makeup, or specially themed garments that remind them of their kintypes. When asked about this species transvestism, they are most likely to say they do it to reduce species dysphoria, but some say that sexuality plays a role. To

more fully embody their kintype on a permanent basis, some otherkin seek body modifications such as tongue splitting, teeth sharpening, or ear shaping.

* It is orthodox opinion among otherkin that being otherkin requires identifying *as* a nonhuman entity and that the propensity to be otherkin is an innate trait, so they've created a set of labels to describe alterhuman identities that don't meet these requirements. These labels differ based on the stated strength of the identity, the degree of agency involved in coming to it, and whether the identity was adopted for emotional ends.

* Otherkin have created a special set of nonbinary gender identities to describe their feeling of being something that falls outside of human notions of gender. These xenogenders may describe their nonhuman kintype (e.g., dragongender) or represent a confluence of nonhumanity and gender (e.g., doegender, buckgender). For xenogenders to not count as gender identities, the construct of gender identity must be restricted to human notions of masculinity and femininity.

* Community surveys reveal that otherkin are far more likely to identify as transgender or have suprabinary gender identities than the general population. In the last decade, transgender identification rates among otherkin

increased about 3% per year. Therians tend to have more concordance between their animal and human genders than they do between their animal gender and human sex. The identities and dysphorias of their animal and human sides may each inform the other, so it can be hard for them to differentiate between the two influences.

* When surveyed about their sexuality, most otherkin admit they are sexually attracted to their kintype or consume porn depicting it, and most say they've been their kintype in sexual fantasies or like being treated as their kintypes in sexual situations. Thoughts of being their kintype can bring on sexual arousal, mental shifts, or phantom shifts. In short, otherkin are sexually attracted both to and to being that which they identify as, consistent with the general pattern seen among autosexual orientations.

TRANSRACE

BEING A PARTICULAR RACE

Born to strict Christian parents and bound to her family's homestead property, Nkechi Diallo (pronounced "en-kay-chee dee-ah-loh") would dream of being elsewhere whenever she got the chance. Hidden in a distant part of her family's garden, she sometimes spread watery mud on her arms and legs to pretend she was an African princess or Bantu woman[1].

She had been introduced to images and stories of African people through the *National Geographic* subscription her grandmother gave her one Christmas. She thought they were beautiful and interesting, so much so that she longed to be one. Diallo saw herself as black and felt she was black too[2].

Later, she encountered black American athletes through issues of *Sports Illustrated*. They captured her full attention:

> "I was enraptured by what I saw. To me, the images of the Black athletes I found on the pages of the magazines were the very height of human beauty. Their complexions, their hair, their features, they were all so captivating to me."[3]

In the pages of these magazines, she was introduced to Darryl Strawberry, Magic Johnson, and Mike Tyson. She was infatuated with all three, which left a lasting impression: "Though all three soon faded from my consciousness, the idealized image of Blackness I'd developed while studying photographs of them never did"[4].

When Diallo was a teenager, her parents adopted four black babies. With their arrival, she finally felt like she truly had a family[5]. As they grew, she taught them what she had learned about black culture and history from the many library books she had read on the subject[6]. Doing so made her feel more connected to black culture. She increasingly felt as though she saw the world through a black perspective[7].

In college, she learned that race was a social construct that wasn't based on genetics. This made her feel less obligated to identify as white[8]. The first time she had her hair fully braided, it was a game changer[9]. She felt more at home in herself and noticed that black people treated her in a more familiar, less guarded way.

After completing her undergraduate degree, Diallo was accepted to grad school at Howard University, the only school she applied to[10]. She married a black man while there, but he didn't like her cross-race embodiment and kept imploring her to be more white[11]. They soon divorced.

Diallo later became the president of the Spokane, Washington, chapter of the NAACP. On June 10, 2015, a local news reporter interviewed her and questioned her racial identity. Overwhelmed by that line of questioning, she abruptly turned off her mic and ended the interview[12].

Within days, news articles depicting her as a white woman pretending to be black filled people's social media feeds[13]. The articles often portrayed her as an object of ridicule. To many, she was a laughingstock. For a minute, she was the talk of the nation simply because she was born to parents of European descent yet identified as black. Her name was Rachel Dolezal at the time.

Diallo's story spurred a national conversation about transracialism. Before her, transracialism usually referred to the cultural experience of children adopted by parents of another race.

But the kind of transracialism that comes from adoption isn't the subject of this chapter. Instead, I'll investigate a type of transracialism characterized by autosexual attraction to being a particular race.

PHYLOPHILIA: RACE-BASED SEXUAL ATTRACTION

Although the existence of race-based attraction is common knowledge, there hasn't been a neutral term for it. It's often called "racial fetishism"[14].

Unfortunately, the "racial fetishism" label seemingly implies that race-based sexual attraction is less legitimate or worthy than other kinds of sexual attraction. To put race-based sexual attraction on equal standing with other dimensions of sexual attraction, I will instead use a Greek construction that adheres to standard naming conventions.

Phylophilia is a race-based sexual attraction ("phylo" means "tribe", "kind", or "race"). For example, if someone were specifically attracted to people of a particular racial appearance, this attraction could be described as phylophilic. Instead of making a separate term for each race, I'll use *phylophilia* as an umbrella term for race-based sexual attraction and leave it at that.

The autosexual counterpart to phylophilia is *autophylophilia*, a sexual attraction to being a particular race.

Anne Lawrence's book contained a narrative from someone who specifically fantasized about being a woman of another race. They reported, "I am an Asian male, but I do not fantasize about being an Asian woman, but rather a Caucasian woman, because I prefer and am most sexually attracted to Caucasian women"[15].

It stands to reason that if race-based attraction exists, then so does attraction to being a particular race. And if attraction to being a particular race exists, then so does a type of trans identity associated with that attraction. That's why I think autophylophilia is the most likely cause of these newer cases of transrace identity that make such big waves in the media.

This newer type of transracialism is *autophylophilic transracialism* because it occurs when a person develops a cross-race identity as a result of autosexual attraction to being that race.

If this theory seems far-fetched, consider a recent prominent case of transracialism, that of Oli London. In June of 2021, they came out as Korean and identified specifically as Jimin, a K-pop star they adore[16]. Although they didn't outright say that their transrace identity had sexual roots, they *did* marry a cardboard cutout of Jimin the year before[17]. More recently, they came out as a transgender woman[18].

MULTIPLE TYPES OF TRANSRACE IDENTITY

One type of transracialism, *adoptive transracialism*, is the product of transracial adoption: when parents of one race adopt a child of another race.

There are also historical examples of people who chose to live as another race because it afforded them better social treatment, such as light-skinned descendants of slaves in America who could pass as white.

These types of transracialism are associated with specific life circumstances, so I'll use *situational transracialism* as an umbrella term for cases of transracialism that are related to life circumstances rather than sexuality. Adoptive transracialism is one type of situational transracialism.

Some cases of transracialism are associated with sexuality (autophylophilic transracialism), while others are associated with life circumstances (situational transracialism). Thus, there are multiple distinct types of transracialism.

INVESTIGATING TRANSRACIALISM

When I initially looked into transracialism, I quickly realized there was little empirical research about it. There were plenty of opinion pieces making fun of it, but very little on what it actually *was*.

Given what I knew about various forms of autosexual trans identity, I suspected that an autosexual version of race-based sexual attraction caused transracialism. After all, there are otherkin who identify as elves and vampires. The ears or teeth of these mythical races may be especially pointy, but they often look quite similar to humans. I figured that if cross-race identification as a mythical humanoid race could stem from autosexuality, cross-race identification as a real human race likely could as well.

I created a transracialism survey[19] to explore this possibility. The online transracialism community is small and understandably wary of outsiders asking questions, but I was still able to collect some responses. At the time of this writing, I'd received thirteen responses from transrace people.

Since I specifically wanted to study autophylophilic transracialism, I excluded four responses from this analysis because they reported a lack of arousal to any forms of cross-race embodiment. A couple of these gave contradictory answers about how often they were their identified race in sexual fantasies, but overall, they reportedly never fantasized about various elements of being their identified race. I will rule them out as being either not autophylophilic, or insufficiently so. Among these four excluded responses, three were female and one was male.

I categorized the remaining nine responses as cases of autophylophilic transracialism. All nine said they were "frequently" or "often" their identified race in sexual fantasies. In contrast, all but one said they were "rarely" or "never" their assigned race[20] in sexual fantasies.

There were two females, both of whom reported a sexual preference for women. Of the seven males, six were transgender or nonbinary. All were under forty years of age. Four respondents were in their early twenties, three were in their late twenties, and two were in their thirties.

In addition to multiple-choice questions, I also asked some open-ended questions in order to get written responses. I've presented most of the written responses here just as I received them. In a few, I made small tweaks to grammar or syntax to improve clarity.

I posted the survey in two transracial subreddits and one transracial Facebook group. Based on submission time stamps, I suspect that seven respondents came from the transracial subreddits and two from the transracial Facebook group.

FIRST SIGNS OF TRANSRACIALISM

To see if the developmental trajectory of transracialism paralleled the trajectory of other types of trans identity, I asked when their first signs of being transracial appeared and what those signs were. I also inquired about how they became aware of their transrace identity.

One of the female respondents wrote about her transrace awakening, which occurred at an age when many females are going through puberty:

"It hit me like a truck. I was thinking about what I should even do since I was no longer satisfied by the immigration fantasy, and I imagined different versions of myself. It was a long time ago so I don't remember exactly what I thought about, but it clicked really fast that 'Asian me' was the real me. I felt like she was beautiful and that's what was missing from me. I knew something was off for a long time and I didn't know what until then. It was like a lightbulb moment."

An MTF explained how her experiences with black female classmates made her aware of her cross-race inclination. It happened at an age when many males start puberty:

"Honestly, [I] became more aware of the feelings when I understood what being transgender meant. Got me thinking about where my envy of the black girls I met in school came from. Realized I was meant to be a black female. Just feel more comfortable identifying that way."

Her sense of kinship with black girls at school helped her realize she wanted to be one: "Mostly a kinship with the black girls in my school. Wishing I looked like them, talked like them, and just had experienced their life more so than my own".

A nonbinary male exhibited the first signs of transracialism around five or six years of age, the earliest of any respondents. They reported the following signs: "Staying out of the sun in an attempt to lighten my skin, never identifying with my birth race, hating the color of parts that were dark. Staying away from people of my assigned race".

Unfortunately, many of the respondents first questioned if they were transracial after encountering media about it, and most of that media was negative.

MEDIA COVERAGE OF TRANSRACIALISM

I asked respondents how they felt about media coverage of transracialism. I wanted their side to be heard, because transracial voices are frequently left out of transracialism discourse.

They were united in perceiving media coverage of transracialism as negative and unfair to them. Most of them also wrote about how it hurt and why. It made one feel like "a weirdo", while another felt "awful, like I'm not even human".

One of the females had been hurt several times in this way: "People's cruelty, hate, and mockery has ruined my day several times. I ugly cried about an article I read about us because it was so wrong about my experience and so hateful".

One MTF shared that it "makes me feel sad and judged. I can't help how I feel inside". Another noted that "they're always making fun of us. Nobody has defended us yet and it hurts to see that I have to be in the closet about this still".

I asked them what they wanted the general public to know about transracialism. In response, survey respondents stressed their common humanity and asked for open-mindedness.

One said, "I didn't choose this". Another reinforced the importance of belonging: "I'm not lying. It is such a privilege to wake up and belong, please keep that in mind". Another said, "We're real human beings with real feelings. We're for real".

One of the transfem respondents remarked that "it's no different than being transgender". A couple of the other transfem respondents made clear their racial identifications were sincere, and they weren't trying to be offensive:

"We're not playing racial dress-up or blackface, we fully intend to live as our identified race all pros and cons included such as enduring racism once we pass, racists won't check your parental lineage before being racist to a darker person."

"We aren't trying to offend people. We want to identify the way we do and we feel comfortable/euphoric. Don't take this away from us. We aren't challenging your identity. We can both exist at the same time."

Overall, the transracial respondents made it clear that being transrace (*trace*) wasn't easy. One asked the public for understanding:

"Please be understanding. Stop mocking people for trying to figure themselves out. Being trace is a curse as it is, we don't need hate on top of that. It's been really hard for me, I imagine it's been hard for others."

Unfortunately, the pain of being ridiculed in the media was far from their only obstacle. They also had to deal with race dysphoria.

RACE DYSPHORIA

Race dysphoria was common in these nine participants. All but one reported strong race dysphoria. Like transgender people, they reported the strongest race dysphoria with respect to their bodies and social roles.

When describing how race dysphoria felt, they didn't hold back. A female respondent spoke to the feeling of hopelessness and entrapment that characterized her race dysphoria:

"It's hell. It's the most uncomfortable thing I experience. I feel hopeless and trapped when I experience it. I feel physically sick when I see my reflection when I'm having it. Sometimes it feels like there is nothing that can be done about it."

A transfem respondent wrote about the overlapping pain of both her types of dysphoria. She described it as "a dreadful emotional weight that I'll be eternally stuck in the body of a white male. It's constantly there and ruins my day".

Another transfem remarked that race dysphoria felt "very similar to gender dysphoria; crushing, depressing", while another said it felt "like you're trapped in someone else's body".

"When I am in the closet," wrote another transfem, "it is as if I have to be a stereotype of the race I was assigned at birth. Whereas when I'm able to express myself as my true race I feel more authentic".

This sense of self-alienation came up in a few responses. "Every time you go outside", reported a nonbinary male respondent, "it's like someone else you don't know is representing you, talking for you instead of you talking". A female respondent even said this sense of separation transcended herself because it was "a disconnect from not only you, but your ancestors".

The emotions these respondents described—feeling trapped, hopeless, disconnected, and depressed—are the same types of feelings that autohet trans people describe when they talk about gender dysphoria.

To get a sense for which situations triggered their race dysphoria, I asked if they had noticed any patterns about the types of situations that caused them to feel dysphoric. One transfem captured the overall pattern when she said a dysphoria-causing situation could be "any in which my assigned race is brought into attention".

Other transracial respondents noted how having their racial identity invalidated, hearing their birth name, or wearing clothes associated with their assigned race could all dampen their spirits:

"Being reminded that I'm white is like a bullet. People calling me white and shit triggers the hell out of me. Same with being told I'm not Asian. If I look in the mirror too long I get triggered too."

"Situations such as being around people of my assigned race, wearing ethnic clothing, looking at old family pictures, hearing or reading your first and last name, and eating food that belongs to your assigned race when other people are around."

One of the transfem respondents mentioned the pain of intersecting race and gender dysphorias, saying, "Every waking moment existing as a white male and not a black female is such a weight". Another said she was hurt by "racialized situations where I get treated as a white person or people that deny my blackness".

Overall, it seemed that any perceived shortcomings of cross-racial embodiment could drag down their mood. Seeing themselves in the mirror, hearing their assigned name, and behaving or being seen by others as their assigned race could all bum them out.

RACE EUPHORIA

Knowing that autoheterosexuals treasure gender euphoria, I asked about race euphoria. I wanted to see if transracial people described similar feelings of comfort, joy, and being at home in themselves. Unsurprisingly, they did.

Just as many respondents noted that race dysphoria created an internal disconnect within themselves, many also said that race euphoria made them feel more in touch with themselves.

A nonbinary male said race euphoria felt "like I'm closer to being myself", while a female respondent said she felt "belonging and present in my body". A transfem reported that when she was feeling race euphoria, "I feel like I am being genuine to myself. And less of a caricature".

One transracial female found race euphoria comforting and acknowledged, "It's not very intense yet since I haven't had anything major done to convert to my desired race, but the little scraps that I get really help".

Various transfem respondents said that race euphoria made them feel "happy with myself and my body", "ecstatic, amazing, joyful", or "like you can be free and yourself for a while".

Another transfem said that during a race euphoria experience, "a sense of calm of self washes over me. Life and my goals become far more clear. As well, just feel more whole".

As with the questions about dysphoria, I asked transracial respondents if they noticed any patterns regarding the specific situations that led them to feel race euphoria. In response, they told me of various ways they attained a sense of cross-race embodiment.

A female respondent remarked on the helpfulness of sartorial embodiment: "Dyeing my hair, dressing a certain way, and doing my make up a certain way can really help me feel better. Also, being honest with people about how I really feel helps a lot, especially if they are supportive".

A transfem spoke to feeling racially embodied through interpersonal interactions: "My partners all know I'm trans black and support me and treat me in a way that acknowledges my blackness when appropriate and even pokes fun at it where appropriate".

A nonbinary male said that "shaving and wearing sunscreen are the two biggest ones". A transfem reported that "getting tan" and "imagination" helped her feel race euphoria. A different transfem noticed gender euphoria from "dressing, acting, and being as close to who I actually am inside", while another said it happened "whenever I can just focus on being myself".

A transfem who had put effort into learning the language of her identified race said that "speaking to others in our language absolutely helps me feel euphoric".

Imagination. Behavior. Fashions. Social interactions. These are the same avenues that countless autosexuals have used to attain various forms of cross-embodiment.

I also asked transracial respondents how they felt when consuming media that helped them get in touch with their transrace identity. They reported "joy", "recognition", and "a sense of belonging, warmth, love, and respect". Another felt "happiness and comfort" and explained, "It's like a light for me in a dark world". Others reported feeling "happiness, confidence, pleasure", or "joy, euphoria, longing, sadness".

Perhaps for historical reasons, a trans-indigenous respondent didn't feel so good about consuming media relating to her transrace identity. She reported feeling grief and elaborated, "I've inherited all of the intergenerational trauma and none of the community".

MEDICAL TRANSRACIALISM

Virtually all the transracial people under analysis here were interested in medical interventions to more closely align their racial appearance with their racial identity.

With the exception of the one trans-indigenous respondent who already passed as her identified race, *all* the other cases discussed here were interested in getting facial surgery to more fully attain their desired racial appearance, and all but one were interested in drugs to change their skin color.

Yet even though interest in these drugs and surgeries was high, only the nonbinary male had already tried drugs to change their skin color, and only a couple of the transfems had received race-affirming surgeries.

RACE-BASED SEXUALITY:
ALLOPHYLOPHILIA AND AUTOPHYLOPHILIA

As noted earlier, all nine cases here "frequently" or "often" pictured themselves in their sexual fantasies as their identified race. In contrast, all but one said they were "never" or "rarely" their assigned race in sexual fantasies.

In order to get more granular about which aspects of cross-race embodiment they found sexually interesting, I presented a set of five questions that asked about arousal at being their identified race, having physical features of it, being seen as it, dressing as it, and behaving as it. I asked these to investigate the presence of core, anatomic, interpersonal, sartorial, and behavioral autophylophilia, respectively.

Six of them said these forms of racial embodiment were at least "somewhat" arousing. Four reported higher levels of arousal—all were transfems.

Among the remaining three, one admitted he was "quite" aroused by imagining himself with the physical features of his race, one said she was "somewhat" aroused by the idea of being seen or treated as her identified race, and one denied all arousal to cross-racial embodiment.

I asked this same set of five embodiment questions about fantasy frequency, and all but one of the autophylophilic respondents gave high-frequency responses ("frequently" or "often") to the majority of the questions. If the patterns here are the norm for autophylophilic transracial people, it seems that it is common for them to embody their identified race in sexual fantasies in body, behavior, dress, and social role.

Their allosexuality with respect to race suggested they were also particularly interested in people of their identified race. Seven of them said they'd prefer if their next sexual partner were of their identified race; just as many said they found people of their identified race more attractive than people of their assigned race. Six had a childhood crush on someone of their identified race.

I also asked how often they looked at porn depicting people of either their identified race or assigned race. Among the five respondents who reported watching porn of their assigned race and identified race at different rates, *all* watched porn of their identified race more often than porn of their assigned race.

AUTOHETEROSEXUALITY AND GENDERED SEXUALITY

Autoheterosexuality was present in autophylophilic respondents at rates far beyond those in the general population: five of nine said they were "frequently" or "often" the other sex in their sexual fantasies, and six of nine said they would be "quite" or "very" aroused by the majority of the scenarios having to do with cross-gender embodiment.

In fact, the only respondent who denied any cross-gender sexuality was a bisexual transfem who reported high attraction to trans people and gave high scores to all questions about cross-race sexual embodiment, so I suspect that her answers to questions about cross-gender fantasy reflected either confusion or a desire to deny autogynephilia.

As expected, signs of autoheterosexuality were strongly associated with having a nondefault gender identity. Five of the six respondents who reported high levels of cross-gender arousal had nondefault gender identities. Similarly, two of the three respondents who reported little or no cross-gender arousal were still using their default gender identities.

Even though seven of nine respondents had heterosexual first crushes, the sample was highly nonheterosexual and highly attracted to androgyny. When asked their sexual orientation, only one person said they were heterosexual, and this same person was the only one who said they weren't strongly attracted to either trans men or trans women.

Both female respondents identified as homosexual and were most strongly attracted to women.

Overall, this sample was highly autoheterosexual, and correlates of autoheterosexuality such as bisexuality and attraction to trans people were also present at elevated rates.

SURVEY SUMMARY

This small exploratory survey presents preliminary evidence that there is a type of transracialism which is accompanied by sexual interest in cross-race embodiment.

All respondents included in this analysis were frequently their identified race in their sexual fantasies, and a solid majority said it would be arousing to embody their identified race in body, behavior, dress, or social role.

Similarly, two-thirds indicated moderate to high arousal to embodying the other sex in body, behavior, dress, or social role. Relatedly, all but one reported a nonheterosexual orientation and a high degree of attraction to trans men or trans women. In addition, all but one of the male respondents were transgender or nonbinary.

Transracial respondents felt warm fuzzy feelings or at home in themselves when embodying their racial identity. By contrast, they felt awful when they perceived shortcomings in cross-racial embodiment. The positive and negative race-based feelings they described bore a strong resemblance to the gender-based feelings that autohet trans people describe. Similarly, many transracial respondents wanted to get drugs or surgeries to more fully embody their racial identity.

The high concurrent rates of autoheterosexuality and autophylophilia suggest that these orientations may both have a similar underlying cause.

LIMITATIONS

My analysis excluded transracial people who did not report any degree of erotic racial embodiment. By design, it did not try to account for all transracial people.

The size and type of the sample is another limitation. Only nine transracial people completed the survey and showed sufficient autophylophilia to be included in the analysis, all of whom were recruited through online transracial communities.

In addition, the sample was too small to analyze with inferential statistics, so the analysis was restricted to descriptive statistics.

Lastly, the scales I used to ask about various forms of embodiment all had fairly abstract, top-level items. Future investigators may want to create scales that focus with greater specificity on the various aspects of cross-race embodiment that appeal to transracial people.

ARGUMENTS FOR TRANSGENDER LEGITIMACY ALSO APPLY TO TRANSRACE IDENTITY

Given that the transracial people I surveyed dealt with race dysphoria and other difficult aspects of being transracial, I doubt they adopted transracial identities in order to feel special or stand out. In fact, about half hadn't told *any* friends, family, or lovers about their racial identities.

Instead, I think these transracial people were dissatisfied with their birth race, yearned to be another race, and found the *transrace* label captured their feelings best. In short, they have feelings about their race which parallel the feelings autohet trans people have about their gender.

These similarities raise an important question in the domain of trans identity: if transracialism can be caused by race-based autosexual attraction, who can authoritatively say it isn't every bit as legitimate as transgenderism that's caused by gender-based autosexual attraction?

If transracial people truly do feel they are a race that differs from their default race, isn't it time to treat people with transracial identities more respectfully? After all, arguments for the legitimacy of transgenderism also apply to transracialism: if one is legitimate, so is the other.

Feminists who have looked into this came to a similar conclusion[21]. In her famous paper "In Defense of Transracialism", Rebecca Tuvel contended:

"Considerations that support transgenderism extend to transracialism. Given this parity, since we should accept transgender individuals' decisions to change sexes, we should also accept transracial individuals' decisions to change races."[22]

People of different races have more shared traits than do people of different sexes. Treating race-crossing as impossible while simultaneously treating gender-crossing as perfectly doable makes no sense.

If it's appropriate to respect cross-gender identities caused by attraction to being another gender, then it's also appropriate to respect cross-racial identities caused by attraction to being another race. It is logically inconsistent to admit one as legitimate and decry the other as illegitimate.

If transgenderism is legit, so is transracialism.

WHY THESE OTHER AUTOSEXUALITY CHAPTERS WERE HERE

This concludes our sojourn through the nongendered dimensions of autosexuality. To close out Part 7 of this book, I want to restate why I included these chapters and why they are important.

These autosexuality chapters are here to bolster the case for autoheterosexuality and the two-type transgender model. I intend them to serve as a series of "outsider tests"[23] so that autohet trans people can test their beliefs about transgenderism from a neutral, outside vantage point.

I want autohet trans people to realize that if dragon-identified people are sexually attracted to dragons and sexually attracted to being a dragon, maybe something similar happens with heterosexuality. And since heterosexuality is the most common sexual orientation, maybe its autosexual version is prevalent enough to be the most common cause of transgenderism.

I took this approach because critiques[24] of autogynephilia and its associated two-type model of MTF transgenderism are abundant and exceedingly popular among autohet trans people. The ubiquity of these critiques enables them to function as reference texts in a propaganda system that precludes many trans people from understanding the truth of their condition.

Given that so many of my kind have been propagandized in this way, I needed a way to sidestep identity-motivated blind spots while also retaining the interest of readers who aren't autoheterosexual themselves.

I hope it worked.

IN SUM

∗ Phylophilia is sexual attraction to people of a particular race. Its autosexual counterpart is autophylophilia, a sexual attraction to being a particular race.

∗ I collected survey data from transracial people in order to explore the possibility that some cases of transracialism were associated with autophylophilia rather than immersive cross-cultural experiences like transracial adoption. Most survey respondents reported autophylophilic fantasies or arousal. I examined these autophylophilic responses in greater detail.

* Autophylophilic transrace respondents talked about race dysphoria in ways that strongly resembled the gender dysphoria of autoheterosexual transgenderism. They battled internal disconnection, depression, and hopelessness. Authenticity came at a cost, but they pursued it anyway. Ultimately, anything in their environment that signified shortcomings of cross-racial embodiment could bring down their mood.

* Autophylophilic transrace respondents spoke of race euphoria in ways that mirror the gender euphoria of autoheterosexuals. When they were in touch with their race, they felt comfortable and at home in themselves. The internal disconnect dissipated, and they saw more clearly. They became more at peace with their body and were more able to feel joyful, free, or ecstatic. These positive feelings were associated with cross-race embodiment through imagination, behavior, dress, or social interactions.

* The transrace respondents analyzed here were all autophylophilic: all of them reported sexual fantasies in which they were their identified race. Similarly, most of

them also reported that it would be arousing to embody their identified race. Their allosexual racial preferences seemed to mirror their autosexual ones: most respondents said they found people of their identified race more attractive than people of their birth race, and most had a preference for dating someone of their identified race. In addition, they tended to watch porn depicting people of their identified race more often than porn depicting people of their assigned race.

* Most autophylophilic transrace respondents had cross-gender sexual fantasies or found the idea of being the other sex arousing. Almost all of them had correlates of autoheterosexuality such as bisexuality, attraction to trans people, or nondefault gender identities.

* Transracial respondents were emotionally hurt by the unfair media treatment they received. They asked for understanding and stressed their common humanity.

* Arguments for the legitimacy of transgenderism also apply to the legitimacy of transracialism. If it's appropriate to respect cross-gender identities caused by attraction to being another sex, then it's also appropriate to respect cross-race identities caused by attraction to being another race.

PART 8

CULTURAL INTEGRATION OF AUTOHETEROSEXUALITY

CULTURALLY INTEGRATING AUTOHETEROSEXUALITY

THE NOVEL SITUATION OF SEXUAL DIFFERENCES IN LOCATION

Autoheterosexuality and the two-type model of transgender-ism will become mainstream knowledge. When that happens, how should society handle it?

To orient thinking on this topic, consider homosexuality.

Homosexuality has been destigmatized to the point that same-sex marriage is legal in many places around the world, and discriminating against people on account of their sexual orien-tation is becoming more socially and legally unacceptable. These are welcome changes. After all, it's a form of sexual discrimination to police which gender someone's sexual partners can be[1].

Homosexuality is also associated with gender-atypical mental traits and behavioral expressions. Although these reach their most vibrant expression in the drag subculture, they are present to a lesser extent in everyday life. When people mistreat gender-atypical homosexuals because of this gender variance, it is another form of discrimination based on sex.

Like homosexuality, autoheterosexuality can also lead to same-sex partner preferences and gender-atypical behavior. Just as it would be wrong to mistreat homosexuals for their partner choices or gender nonconformity, it would be just as wrong to mistreat autoheterosexuals for the same.

However, autoheterosexuality isn't exactly the same situation. Homosexuality differs from heterosexuality in the dimension of *gender*, whereas autoheterosexuality differs in terms of *location*. The sexual dimension of location is a new one for people to consider.

Even though neither of these gender-based sexual orientations are intrinsically harmful, it will require some new thinking to settle on the appropriate norms regarding autoheterosexuality and autosexuality more broadly.

FREEDOM OF DRESS

What are the acceptable bounds for autoheterosexual expression?

Some people have argued that crossdressing in public is unacceptable for autoheterosexuals on the grounds that it's analogous to involving bystanders in a kink or a fetish. But I think this is wrongheaded for a few reasons.

In Western countries like the US, it's common for people to kiss, hug, or hold hands with someone of the other sex in public[2]. It seems that most people are fine with public displays of affection. In fact, some people even like to see these signs of love in everyday life.

Most of the autogynephilic transfems I've seen out in public are shrouded in the transvestic equivalent of hand-holding or a peck on the cheek. It's tame. It's rare that I see a truly saucy outfit on others of my kind out in the wild. And even when I do, I don't see any tangible harm from it.

If anything, the greater harm would be to prohibit people from such behavior. Restricting clothing choices based on the sex of the person wearing them is a form of sexual discrimination.

Do we want to live in a society where females are forbidden to wear pants, and males forbidden to wear dresses? This sort of prohibition reinforces antiquated approaches to gender roles that restrict people to certain narrow norms of behavior and expression based on their sex or gender: women can do *this*; men can do *that*.

Feminists fought hard to create cultural norms that enable females to wear pants. A whole rainbow of queer people fought hard for the ability to deviate from gender norms through same-sex relationships and alternative gender expressions.

Prohibiting people from wearing clothing associated with the other sex would go against the spirit of this gender liberation. It would also make everyone less free to express themselves in their everyday lives.

PRONOUNS

When someone wears clothing associated with the other sex, it does not require any participation from other people.

Pronouns, however, are different.

When a trans person has pronouns that don't match those that others would attribute to them by default, other people must put effort into remembering those pronouns in order to avoid misgendering. The incongruence between the gender people *see* and the pronouns they are expected to *say* can make some people uncomfortable. It's like a small taste of the internal gender incongruence that trans people experience.

Unsurprisingly, a lot of people don't like this feeling. Some resent the expectation that they should override what their brain is telling them in order to cater to someone else's gender feelings.

In his stand-up special *The Closer*, Dave Chappelle asked a question that gets to the heart of the pronoun issue: "How much do I have to participate in your self-image?"[3].

It's a valid question.

To complicate matters, most transgender identities are a downstream effect of autosexual orientations, and interpersonal autoheterosexuality can cause someone to get gender euphoria or arousal when treated as the other sex. Therefore, it could be argued that when autohet trans people request that others use their cross-gender pronouns, they're involving bystanders in their sexuality.

Focusing on eroticism, however, would largely miss the point.

It's uncommon for autoheterosexuals to socially transition simply to get off sexually. Most transition because they have strong feelings about wanting to live as another gender that transcend eroticism. For many, the prospect of transitioning is terrifying, but they do it anyway.

In the case of trans women, the drugs they take to lower their testosterone tend to drastically reduce their propensity for erotic response. And on the odd occasion they do get aroused by being addressed with feminine pronouns, it's often upsetting to them because it conflicts with their idea of femininity.

In general, when trans people ask others to use their pronouns, they're not doing so to seek arousal. Many hate feeling like they're imposing on other people by even making a pronoun request in the first place.

Trans people usually ask people to use certain pronouns for identity reasons. It's perfectly acceptable for them to request that others use their pronouns, and I believe it's also reasonable to honor that request if they're using one of the commonly used pronouns (she/they/he).

Sometimes people are against using trans people's pronouns, however, and they may argue that forcing them to do so is compelled speech. As a freedom-lover, I'm somewhat sympathetic to this argument. Legal mandates to use particular pronouns would conflict with the principle of free speech, so such laws would be a terrible idea.

However, cultural norms are another matter entirely. Cultural norms are guidelines for behavior, not mandates backed by the threat of state violence.

To ponder this cultural question, it can be helpful to have a little distance.

If you were to be born into a society but couldn't know ahead of time what sort of traits you would have (sex, health conditions, sexual orientation, race, etc.), what sort of society would you like to be born into?

There's some risk of being born with a sexual predisposition that causes gender issues. Knowing that risk exists, would you want to be born into a culture in which it was customary to use people's preferred pronouns, or one that didn't?

If you reproduce, your offspring may be born with a sexual orientation that leads to gender issues. If you had a kid who suffered when reminded of their sex, what type of society would you want for your kid?

Personally, I'd prefer to live in a society that honors people's preferred pronouns for the most part. I believe a society that makes such accommodations to help reduce gender-based suffering is more thoughtful and kind than an otherwise equivalent society that doesn't do so.

WHICH KINDS OF TRANS IDENTITIES CAN FIT INTO SOCIETY?

I think it's great that transgender people have raised awareness of their situation and improved public understanding of their condition. With greater understanding, they are better incorporated into broader society. I'm also strongly in favor of an adult's right to modify their body how they wish and for trans people to live as the gender they feel themselves to be.

The recent gender liberation spearheaded by trans people also allows nontrans people to have more leeway in their gender behaviors. Gender roles have become less strict, which increases freedom for everyone, not just trans people.

However, transgender identity isn't the only type of trans identity—transrace, transabled, transspecies, and transage identities exist too. At some point, people will have to decide which types of trans identities can (or ought to) be accommodated by society, and which cannot.

Due to the allosexual attractions associated with these types of cross-identity, I suspect that transracialism and transableism have a chance at acceptance, but transspecies and transage identities don't. People of various races and disabilities can consent to sexual activity, but children and nonhuman animals can't. Children aren't developed enough to adequately advocate for themselves, and nonhuman animals can't speak human languages.

Sexual interest in children is the most heavily stigmatized type of sexuality because of the immense damage caused by acting upon it, so anything even *associated* with that kind of attraction faces immense headwinds. If transageism fits the pattern seen with other types of trans identity, most transage people experience sexual attraction to minors.

But even if transage people don't fit that pattern, how would transageism fit into everyday life? Adults who outwardly identify as eight years old don't belong in third grade, let alone the broader K–12 school environment.

Sexual attraction to animals is also heavily stigmatized, so transspecies identity faces similar obstacles to acceptance. Yet even if stigma weren't an issue, where do wolf and dragon identities fit into society? Perhaps I'm just sheltered, but I have yet to encounter a dragon in real life.

These issues make it clear that transage and transspecies identities face significant hurdles to acceptance. The prospect of integrating transableism or transracialism into society, however, is much more plausible.

There are preexisting legal and architectural accommodations for disabled people that could just as well be used by "post-op" transabled people. And transableism is quite rare, so transabled people probably won't make a noticeable dent in the resources available to conventionally disabled people.

Although currently contentious, I expect that transrace identity will ultimately attain a moderate degree of societal acceptance as well. For the most part, fitting transracialism into society requires taking someone's word for it if they identify as a particular race.

When the time comes, there will be debates over transrace inclusion in scholarships and awards meant for people of certain races. There will also be debates over whether transrace people should have race-affirming medical care covered by insurance.

There are undoubtedly obstacles to transrace and transabled acceptance. However, I suspect both groups will ultimately overcome these barriers, and I wish them the best of luck.

THE VANILLA DEFINITION OF SEXUAL ORIENTATION IS OBSOLETE

The conventional definition of a sexual orientation only describes sexual preferences for adults based on their gender. It's usually something like, "an enduring pattern of sexual or romantic attraction to women, men, or both".

This is the vanilla definition of sexual orientation, and it's too limiting. Frankly, it's obsolete. It excludes *all* autosexual orientations. It also excludes nongendered dimensions of attraction such as race, age, body integrity, and species.

These other forms of attraction may not be the norm, but they have a similar capacity to create strong attachments, alter identity, and shape sentiments such that people build their lives to accommodate them.

If a person is consistently most aroused by one of these types of attraction, and it's their strongest source of sexual and romantic fulfillment, who can say it doesn't count as their sexual orientation?

Someone might argue that nonvanilla sexual orientations don't count as orientations because they're too rare or too weird. Rarity and weirdness, however, do not determine if a form of sexuality counts as a sexual orientation. And even if they did, autoheterosexuality itself would still count as a sexual orientation.

It's about as common as homosexuality, so it's not too rare. And it's a type of heterosexuality, so it's not too weird.

When it comes to nonvanilla sexual orientations, the real question is *which of these attractions are acceptable or ethical to act upon, and under what circumstances?*

Pedophilia can be a sexual orientation, but it's not morally permissible for adults to have sex with children under any circumstances. And although autozoophilic people may love puppy play and want to be in dog mode 24/7, it's not appropriate for them to mark their territory in the pet aisle at Walmart.

As a culture, we need to collectively hammer out the acceptable range of behavior for different types of sexuality instead of declaring that a whole bunch of sexualities with the same propensity for attraction and attachment as vanilla sexual orientations somehow don't actually count as sexual orientations.

This old way of framing sexuality collectively holds us back from having a more nuanced, advanced level of discourse about human sexuality by artificially deciding that anything described as "sexual orientation" is acceptable, but anything else is less important or fundamentally different in nature.

It's time to expand the definition of sexual orientation. As a start, I suggest the following:

Sexual Orientation—an enduring pattern of preferential sexual or romantic interest in a particular type of entity, embodiment, or method of interaction.

Under this definition, a person who has the strongest interest in adults of the other sex has a heterosexual orientation.

Likewise, someone who is most strongly attracted to animals would have a zoophilic sexual orientation, and someone whose primary sexual interest is being degraded and physically hurt would have a masochistic sexual orientation.

TECHNOLOGY TO CHANGE SEXUAL ORIENTATION

It would be a net good if it became possible to change human sexual orientation. If a safe, reliable technological method of changing human sexual orientation existed, it could avert a great deal of suffering.

The primary benefit of this technology would not be its ability to turn gay or bisexual people straight. Gender-based attractions like these are fine. Instead, other dimensions of sexual orientation such as *age* and *species* would be the best targets for change.

Consider pedophilia, the most vilified sexual orientation. When pedophilic people act on their sexual attraction to children by molesting them, it causes serious psychological harm. If technology existed to make these child-attracted people attracted to adults instead of kids, it would protect millions of minors from sexual harm. It would even help pedophilic people who abstain from sexual contact with children by removing a part of themselves that brings upon shame, vilification, and a desire that can't be met.

A similar rationale applies to changing species-based attractions. Animals cannot consent to sexual contact with humans, so it would prevent both animal and human suffering if it were possible to change a zoophilic person's sexual orientation to instead be attracted to adult humans.

Changing sexual orientations in the dimension of *location* could also help reduce suffering.

There are many autoheterosexuals who wish more than anything that they could be regular heterosexuals. There are also plenty who suffer intensely from gender dysphoria.

If the *location* dimension of sexual orientation could be changed, it would be possible to directly address the root cause of not only autohet gender dysphoria but also autophylophilic race dysphoria, autoacrotomophilic body integrity dysphoria, autopedophilic age dysphoria, and autozoophilic species dysphoria. All of the forms of autosexual dysphoria could be alleviated.

To be clear, I think humanity is nowhere near creating technology that can safely and reliably change sexual orientation. However, such technology has the potential to greatly reduce sexuality-related suffering, so its development should not be forbidden.

SEXUAL PREFERENCES ARE NOT TRANSPHOBIC

It isn't transphobic to lack sexual interest in transgender people.

It's flat-out unacceptable to suggest to someone that they might be transphobic (or that transphobia informs their sexual preferences) simply because they don't want to have sex with trans people.

Evolution has shaped human sexual orientation to optimize the union of sperm and egg, so attraction to physically typical adults of the other sex is the most common sexual orientation. Most people won't be attracted to people who possess a mixture of female and male sex traits.

The "born this way" framework for understanding sexual preferences that has helped destigmatize both same-sex sexuality and transgenderism is incompatible with the notion that sexual disinterest in trans people is a moral failing, or in any way political. When someone is not attracted to trans people or doesn't want to be sexual with them, it does not indicate a moral shortcoming.

People are allowed to decide who they want to get with and who they don't. If someone can't say "no", *free from coercion*, then they can't truly consent. Any deviation from this absolutely basic principle of sexual autonomy betrays the spirit of consent.

Just because a trans person's gender identity is supposedly compatible with another person's stated sexual orientation, it doesn't mean that person must be open to having sex with them. Straight dudes aren't obligated to be sexually open to trans women, and straight women aren't obligated to be sexually open to trans men. Most people are heterosexuals who want to have sex with people of the other sex that aren't trans[4], and that's okay.

If a lesbian doesn't want to have sex with trans women but feels pressured to do so because she's worried about being seen as transphobic for only being attracted to females, that's coercive bullshit. Lesbians, like any other group of people, should be free to say no to sleeping with trans women. They should be able to freely state their sexual boundaries and have them respected without bargaining, guilt trips, insinuations of transphobia, negative social consequences, or any other coercive tactics.

If a gay man doesn't want to hook up with a trans man, he is not transphobic for being true to his sexual preferences. A lot of gay men only want to get with males. They didn't choose to like that, it's just what they like. And that's okay.

It has to be, if consent is something we truly value and want to continue striving for.

IN SUM

* Many of the considerations that extend to homosexuality also extend to autoheterosexuality. It is a form of sexual discrimination to force people to adhere to gender norms or have sexual partners of a particular gender. Neither homosexuals nor autoheterosexuals should be subjected to these forms of sexual discrimination.

* Restricting the types of clothes someone may wear on account of their sex is a form of sexual discrimination that goes against the spirit of sexual and gender liberation inherent to the gay rights and feminist movements. Even though dressing as the other sex can be erotic for

autoheterosexuals, in practice it's usually as tame as heterosexual public displays of affection such as hugging and holding hands—both of which have widespread cultural acceptance.

* When a trans person prefers pronouns that differ from those usually attributed to them by default, other people must put effort into remembering those pronouns in order to avoid misgendering. The conscious effort required to do so can make people uncomfortable. There is a legitimate tension between people who want to prioritize sex over gender and people who want to prioritize gender over sex.

* It's possible to act on sexual attractions in the dimensions of gender, race, or body integrity because the targets of these attractions can consent, but children and animals cannot. This ability to be an independent agent capable of giving consent is also what separates the types of cross-identities that may be embodied full-time and integrated into broader society (transgender, transracial, transabled) from those that cannot (transage, transspecies).

* The definition of sexual orientation should be expanded to include any enduring pattern of preferential sexual or romantic interest in a particular type of entity, embodiment, or method of interaction. Ethical concerns over which sexual orientations are acceptable to act upon

are completely irrelevant to the question of whether various forms of sexuality count as sexual orientations.

* It would be beneficial if technological methods to change sexual orientation were developed—not to change gender-based sexual orientations, but to change other dimensions of sexual orientation such as age, species, and location. Children and animals are not ethically viable erotic targets, so the ability to eliminate attractions to them would reduce sexual abuse. In addition, many autosexuals have autosexual dysphoria and would gladly change their orientations if it meant they would suffer less.

* It's not transphobic to lack sexual interest in trans people. Sexual preferences largely result from inborn developmental factors and are thus highly individual. Although societal forces may influence their expression, sexual orientations do not yield to the dictates of society. People like what they like, and that's okay. It's not acceptable to insinuate that someone is transphobic if their sexual preferences don't include trans people. In order to stay true to the sexual principle of consent, people must be free to say "no"—free from coercion—to any sexual interactions in which they do not wish to participate.

JUVENILE TRANSSEXUALISM
YOUTH GENDER TRANSITION

As transgenderism has become more widely understood and destigmatized, the number of children and adolescents seeking treatment at gender clinics has surged. To meet the needs of this rapidly growing population, gender clinics are proliferating.

Some of these clinics give kids drugs that strip their bodies of hormones to forestall their default puberty. People in favor of this approach argue that suppressing puberty will give the children and their clinicians more time to decide whether medical transition is right for them. In reality, however, almost all children who start taking puberty blockers for their gender issues will continue onto cross-sex hormones at a later date.

In the matter of juvenile transsexualism, there is a genuine conflict between conventional ethical considerations and the realities of human biology. Puberty happens before kids are mature enough to truly grasp the implications of their decision to transition. Some of these child transitioners will consider medical transition to be the best decision they ever made, but others will deeply regret it.

It's impossible to know for sure whether a would-be transsexual child will derive overall benefit or harm from medical transition[1]. The long-term outcomes of medical transition in minors are still unknown, and studies in this realm tend to be of low quality[2].

The practice of medically transitioning youth has spread rapidly. It's also heavily politicized. Driven by the urge to do good, inexperienced clinicians will help some kids have a good life—and lead others to ruin.

When all is said and done, there will be stories of medical malpractice wherein clinicians gave kids puberty blockers, hormones, and surgeries despite obvious warning signs that such treatment was inadvisable. There will also be stories from grateful transsexuals who overflow with gratitude for the doctors who took a chance on them.

It's truly a mixed bag.

It's also unknown whether doctors currently facilitate medical gender transition in youth in a way that leads to net benefits instead of net harm. If, hypothetically, child transition as currently practiced is harmful overall, is it possible to instead do it in a way that leads to overall benefits? And if so, what exactly would that set of clinical guidelines, methods, and medical interventions look like?

It worries me that kids are going through medical transition well before they would otherwise be able to give consent for such serious medical interventions. Worse yet, there is not yet a solid body of high-quality evidence demonstrating the efficacy of juvenile transsexualism. Youth gender transition is still quite new and experimental, and its long-term outcomes are unknown[3].

There are two aspects of juvenile transsexualism, however, that I feel confident enough about to say something here. One is the need to curtail the use of puberty blocker monotherapy because being hormonally sexless wreaks havoc on the human body. The other is the need to expand the scope of data collection to improve trans health care outcomes for future generations.

I'll start by elaborating on the need for more robust data collection in transgender health care.

COLLECT MORE DATA, AND FOLLOW UP FOR LONGER

Trans people would benefit in the long term if clinicians coordinated their efforts to achieve large-scale, systematic collection of data from gender-dysphoric people of all ages. The best way to learn from the mistakes and successes happening now is to measure them.

For decades, Dutch and Canadian gender clinics administered questionnaires to gender-dysphoric people and stored their responses in databases. This data formed the basis for dozens of studies, including Blanchard's famous studies that empirically demonstrated the validity of the two-type MTF model.

Other clinicians operating today should follow this example. By forming cooperative networks such as the European Network for the Investigation of Gender Incongruence (ENIGI)[4], clinicians can gather data on a larger scale and thus enable deeper investigation.

With more data, clinicians could better predict whether someone is a good candidate for gender transition. By publishing better studies, researchers could help the transgender health community improve treatment outcomes.

Technological advances can facilitate these changes. Electronic medical records can follow patients better than the paper records of the past, so it's more possible than ever to obtain long-term data on outcomes. If medical organizations coordinated their actions to collect data from trans people throughout their lives, it would improve transgender health care.

As it stands now, too many transgenderism studies record a snapshot of time, and too few examine outcomes over a long period of time. Making a systematic, long-term effort to gather longitudinal data can help correct this shortcoming in the transgender literature.

Transsexualism is a long-term decision. Its study requires long-term follow-through.

HORMONES, BLOCKERS, AND MITOCHONDRIA

Over the next several pages, I'll show that sex hormones are essential for maintaining physical health, and that while using drugs to strip the body of sex hormones is likely to harm humans of any age, it's especially bad for pubescent youth.

I'll also show that social transition and puberty blockers each greatly increase the odds of kids staying on the transsexual path—these interventions cannot be considered neutral.

To understand why puberty blockers can wreak havoc on human health, it's important to understand some basics about how hormones work, as well as how they act upon mitochondria and thus impact cells throughout the human body.

SEX HORMONES IMPACT ALL BODILY SYSTEMS

Sex hormones affect the creation, maintenance, and function of our tissues and organs by binding to receptor sites. The impact of sex hormones is systemic and not limited to reproductive or sexual functioning.

Sex hormone receptors are found throughout the tissues and organs of the human body. This means they play a regulatory role throughout the body and directly or indirectly impact *all* of its processes.

Scientists have found receptor sites for sex hormones in the brain[5], heart[6], gastrointestinal system[7], immune system[8], liver[9], eyes[10], vocal folds[11], fat cells[12], skin[13], muscles[14], joints[15], bones[16], and more. These receptor sites are everywhere.

Hormones are especially influential in determining the strength of bones. For females and males alike, a shortage of sex hormones leads to loss of bone mass and strength[17].

Sex hormone receptor sites are also found in mitochondria[18], the organelles inside our cells that produce adenosine triphosphate (ATP), the form of chemical energy that cells require to function. Due to their essential role in energy production, mitochondria exist in cells throughout the human body, which means hormones influence a wide variety of tissues by changing how mitochondria function.

MITOCHONDRIA

When the mitochondria within a cell produce insufficient energy for the cell to keep living, that cell will die. Proper mitochondrial function is essential.

If our mitochondria stop, we stop. (This is the mechanism by which cyanide kills).

As mitochondria produce their chemical energy, they sometimes create reactive oxygen-based molecules known as *reactive oxygen species*, which damage DNA, proteins, and other molecules in the body. This damage is *oxidative stress*, and the chemicals that help combat this damage are *antioxidants*.

Although it's normal for mitochondria to produce some oxidative stress, when enough of this damage accumulates, it can lead to *mitochondrial dysfunction*, a state in which mitochondria deteriorate in form and function, becoming less efficient at producing energy and releasing even more reactive oxygen species.

When mitochondria aren't functioning properly, disease states are likely to follow—especially in energetically expensive organs like the brain and heart. In an influential paper that's been cited over six thousand times, the authors concluded that "mitochondrial dysfunction and oxidative stress occur early in all major neurodegenerative diseases, and there is strong evidence that this dysfunction has a causal role in disease pathogenesis"[19].

Unsurprisingly, mounting evidence suggests that mitochondrial dysfunction plays a role in the development of depression and bipolar disorder[20]. Mitochondrial dysfunction is implicated in heart disease too[21].

Mitochondrial dysfunction is one of the hallmarks of the aging process[22], and the accumulation of oxidative damage is thought to be one of the primary causes of the aging process[23].

ESTRADIOL PROTECTS AGAINST MITOCHONDRIAL DYSFUNCTION

Estradiol, a form of estrogen and the primary female sex hormone, acts both directly and indirectly upon mitochondria to change how they function[24]. Estradiol has a protective, antioxidant effect on mitochondria in the brain[25]. It helps protect cells by improving mitochondrial efficiency and reducing the production of reactive oxygen species[26].

These effects are so pronounced that it leads to measurable differences in mental performance. Experiments on estrogen deprived rhesus monkeys found they performed worse on a test of working memory than those who received estrogen therapy, and the mitochondria in the corresponding part of their brain were also more likely to be misshapen—a sign of oxidative stress[27]. This finding demonstrated that the health of mitochondria directly relates to mental performance outcomes[28].

Authors of a study examining the brain mitochondria of rats whose ovaries had been removed came to a similar conclusion. A single dose of estrogen significantly improved mitochondrial function, a change the authors described as "a systematic enhancement of brain mitochondrial efficiency"[29].

GONADOTROPIN-RELEASING HORMONE (GnRH) AND SEX HORMONES

The pituitary gland secretes hormones called *luteinizing hormone* (LH) and *follicle-stimulating hormone* (FSH), both of which interact with tissues in the gonads to drive the production of estrogens and androgens. Since LH and FSH stimulate activity in the gonads, these hormones are known as gonadotropins.

Accordingly, the hormone that signals their release is called *gonadotropin-releasing hormone* (GnRH).

When working properly, these various hormones signal to each other in ways that keep physiological systems in balance. The release of GnRH leads to the release of LH and FSH, and these induce the release of estrogens and androgens which then provide attenuating feedback that moderates the later release of GnRH.

During childhood, GnRH levels are low. But as GnRH activity ramps up during the onset of puberty, so does the production of sex hormones. It's at this time that some gender-dysphoric kids want to get on GnRH agonists (aka puberty blockers).

GnRH agonists work by binding to GnRH receptors. But unlike the natural functioning of GnRH, which occurs in pulses, GnRH agonists constantly activate GnRH receptors. The body then responds to this overstimulation by reducing the number of GnRH receptors.

With far fewer GnRH receptors around, the release of LH and FSH drops dramatically. In this state, the body produces almost no estrogens or androgens. People who take GnRH agonists without supplementing with sex hormones will exist in a sexless hormonal state that leaves their body without the protective, regulating effects of estradiol and other sex hormones.

In a sexless hormonal state, tissues and organs with sex hormone receptors won't receive the important hormonal signals that help keep them in good working order. Hormone levels are especially relevant when it comes to bone health—both males and females lose bone mass and bone strength when they have a shortage of sex hormones[30].

This effect is even more relevant during puberty. Bone mass typically doubles over the course of puberty and reaches its peak density near the end of adolescence[31]. If people don't have adequate hormone levels during puberty, however, their bones won't grow as strong. This leaves them at greater risk of osteoporosis and other bone ailments.

GnRH AGONISTS HAVE HELLA SIDE EFFECTS

Doctors prescribe GnRH agonists such as leuprorelin and trip-torelin to children in order to delay puberty—either because they are on the transsexual path or because their puberty came too early. Females hit puberty earlier than males, so they receive puberty blockers for precocious puberty more often.

Doctors give GnRH analogues to adult males for testosterone suppression during prostate cancer treatment. Doctors also give GnRH agonists to adult females for the purpose of reducing gynecological issues such as endometriosis or uterine fibroid tumors.

More studies have been conducted on the effects of GnRH agonists in females, so I'll primarily draw upon that research. It's worth noting, however, that research on males who receive GnRH agonists as part of prostate cancer treatment shows they lose more bone mass and have more bone fractures than males who aren't testosterone-deprived[32].

Among females, side effects from GnRH agonists seem not only more common but also more widespread within their body systems. Overall, these side effects support the idea that estradiol-deprivation-induced mitochondrial dysfunction plays a key role in their genesis.

Despite widespread side effects in females, doctors still prescribe GnRH agonists such as leuprorelin for the treatment of endometriosis and uterine fibroid tumors.

In one study that followed 3,153 adult females taking prescribed leuprorelin, an astounding *77% of them* reported joint pain[33]. In addition, about 36% reported increased propensity toward negative emotions, 43% reported memory loss, and 48% reported irritability[34]—all of which suggested that leuprorelin had negative impacts on their neurological functioning.

Adult females who have taken GnRH agonists commonly report overt neurological issues like headaches and migraines, or energy-related issues like sleepiness, fatigue, and insomnia[35]. Psychiatric symptoms like depression, anxiety, and susceptibility to changing moods are common, as are connective tissue-related symptoms like joint pain, muscle pain, and cracked teeth.

These negative effects on memory and mood are typical. Other studies that directly tested the working memory of adult females on leuprorelin treatment have found that it's associated with memory deficiencies and declines in mental health[36].

Females who halt their precocious puberty with GnRH agonists show a decline in general intelligence over the treatment period[37]. As adults, many report long-term neuronal and bone-related health issues[38]. Psychiatric symptoms are common too.

Altogether, these side effects point to the central role that hormones play in maintaining proper mitochondrial function[39] as well as the health of bones and other connective tissues[40].

PUBERTY BLOCKER MONOTHERAPY WEAKENS BONES IN TRANSSEXUAL MINORS

Under the influence of sex hormones, bones strengthen significantly during puberty. But kids on puberty blockers lack these hormones, so their bone strengthening slows or halts, leaving them behind their pubescent peers.

Several studies have found that even prior to taking puberty blockers, MTFS lag behind other males in terms of bone mineral density[41], and FTMS who start blockers in early puberty lag behind other females in terms of overall bone mineral density[42].

When they go on blockers without cross-sex hormones, biochemical markers of bone growth drop in both FTMS and MTFS, signaling that bone growth has stalled[43]. Their bone mineral density, a key measure of strength, also drops[44]. In this sexless hormonal state, their waist-to-hip ratio demasculinizes, their lean body mass drops, and their body fat percentage increases[45].

Once cross-sex hormones are added, though, transsexual minors start shifting toward other-sex norms for all these characteristics[46]. Their bones begin strengthening too. After two to three years of receiving cross-sex hormones, bone mineral density in FTMS approaches or reaches norms for their sex, but MTFS still lag behind[47]. A study that measured bone stats even later in life, at age twenty-two, found a similar pattern[48].

When interpreting these findings, it's important to consider that males tend to have more bone than females[49]. Much, but not all, of this difference is because males are bigger. Even when accounting for size differences between sexes, however, males still have more bone[50].

With this sex-based difference in mind, it makes sense that trans men showed less bone deficiency than trans women when compared to others of their sex. FTMS were given hormones of the sex that has stronger bones and compared to the sex that has weaker bones. Likewise, MTFs were given hormones of the sex that has weaker bones and compared to the sex that has stronger bones.

In sum, the negative effects of puberty blockers on bone density are most apparent in transsexual kids who take them without also taking sex hormones that could help them retain and build bone strength.

PERSISTENCE, DESISTANCE, AND SEXUAL ORIENTATION

Historically, most gender-dysphoric children who presented at gender clinics did not ultimately follow through on medical transition—they *desisted* from the transsexual path. In contrast, those who medically transitioned *persisted*.

Rising cultural awareness and acceptance of transgenderism has increased the rate of persistence. So has the use of puberty blockers.

In order to show the differences in persistence and desistance based on sexual orientation, I'll use four studies. Two are from the Dutch clinic[51], and two are from the Toronto gender clinic[52]. Almost all the data in these studies was collected before the social media revolution.

In these four studies, persisters were usually homosexual. Desisters had a more even mix of homosexuals and nonhomosexuals but leaned toward the latter.

At the Dutch gender clinic, approximately 36–50% of females and 70% of males desisted[53]. All, or virtually all, female desisters had nonhomosexual orientations. Approximately 44–60% of the male desisters had nonhomosexual orientations.

By contrast, those who persisted in their desire for medical transition were far more likely to be homosexual. In both of the Dutch studies examined here, virtually all persisters were homosexual[54].

The other data on persistence and desistance in childhood gender dysphoria comes from Toronto, Canada. It's split into two studies—a small one on females in which 22 of 25 (88%) desisted[55], and a large, thorough one on males in which 112 of 129 (87%) desisted[56]. These desistance rates are much higher than those found in the Dutch studies.

Among the Canadian desisters, 81% of females[57] and 58% of males[58] (see endnote[59]) had a nonhomosexual orientation.

As in the Dutch studies, the Canadian studies showed that persisters were overwhelmingly homosexual. Among the three female persisters, two were homosexual. The third was asexual, reported no fantasies, and said he was "dead sexually"[60]. Among the male persisters, 15 of 17 (88%) were homosexual[61].

This association between sexual orientation and persistence/ desistance works in the other direction too. Depending on whether groups of children are homosexual or nonhomosexual, they have much different rates of persistence and desistance. Homosexuals are more likely to persist.

Both Canadian studies reported sexual orientation and whether it persisted for each individual case, which let me calculate precise persistence rates based on sexual orientation. A third of homosexual females persisted, but only 5% of nonhomosexual females did so[62]. The males showed a similar pattern: 24% of homosexual males persisted, but only 3% of nonhomosexual males did so[63].

The Dutch studies didn't report the sexual orientation of all the patients, but they did report it for most of them. I used their figures for sexual fantasy to make similar estimates. Among females, approximately 87% of homosexuals and 6% of nonhomosexuals persisted. Among males, approximately 56% of homosexuals and 4% of nonhomosexuals persisted.

Taken altogether, these studies on childhood gender dysphoria back up the conventional wisdom among gender clinicians that early-onset gender dysphoria is usually of homosexual etiology. Almost all persisters had homosexual orientations. Among desisters, however, nonhomosexual orientations were the norm.

Their country of residence made a difference too: most of the gender-dysphoric homosexuals in the Dutch clinics continued on to transition, but only a minority did so in the Toronto clinic. However, both clinics had single-digit percentages of persistence among nonhomosexuals of both sexes.

Although it's impossible to know for sure ahead of time which individual children will benefit from medical transition[64], these results show that sexual orientation is an important consideration in making the call about which children are likely to persist in their pursuit of medical transition.

THE DUTCH PROTOCOL

In 1998, Dutch researchers published the first case report of puberty suppression in a gender-dysphoric child. He reported satisfaction with his subsequent masculinization and adjusted easily to a male social role[65].

In the subsequent decade, clinicians at this gender clinic developed a selection process for suppressing puberty that came to be known as the "Dutch Protocol". To qualify, children had to be at least twelve years of age and show physical signs of puberty. They also had to have the following:

1. Persistent gender dysphoria that began in early childhood
2. Greater dysphoria as puberty started
3. No co-occurring psychiatric issues that complicate the diagnosis or treatment process
4. Mental and social support during treatment
5. A thorough understanding of the effects and repercussions of hormones, surgery, and sex reassignment[66]

These Dutch researchers portrayed puberty suppression as "fully reversible" and argued that puberty blockers would give gender-dysphoric children and their parents time to carefully consider whether medical transition was right for them.

If careful consideration about the decision to transition *did* happen, though, there's no way of knowing: all the children who started puberty blockers kept taking them, and they all ended up taking cross-sex hormones too[67].

PUBERTY BLOCKERS SOLIDIFY COMMITMENT TO MEDICAL TRANSITION

The vast majority of children who go on puberty blockers for gender dysphoria ultimately continue onto cross-sex hormones.

Researchers from the Dutch clinic found that only 4.1% of MTFS and 0.7% of FTMs[68] who started on blockers did not proceed to taking cross-sex hormones. Another Dutch study, one from a newer gender clinic, found that only 3.5% of patients who went on puberty blockers ultimately decided against going on cross-sex hormones[69].

These gender-dysphoric Dutch youngsters weren't alone in their tendency to continue onto cross-sex hormones after starting puberty blockers. American clinicians also report low levels of desistance after the start of puberty blockers.

Norman Spack, a Boston-based pediatric endocrinologist, reported in 2016 that of the hundreds of children to whom he gave puberty blockers, all continued onto cross-sex hormones— "no one changes their mind", he said[70].

Johanna Olson, a Los Angeles–based pediatrician who specializes in transgender health, reported, "In my practice, I have never had anyone who was put on blockers that did not want to pursue cross-sex hormone transition at a later point"[71].

This pattern holds for Brits too: gender clinicians working in the United Kingdom reported of their sample that "no patient within the sample desisted after having started on the [puberty] blocker"[72]. By contrast, "90.3% of young people who did not commence the blocker desisted"[73]. The web page that originally stated these findings so clearly and succinctly has since been taken down.

These soaring persistence rates go far beyond what was seen before puberty suppression was offered by gender clinics.

Considering how gender patients view puberty blockers, however, this high rate of persistence is no surprise. Researchers have asked parents and patients about their views on puberty blockers and found that "all of them saw it as the first step in treatment"[74].

SOCIAL TRANSITION INCREASES COMMITMENT TO THE CROSS-GENDER PATH

It's becoming more common for gender-dysphoric children to undergo social gender transition at a young age, and those who do are more likely to follow through on medical transition down the line.

Dutch researchers found that whether male children dressed or socially presented as girls strongly predicted whether they persisted in the desire to transition[75]. Among male persisters, 43% already dressed or lived as a girl, but only 4% of male desisters did so. On the other hand, the rates of females dressing as boys didn't vary much between persister and desister groups, and only one female, a persister, already lived as a boy[76].

Recent research on children who socially transitioned at a young age suggests that most kids who socially transition before puberty will ultimately proceed onto puberty blockers and cross-sex hormones[77]. This study tracked 317 youth who first transitioned an average of five years prior and found the vast majority maintained nondefault gender identities: 94% of the kids still had binary transgender identities and 3.5% had non-binary identities[78]. In contrast, only 2.5% had reverted to their default gender identities.

This high rate of persistence among social transitioners closely resembles the high rate of persistence among kids who start puberty blockers. Both interventions greatly increase the odds of staying on the transsexual path.

A POLITICAL FIGHT OVER AN EMPIRICAL QUESTION

Childhood gender transition has become a battleground in the ongoing culture war.

The two biggest camps on the anti-transition side are 1) social conservatives who feel a traditionalist imperative to preserve the gender binary and 2) a subset of feminists who prioritize sex over gender and regard gender as a method of oppressing females. Many of these social conservatives and feminists have ideological blinders which keep them from acknowledging that some kids will benefit from avoiding their default puberty with medical transition.

People on the pro-transition side are often motivated by ideology too. In particular, many are motivated by a fusion of critical theory and postmodernism most commonly known as "wokism" or "wokeness"[79]. Among its many flaws, wokism rejects the idea that liberal science is the best method for creating knowledge that corresponds to reality.

Another big group on the pro-transition side comprises well-meaning progressives. They often want trans people to be treated well and see childhood gender transition as part of that. These progressives are likely to go along with whatever they see trans-gender people advocating for.

This is a problem: prepubescent gender-dysphoric youth are mostly of homosexual etiology, but many of the fiercest advocates for youth gender transition are autohet transsexuals who transitioned as adults and wish they had been able to transition younger.

Since autoheterosexual and homosexual orientations are opposites in both gender and direction, it is unlikely that late-transitioning autohet transsexuals have special insight into the experiences of children with early-onset homosexual gender dysphoria. These are fundamentally different situations that should not be conflated.

The intense political battle over youth gender transition makes it harder for clinicians to do their job of answering the practical questions at the heart of this issue:

* Is it possible to know which kids will benefit from medical transition and which will be harmed by it?
* If so, how can we tell them apart?

These questions are ultimately empirical in nature. The real, workable answers will come from clinical experience and scientific study, not ideology.

CAN KIDS CONSENT TO TRANSSEXUALISM?

Can kids meaningfully consent to going down the transsexual path?

Skipping default puberty by going on puberty blockers and cross-sex hormones renders a child sterile, and those who remove their gonads become hormonally dependent upon the medical industry for the rest of their lives.

Can a fourteen-year-old kid fully grasp the consequences of this decision? What about a ten-year-old kid?

To make matters worse, public understanding of transgenderism and transsexualism is in a truly sorry state. For example, it is not yet common knowledge that there are two fundamentally different types of transgenderism.

If adults lack such basic, rudimentary knowledge, how much can the kids know? In this state of ignorance, can kids even *begin* to make informed decisions about transition?

Kids are also not being told about the limitations of transsexualism. It is not currently possible for humans to change sex. Kids ought to know that medical transition makes people more closely resemble the other sex, but it does not literally make them that sex.

Youth gender transition is backed by several large medical organizations, and it's often portrayed as a safe, efficacious treatment. In truth, the efficacy of youth medical transition is still unknown. It's important for gender-dysphoric kids and their parents to know that medical transition remains an experimental treatment, and there is no way to know for sure whether any particular individual will ultimately benefit from medical transition.

GIVING CROSS-SEX HORMONES EARLIER AS HARM REDUCTION

The original justification for using puberty blockers in transsexual youth was to give them time to think through the decision to transition. But studies show that almost all transsexual youth who start puberty blockers continue onto cross-sex hormones, so the original justification does not hold up.

Portrayal of puberty blockers as safe and reversible is also misleading. If a child takes blockers to forestall puberty and decides to go off of them and resume their natal puberty, it is not as though nothing has happened.

Puberty blocker monotherapy in pubescent kids stalls bone growth during a developmental stage in which bone strengthening is typically rapid and pronounced. Stripped of hormones, people are more susceptible to developing neurological issues suggestive of mitochondrial dysfunction such as joint and muscle pain, cognitive impairment, and mental health issues—all of which lower quality of life.

Given that puberty blocker monotherapy causes such intense side effects and is used primarily to forestall puberty until the calendar says a kid can consent to taking cross-sex hormones, this use of puberty blockers should be reconsidered.

I have a proposal. Instead of giving puberty blocker monotherapy to juvenile transsexuals, give them what they actually want: cross-sex hormones. These could be administered instead of puberty blockers, or in combination.

This proposal might seem extreme, but is giving pubescent kids cross-sex hormones any more extreme than several years of puberty blocker monotherapy followed by giving them those same hormones?

One potential snag to this approach is that it's probably less feasible for FTMs. Females hit puberty earlier than males and testosterone is arguably more intense than estrogen, so cross-sex hormone administration after the onset of puberty is less risky for MTFS.

In general, I am quite wary of youth gender transition. It is still new and its long-term efficacy unknown.

I also doubt most gender clinicians working today can identify the kids who would benefit from medical transition reliably enough to make the enterprise of youth medical transition ethical overall.

In addition, transsexualism studies have low follow-up rates that call into question the validity of the findings, and there are more detransitioners with each passing day.

However, I believe some kids stand to benefit from youth medical transition. I don't know the proportion or how to reliably identify them, but some surely exist. For the subset of kids who stand to benefit from medical transition, which option is better?

1. Having a cross-sex puberty at a developmentally normal age
2. Being held in developmental stasis by a drug with global side effects and lagging behind peers for several years, then going through cross-sex puberty

In both scenarios, the kids end up permanently sterile. In both, they consent to experimental medical treatment before they are truly able to.

However, if virtually all gender-dysphoric kids who start puberty blockers ultimately go on to take cross-sex hormones anyway, isn't it likely that puberty blocker monotherapy is causing a great deal of harm for very little benefit?

IN SUM

* The onset of puberty generally arrives before people are old enough to legally consent to serious, irreversible medical interventions. To get around this issue, clinicians sometimes give gender-dysphoric minors puberty blockers to halt puberty until the calendar deems them capable of consent.

* Although youth gender transition is an experimental treatment, recipients of this treatment are not being tracked long term. This hinders the ability of clinicians to improve transgender health care. Without data on

treatment outcomes, it will not be possible to arrive at optimal clinical practices. This ignorance will harm future generations of trans people.

* Sex hormones impact the whole body by acting at receptor sites in tissues and organs. They also act through receptor sites in mitochondria—organelles found in nearly all human cells which produce the chemical energy that keeps us alive.

* Estradiol helps maintain mitochondrial health. Devoid of sex hormones, people are more susceptible to developing mitochondrial dysfunction. Puberty blockers strip the body of sex hormones, so their use contributes to systemic mitochondrial dysfunction. Since puberty blocker monotherapy is so detrimental, it might be less harmful to give cross-sex hormones earlier, at a more developmentally appropriate time.

* GnRH agonists (puberty blockers) have intense, widespread side effects. People on these drugs commonly report serious neurological or physical issues such as memory loss, neuroticism, headaches, fatigue, joint pain, muscle pain, or bone deterioration. Puberty blocker monotherapy weakens the bones of transsexual minors by stalling bone growth during a developmental phase in which bone growth and strengthening is generally rapid.

* Prior to the social media revolution, persistence and desistance rates among dysphoric youth differed drastically based on sexual orientation. Children whose wish for medical transition persisted were overwhelmingly homosexual, while those who desisted were mostly nonhomosexual.

* Puberty blockers solidify commitment to gender transition. Social transition does too. The transsexual path involves highly consequential surgeries and lifelong reliance on synthetic hormones, so social transition and puberty blockers are not neutral interventions.

* Ideologically motivated stances on youth gender transition are unlikely to reflect what is actually best for transsexual youth. It's still unknown whether it is possible to adequately differentiate kids who would be harmed by medical transition from those who would achieve a net benefit. Clinical experience and empirical studies will ultimately provide insight into the best practices for dealing with juvenile gender dysphoria. Ideology will not.

ENDING THE COVER-UP

HELPING AUTOHETEROSEXUALS INTERPRET THEIR EXPERIENCES

The evidence for the existence of autoheterosexuality is over-whelming: it *obviously* exists.

If millions of people are autoheterosexual, is it even *possible* to continually suppress knowledge of it on a long-term basis? And if it is possible, is it *ethical*?

Autoheterosexuality is the most common driver of transgen-derism. Given this fact, shouldn't autoheterosexuals have access to knowledge about their orientations so they can properly interpret their experiences and make informed decisions regarding gender transition?

Ideally, yes. But that's not what's happening.

In the early 2000s, a misguided group of transgender activists worked together to suppress awareness of autoandrophilia and autogynephilia[1]. This set in motion a suppression impulse that continues to the present day. Online, there is a strong social norm among trans people to downplay the relevance of these concepts or outright dismiss them as transphobic and pseudoscientific whenever they get brought up.

This socially enforced ignorance among autohet trans people makes it harder for the broader autoheterosexual population to interpret their feelings and comprehend their situation.

This is an injustice pertaining to knowledge—a type of injustice known as *epistemic injustice*. It is an epistemic injustice when people are unable to adequately interpret their own experiences because the essential concept to grasp is hidden from them[2].

As it stands now, some autohet trans people are prioritizing their desire to *see themselves a particular way* over the desire that other autoheterosexuals have to *properly interpret their own experiences and feelings.*

Many autohets don't even know a name for the orientation that drives their gender feelings. And when they do finally learn a name for it, they often encounter misleading information that damages their ability to interpret their situation.

This epistemic injustice has harmed me and countless others. It is unfair and unnecessary, so it must end.

Activists have successfully suppressed knowledge of autoheterosexuality and its connection to transgenderism so far, but eventually the truth will get out.

When it does, gender-critical feminists (aka "trans-exclusionary radical feminists" or "TERFS") and socially regressive political groups will disparage autoheterosexuality and push the narrative that suits their ideological goals. They already do.

However, if the trans people who are supposedly safeguarding trans rights are obviously wrong about autoheterosexuality, they won't be taken seriously.

To end the epistemic injustice caused by the autohet cover-up, autoheterosexuals must understand their orientations so they can speak about them clearly.

It needs to be socially acceptable within the trans community to identify as autogynephilic, autoandrophilic, or an equivalent label. As it stands now, autoheterosexuals can lose friends and get excluded from LGBTQ groups for being honest, informed, and open about their sexual orientation.

This state of affairs is obviously insane: one of the central aims of LGBTQ organizations is to fight against stigmatization of uncommon gender-based sexual orientations and to advocate for the people who have them.

Why is there an exception for autogynephilia and autoandrophilia?

Why are so many new identities invariably deemed *valid*, yet identifying as autogynephilic or autoandrophilic brings hostility? Pretty suspicious, right? This hypocritical bias is just one more sign that these orientations exist and are the norm among trans people.

The current widespread dismissal of autoheterosexuality among autohet trans people leaves them unprepared to contest false claims about the orientation that birthed their gender identities. With their heads buried in the sand, their asses are ripe for a kicking.

When autoandrophilia and autogynephilia go mainstream, there will be some backlash against gender-variant people. The sooner trans people destigmatize these orientations among themselves, the better the odds of successfully combating political backlash.

Fortunately, it's possible to destigmatize autoheterosexuality through honest and skillful communication. Describing autoandrophilic and autogynephilic orientations collectively as "autoheterosexual" allows us to speak about them *as clearly as possible*, in a way that sounds *as normal as possible*.

Many of the same strategies that proved effective in destigmatizing same-sex attractions can be repurposed to destigmatize attractions to being the other sex (e.g., coming out, "born this way").

The place to start is *within* the LGBTQ community, by coming out to each other.

If autoheterosexuality exists and is the most common cause of transgenderism, don't autoheterosexuals inevitably need to come out at some point? Why wait?

Most people will learn of autoandrophilia and autogynephilia *before* transgender people attain the legal protections they deserve. Waiting isn't realistic.

These autohet orientations are outside of mainstream aware-ness for now, but that's about to end. Although I intend to main-stream them, they're already on their way there. Awareness is building. The tipping point is near.

When the broader public becomes aware of autoheterosexual-ity, how would *you* like it portrayed?

* As an acceptable way to exist that isn't intrinsically harmful and can be integrated into open society?
* As "just a fetish", a mental disorder, or a threat to others?

For the former to happen, autoheterosexuality needs to lose its stigma among sexual and gender minorities. If they can't destigma-tize it among themselves, what hope is there for the rest of society?

That's why progress has to start at home, by coming out to each other.

TRULY INFORMED CONSENT

To many trans people, the concepts of autogynephilia and autoandrophilia feel invalidating or bring up feelings they don't want to address. It doesn't help that in the ongoing culture war over transgenderism, these concepts have been frequently invoked in ways intended to hurt or belittle trans people.

Still, that doesn't make it acceptable to misrepresent autohet-erosexuality—*especially* to people who are trying to figure out their gender situation (i.e., if they're trans).

Autoheterosexuality is too important to be lied about or consistently misrepresented. Gender transition is a fucking serious decision that ought to be informed to the greatest extent possible.

Covering up the central role that autoheterosexuality plays in most instances of transgenderism in Western countries does a disservice to trans people. It robs them of their ability to make truly informed, consensual decisions regarding gender transition.

If an autohet person wants to transition but doesn't even know the *name* of the sexual orientation underlying their desire to be the other sex before they start taking hormones, how is that *informed*? How is that *consensual*?

TEACH AUTOHETEROSEXUALITY IN SEX ED

Both autoheterosexuality and the two-type model of transgenderism belong in the sexual education curriculum.

Kids who are old enough to learn about homosexuality and bisexuality are also old enough to learn about autoheterosexuality (at an age-appropriate level of detail, of course).

It doesn't have to be graphic or complicated. Explaining the gist can be quite simple:

Some girls and boys who like the other gender also enjoy being the other gender. Some of them even choose to live as that gender.

See? The basic idea isn't that complicated.

The two transgender types represent fundamentally different situations. It's important for people with these orientations to know specifically which one they have, so they can best interpret their situation and plan accordingly.

Kids can't do the kind of mature, long-term thinking that ought to precede transsexualism, so it's also important that adults disabuse them of the magical notion that sex change is literally possible. Gender transition allows males to live as women and females to live as men, but it's not possible to truly change sex. Kids who want to live as the other gender ought to understand the limitations and trade-offs inherent to the cross-gender journey.

By receiving reliable knowledge about the causes of transgenderism, gender-variant kids can avoid endless agonizing over whether or not they're "actually trans". Instead, they can immediately recognize if they are autoheterosexual or homosexual and start thinking about how they want to handle their gender situation.

Many post-transition autoheterosexuals wish they had transitioned before they went through "the wrong puberty". Teaching the causes of transgenderism in school is the best way for them to comprehend their gender situation as early as possible. It's in their best interest.

Put autoheterosexuality and the two-type transgender model in sex ed. Leaving them out is lying by omission.

The evidence is in.

Teach it.

THE INCOMPATIBILITY BETWEEN ACTIVISM AND TRUTH-SEEKING

Sometimes people are wrong about themselves. It's rude to point out in social situations but true nonetheless. No one has perfect knowledge of themselves.

Since people can be wrong about themselves, "lived experience" is not a reliable foundation for knowledge[3]. We don't create true knowledge by uncritically accepting people's testimony of themselves.

Humans are innately fallible, which is why we have collectively benefited so much from scientific approaches to knowledge production. Autogynephilic writer Zack M. Davis explained:

"If introspection were sufficient to reveal the true structure of human psychology, it's not clear why we would even *need* to do science; we would just *know*. It's precisely *because* careful observation and experiments can tell us things about ourselves that we didn't already know, that science is useful."[4] [emphasis in original]

This need to look beyond subjective experience is especially important in matters of sexuality.

If someone's sexuality is displeasing to their idealized self-image, they may lie about it. They could also simply be unaware of it. Regardless, their self-reports wouldn't reflect reality.

When this phenomenon occurs on a group level, it leads to a bunch of people lying to each other and telling each other what they want to hear. When researchers set out to help these identity groups and advocate for them by studying them, the resulting research is warped by the dictates of identity politics.

Ray Blanchard wrote about this dynamic:

"People lie about their sexuality. They lie to themselves; they lie to others. They are also sometimes genuinely ignorant of their own predilection until a chance circumstance reveals it to them. It is not only bad people who do this; it is all kinds of people, including good, intelligent, and generally honest people. I realize that this notion will be anathema to those who think that a responsible clinician is one who believes everything that the patient has to say, or that a responsible researcher is one who produces only data that furthers the goals of identity politics."[5]

That last point about research and identity politics is crucial to understand.

In the science game, activism and truth-seeking are fundamentally at odds[6].

The pursuit of truth requires not knowing the conclusion before data collection has even begun. It requires publishing findings even if they're politically problematic.

Just as individuals can be wrong about themselves, groups of people can be collectively wrong about their group—especially if an inconvenient truth sullies their collective self-image. Researchers who strive to validate the preferred narratives of groups they study inevitably corrupt the truth-seeking mission with their desire to do right by that group.

This epistemic malpractice obscures the path to new knowledge and cripples the knowledge-production process. It also damages the ability of individuals in those groups to learn true, actionable knowledge about themselves.

Researchers can't seek truth and do activism at the same time. They must pick one.

IN SUM

* Autoheterosexuality is the most common cause of gender dysphoria, yet many autohet trans people continue to suppress knowledge about their sexual orientation. This cover-up damages autoheterosexuals' ability to properly interpret their experiences and give truly informed consent to gender-affirming medical interventions.

* In order to fix the epistemic injustice created by the cover-up of autoheterosexuality, autohets must become knowledgeable about their orientations, come out, and pass on their knowledge to others like them. If sexual minorities cannot destigmatize autoheterosexuality among themselves, there is little hope of destigmatizing it among the general public.

* Transsexualism is increasingly available on an "informed consent" basis that leaves the patient to be their own gatekeeper. But if a would-be transsexual can't even articulate which of the two known types of gender dysphoria they have, they are not informed and thus are not truly able to give informed consent.

* Autoheterosexuality belongs in the sexual education curriculum alongside instruction on other gender-based sexual orientations. Lessons on transgenderism and gender identity should incorporate the two-type model of transgenderism. By learning about autoheterosexuality and the two-type model in sex ed, homosexual and autoheterosexual youth could comprehend their gender situation as early as possible and thus have more agency in shaping their gender destiny.

* Humans are inherently prone to errors in understanding themselves and the world around them. To reduce the impact of human fallibility in the search for knowledge, our species developed the process of liberal science. For this process to function properly, truth-seeking must take priority over political concerns. Activism and truth-seeking are fundamentally at odds. Researchers cannot do both at the same time.

A CALL FOR REVOLUTION

UPGRADING TO THE NEXT PHASE OF TRANSGENDER RESEARCH

When scientists do research, they operate under a shared intellectual framework. This collection of concepts, past research findings, and theories is known as a *paradigm*[1].

Scientific paradigms direct research by offering the scientific community a common framework to work within. They make clear which research problems seem to have been solved and which remain.

For example, biologists operate within an evolutionary paradigm that understands biological evolution to be the process that creates and shapes biological life. Particle physicists operate under the Standard Model, which can currently describe all of the elementary particles and three of the four elementary forces.

Science advances in complexity and depth through a series of paradigm revolutions. As the contradictions and inadequacies of one paradigm grow too numerous, the opportunity for a new paradigm to assert its superiority presents itself.

In transgenderism research, the cracks are starting to show. It's ripe for a paradigm revolution.

Transgenderism researchers currently operate under a *gender identity paradigm.* In this paradigm, people possess a gender identity. Most people have a gender identity that matches their sex, but some don't. The ones who don't are called transgender.

The gender identity paradigm doesn't sufficiently explain where gender identity and gender dysphoria come from. This glaring shortcoming needs to be addressed.

Scientists working within the gender identity paradigm usually portray transgenderism as some sort of neurological intersex condition in which a person's brain develops in a way that is more like the other sex in some ways. The resulting conflict between brain and body leads to cross-gender identity and suffering in the form of gender dysphoria. For transgender people of homosexual etiology, there's some truth to this[2].

But the gender identity paradigm doesn't account for the majority of trans people, many of whom have heterosexual relationships, marriages, or children before they come out—some in their thirties, their forties, or even later. Their gender nonconformity is usually not as obvious, so their announcement of a transgender identity often comes as a surprise to friends, family, and acquaintances.

Are we to believe that these markedly different types of gender variance have the same cause and are ultimately the same phenomenon at root?

No, of course not—they're obviously different.

THE POWER OF ETIOLOGICAL UNDERSTANDING

The gender identity paradigm doesn't account for the obvious differences between same-sex-attracted trans people and the rest. If anything, researchers working in that paradigm go out of their way to pretend these differences don't exist. Its construct of gender identity is somewhat fuzzy too.

In the gender identity paradigm, gender can be both fluid and a fixed aspect of someone's psychology—ever-changing, yet also unchangeable. Contradictions abound.

The autoheterosexual explanation offers a way out of these apparent contradictions.

Autoheterosexuality can also be measured more directly than gender identity. There isn't yet a way to directly measure the gender someone feels themselves to be, but it *is* possible to measure physical arousal. Sexologists do it all the time.

The two-type model is also more straightforward. Sexual orientations are behind both types of transgenderism. One orientation points toward others of the same sex; the other points toward oneself as the other sex. Although opposites in both gender and direction, these orientations are both associated with gender discomfort and a propensity for sustained cross-gender expression.

The gender identity paradigm lacks this straightforward, elegant symmetry. Its research also continues to produce subpar results. In fact, researchers working within that paradigm who do find patterns may not even notice them.

Recall the massive European longitudinal study that tracked transgender people's sexual orientation over three years[3]. Researchers found that neither hormones nor surgeries had an effect on sexual orientation changes, and in their write-up, they gave no clear explanation for these changes.

However, the interpretive lens of the two-type model enabled me to see an obvious pattern in their results. When a large number of trans people started to play a sex role typically associated with their birth sex within their sexual fantasies, same-sex attraction dropped and other-sex attraction went up: *meta-attraction was behind the reported shifts in sexual orientation.*

Seeing this didn't require fancy statistics, only a better model.

It's time for the scientific community to adopt this superior framework for understanding transgenderism.

The old one is obsolete.

IT'S TIME FOR A PARADIGM REVOLUTION

It's time to transition to an etiological paradigm of transgenderism.

In this paradigm, there are different causal pathways (etiologies) leading to transgenderism. So far, we know two exist.

One is associated with homosexuality and the other with autoheterosexuality.

In this paradigm, the ultimate cause of cross-gender identity and gender dysphoria can be found in either autoheterosexuality or homosexuality.

By independently studying these different types of dysphorias and identities, scientists can better understand the factors that influence the development of gender issues and a desire to transition. There *might* be more etiologies, but until researchers identify study participants by etiology and group them accordingly, it won't be possible to discern what these rarer etiologies may be.

Adopting the etiological paradigm is long overdue. It was prematurely discarded for reasons that were political rather than scientific.

It wasn't debunked, disproven, or falsified.

It remains relevant.

The etiological approach to understanding transgenderism has already produced a fairly solid picture of how autoheterosexual dysphoria and cross-gender identity comes about in males. Building on this foundation, research on female autoheterosexuality could produce knowledge about the similarities and differences in autoheterosexuality between the sexes.

It's also imperative to directly study autoheterosexuality in a stand-alone way that's outside the transgender context. Homosexuality has been studied in this manner, and autoheterosexuality deserves similar consideration.

If autosexual orientations are the mirror image of allosexual orientations, then autoheterosexuality research would also deepen our understanding of alloheterosexuality, the most common sexual orientation.

There used to be more research on homosexual dysphoria and cross-gender identity back when most clinicians and researchers considered it to represent true transsexualism, but research on homosexual transgenderism has been scarce in recent years. Both types of transgenderism have been mixed together under the "transgender" label.

Differentiating between these two types in research will be essential for discovering new, actionable knowledge that can help trans people understand themselves and decide how best to navigate their gender feelings.

Researchers have already formally established the superiority of the etiological paradigm for males. They've also established the existence of a homosexual etiology for females, but formal research hasn't yet caught up with the fact that autoandrophilic transgenderism is common among FTMs.

The etiological paradigm of transgenderism is where the next, more advanced stage of transgenderism research will unfold.

By separating participants by etiology and sex, researchers will obtain a more precise idea of what separates people who have severe gender issues from those who don't—and what makes transitioners different from desisters, detransitioners, and those who don't want to transition.

This more advanced research will discern whether rapid-onset gender dysphoria represents a distinct etiology—and if mental conditions such as autism, schizophrenia, or dissociation can, in rare cases, lead to transgenderism independent of homosexuality or autoheterosexuality.

Further research may find that the two-type model is insufficient and that there are more etiologies of transgenderism. If that happens, the etiological model will need to be updated to incorporate these other etiologies.

Still, the existence of multiple distinct etiologies of transgenderism has long been established. The etiological framework for understanding transgenderism is more accurate and precise than the gender identity paradigm. It's strictly superior.

RESEARCHERS MUST SEPARATE BY ETIOLOGY AND SEX

Not separating study participants by etiology damages the ability to generate findings particular to each etiology. This epistemic negligence especially harms trans people of homosexual etiology, as they are dwarfed by the much larger autoheterosexual population.

How can researchers generate findings relevant to trans people of homosexual etiology if they're mixed in with autoheterosexuals and outnumbered by them? Likewise, how can researchers generate sufficiently precise findings for autoheterosexual trans people if they're being mixed in with those of homosexual etiology?

It's important to separate by sex too. Physical and mental differences between sexes lead to different social realities and psychological tendencies. Sex makes an enormous difference.

With these two etiologies and two sexes, there are four total groups to compare and contrast in order to infer the relative impacts of etiology and sex. By distinguishing between groups of trans people based on their sex and etiology, researchers can arrive at knowledge specific to people in these groups.

These groups arise due to inborn developmental factors that recur across generations, so studies that differentiate between them will have more lasting value (and garner more citations).

It's time for a paradigm revolution that leaves the gender identity paradigm in the past where it belongs.

It's time to move forward.

It's time to use what actually works.

IN SUM

* The scientific process is conducted within a shared intellectual framework—a paradigm. This collection of concepts, past research findings, and theories orients research by making clear which research problems seem to have been solved and which remain. As the flaws and inconsistencies in a given paradigm accumulate, it becomes susceptible to paradigm revolution—replacement by a new paradigm that better explains the data.

* Most transgenderism research is currently conducted within a gender identity paradigm in which most

people have a gender identity corresponding to their sex, but some don't. The ones who don't are called transgender.

* The gender identity paradigm lacks a coherent, evidence-based explanation that can account for most people who have mismatches of sex and gender. It doesn't even have an answer for what causes gender dysphoria and cross-gender identity in the first place. Researchers in this paradigm sometimes suggest that trans people's brains have some sort of cross-sex shift, but this mainly applies to homosexual trans people.

* In the etiological paradigm, there are distinct types of transgenderism with distinct causes known as etiologies. Both known etiologies—homosexual and autoheterosexual—account for virtually all cases of transgenderism. These atypical gender-based sexual orientations are opposites in both gender and direction, but they can both culminate in gender dysphoria, cross-gender identity, and gender transition.

* Transgenderism researchers need to start separating by etiology because the two etiologies are fundamentally different psychological, social, and sexual situations. It's important to separate by sex as well, because females and males have large differences in mental and physical traits that lead to significantly different social realities and life experiences.

* By separating participants into four groups according to etiology and sex, researchers will generate knowledge that has a much higher chance of being relevant to the people in these groups. They will also form a more precise idea of the other factors that separate people who have severe gender issues from those that don't—as well as what differentiates transitioners from desisters, detransitioners, and those who choose not to transition.

PART 9

LOOKING BACK, MOVING FORWARD

CLOSING THOUGHTS

RETRACING STEPS WITH AN
EYE TO THE FUTURE

I wrote this book to solve a problem: autoheterosexuality is the most common driver of transgenderism and about as common as homosexuality, but almost nobody understands it. This widespread ignorance harms autoheterosexuals by damaging their ability to properly interpret their situation, be understood by others, and give truly informed consent for hormones or surgeries.

I began by sketching the outlines. Chapter by chapter, I filled in sections until a detailed picture of autoheterosexuality emerged. I then zoomed out to the broader autosexual context and showed that for each type of external attraction to others, there exists an internal attraction to a type of being.

With the general form of autosexuality now clear, I touched on some aspects of integrating autoheterosexuality into society and gave special attention to the ethically fraught issue of youth gender transition. I also argued that epistemic injustice unfairly keeps autoheterosexuals in the dark about their situation and proposed a systemic solution to this problem: implementing the etiological paradigm of transgenderism.

To wrap things up, let's retrace these steps in greater detail and then end with some thoughts on meaning and direction for autoheterosexuals.

OUR PATH THUS FAR

We began by learning about the two-type model of transgenderism and the concept of autoheterosexuality. We learned how to sort trans people into homosexual and autoheterosexual groups using the two-type typology, and why this sorting method is currently controversial within transgender subcultures.

I listed some common autohet patterns of thought and sexuality, so you could determine if you were autoheterosexual, and then recommended that you avoid making hasty or rash decisions in light of this knowledge.

We then explored the five known subtypes of autoheterosexuality: anatomic, physiologic, behavioral, sartorial, and interpersonal. I proposed that a sixth subtype—psyche autohet—underlies mental shifts and the internal sense of cross-gender identity that autoheterosexuals experience.

Next, we learned about meta-attraction, the gender-affirming attraction to others that can make autoheterosexuals have any type of partner preference and therefore identify as any of the letters in the LGBTQ political coalition. We also saw how this colorful coalition largely breaks down into just two sexual proclivities: same-sex sexuality and cross-gender sexuality—nonhet and autohet.

I concluded the introductory chapter by arguing that *autoheterosexual* is the correct word to describe an attraction to being the other sex, and that politically, this term has protective qualities due to the widespread acceptance of heterosexuality.

In Chapter 1.1, we briefly reviewed sex, gender, and transgenderism in order to provide the context needed to properly understand autoheterosexuality.

In Chapter 1.2, we learned about sexual orientation: what it is, how scientists measure it, and some factors that influence its development.

In Chapter 2.0, we touched on the connection between autogynephilic gender feelings and MTF cross-gender development. We also learned about autogynephilic subtypes and modern expressions of autogynephilic sexuality, and we explored the connection between mental shifts and trans identity using the Hungarian physician's case as an example.

In Chapters 2.1–2.5, we reviewed the overall form of autogynephilic interests one subtype at a time. Each subtype had its own chapter filled with historical examples.

In Chapters 3.0 and 3.1, we followed a similar approach to learning about autoandrophilia, which started with gender feelings and cross-gender development, led to discussion of autoandrophilic subtypes, and described various autoandrophilic interests in terms of these subtypes.

In Chapter 4.0, I argued that traps are not gay.

In Chapter 4.1, we covered gynandromorphophilia (GAMP), the attraction to MTFS that often coexists alongside autogynephilia. We saw how Samoan GAMPs and American GAMPs have similar sexual preferences, which suggests that gynandromorphophilia is an innate disposition that arises across cultures. To close out, I argued that GAMPs deserve a more respectful term than "chaser" for their sexuality, and that they rightfully belong in the LGBTQ political coalition.

In Chapter 4.2, we saw that mental disorders are highly heritable and trans people have them at higher rates, which suggests that even though societal mistreatment contributes to transgender suicidality and mental health issues, genes are probably the single biggest contributor to these difficult aspects of being trans.

In Chapter 4.3, we saw that autism contributes to gender variance in several ways and that it's especially prevalent in trans populations.

In Chapter 5.0, we learned about the population prevalence of transvestism, autoheterosexuality, and same-sex attraction. Using these figures, we saw that males are roughly twice as likely to be either gay or autohet and that there are about three autoheterosexuals for every four homosexuals.

In Chapter 5.1, we saw that ancient Islamic legal scholars differentiated between two types of effeminate males who resemble the two types of MTFS we know of today. We then retraced the path that Western science took to ultimately arrive at the two-type model of MTF transgenderism.

In Chapter 5.2, we looked into the sexual orientation changes that many transgender people report after transitioning. We saw a clear pattern: when fewer trans people reportedly played cross-gender sex roles in their sexual fantasies, they reported less same-sex sexuality. This pattern suggested that meta-attraction influenced these reported changes to sexual orientation.

In Chapter 5.3, we saw that autohet trans is the most common type of trans in Western countries. By applying the two-type typology to data from massive, institutionally popular surveys of transgender Americans, we arrived at an estimate that about 75% of transgender Americans are of autoheterosexual etiology.

In Chapter 5.4, we saw that in recent years, the demographic makeup of gender clinic referrals has drastically shifted toward females. By comparing the etiological makeup of the US transgender population to the makeup of the broader etiological population, we could infer that being either female or autohet increases the odds of gender transition within the broader etiological population.

In Chapter 6.0, we explored the cross-gender development process in which autoheterosexuals develop affinity for being the other sex and disdain for being their own, and saw that reinforcement shifts their gender sentiments over time. We also saw how this process can culminate in transformative gender identity shifts and the desire to live as the other sex.

In Chapter 6.1, we learned more deeply about gender euphoria, the lovely, comforting feelings of rightness that help autoheterosexuals feel at home in themselves. We saw how this internal relationship with the cross-gender self can lead to deep attachment culminating in gender transition—that for autohets, gender transition is about becoming what they love.

In Chapter 6.2, we embarked on a long, dismal journey through the lands of gender suffering and saw how autoheterosexual gender dysphoria can manifest as dissociation, gender envy, depression, anxiety, or suicidality. We also learned about ego-dystonic arousal and shame, as well as the repression that often results from it.

In Chapter 6.3, we explored the question at the heart of the controversy: does autoheterosexuality cause cross-gender identity, or does cross-gender identity cause autoheterosexuality? In the end, the verdict was that autoheterosexuality comes first and cross-gender identity is a potential downstream effect of it.

In Chapter 7.0, we encountered the general form of autosexual trans identity: attraction to being a particular type of entity can make people feel good or bad feelings about how well they embody that entity, and these reinforcing feelings nudge them toward greater identification with that entity over time. We also learned about the etiological theory that explains these autosexual orientations as variations of erotic target location in which the location is one's own body instead of the bodies of others.

In Chapter 7.1, we saw how attraction to being an amputee can lead to transableism in the forms of body integrity dysphoria, transabled identity, and the desire for limb amputation.

In Chapter 7.2, we observed that attractions to being a minor can lead people to embody youth through dress (diapers and children's clothing), behavior (age regression), or social interaction (caregiver/little roleplay). We also learned about age dysphoria, cross-age identity, and other aspects of transageism.

In Chapter 7.3, we began a lengthy exploration of transspecies identity that started with furries. We saw that furries are usually sexually attracted to anthropomorphic animals and also attracted to the idea of being one themselves. We also touched on research suggesting that furry roleplay is associated with a weaker sense of human embodiment and more negative sentiments toward humanity.

In Chapter 7.4, we went deeper into nonhuman identity by learning about therians—people who feel a deep integral connection to an animal species and often identify as an animal themselves. We saw that therians may embody their animal side through mental shifts, phantom shifts, roleplay, or engaging in animalistic behaviors. By looking at community surveys of therians, it became apparent that many therians are sexually attracted to the same type of species they identify as.

In Chapter 7.5, we delved into the broader collection of nonhuman identities that fall under the alterhuman umbrella by learning about otherkin, people with nonhuman identities. We saw that otherkin commonly embody their kintype through xenogenders, body modifications, or body adornments that call forth their inner nonhuman self. By looking at results from a community survey of otherkin, we saw that most otherkin report signs of sexual attraction to being their kintypes. We also saw that otherkin identify as transgender at rates that greatly exceed population norms—an overlap suggesting that cross-gender identity and nonhuman identity share a similar underlying cause.

In Chapter 7.6, I proposed the existence of autophylophilic transracialism: transracialism caused by sexual attraction to being a particular race. I conducted an exploratory survey of transrace people and found that most respondents reported sexual attractions both *to* and *to being* their identified race. Further analysis of this autophylophilic subset revealed they had good and bad feelings about their perceived racial embodiment akin to the gender feelings of autoheterosexuals. Fittingly, most were also autoheterosexual or transgender. Following in the footsteps of feminists, I asserted that arguments for the legitimacy of transgenderism also apply to transracialism.

In Chapter 8.0, we examined some of the potential sticking points for integrating autoheterosexuality into society. I addressed freedom of dress, the issue of pronouns, and broadening the definition of sexual orientation. I also questioned which forms of trans identity can potentially be integrated into society and argued that if safe and reliable technological methods existed that could modify nongender dimensions of sexual orientation such as age, species, and location, it would reduce human suffering. Finally, I argued that it's not transphobic to lack sexual interest in trans people, and that insinuating otherwise is coercive and betrays the spirit of consent.

In Chapter 8.1, we waded into the controversial waters of youth gender transition and found that puberty blocker monotherapy in transsexual minors is widespread yet poorly tracked. After reviewing research on nontrans people, we saw that puberty blocker monotherapy creates a sexless hormonal state associated with a wide array of serious side effects indicative of mitochondrial dysfunction. In light of this evidence, I argued that giving cross-sex hormones to transsexual youth at an earlier age is likely to cause less bodily harm than years of puberty blocker monotherapy followed by cross-sex hormones.

In Chapter 8.2, I argued that suppressing awareness of autoheterosexuality harms autohets by making it harder for them to properly interpret their experiences and make truly informed decisions about how to navigate their gender issues. I proposed two strategies for addressing this epistemic injustice: include autoheterosexuality in sexual education curriculums, and come out.

In Chapter 8.3, I argued that the gender identity paradigm of transgenderism needs to be replaced because it's strictly inferior to an etiological paradigm that incorporates the two known types of transgenderism—and that to implement this change, transgender researchers must start sorting study participants by etiology and sex in order to arrive at findings relevant to each group.

To close out, I'm going to touch on some mental approaches to living with autoheterosexuality:

1. Cultivate an unapologetic disposition toward autoheterosexuality that incorporates both self-awareness and self-acceptance (own it, rock it, be based)
2. Channel the cross-gender drive into embodying virtues associated with the other sex in order to become a better version of yourself and live a more meaningful life

I first came across positive, adaptive ideas like these in Anne Lawrence's work. I'm including them here for readers who know they're autoheterosexual but are unsure of what to do with this knowledge.

They're meant to be a nudge in the right direction, but they aren't the whole map.

THE BASED PATH TO SELF-ACCEPTANCE

In spiritual subcultures, it's common for people to use spiritual ideas and practices in order to avoid addressing their unresolved issues—a phenomenon known as "spiritual bypass"[1]. This behavior has a serious flaw, however: by trying to hitch a ride to the transcendent tip of Maslow's pyramid via spiritual bypass, spiritual seekers ultimately leave their inner conflicts and wounds intact.

Something analogous seems to be happening among autoheterosexuals who aren't self-aware about their orientation, except the dynamic involves identity instead of spiritual enlightenment.

Rather than directly confronting its sexual origins and working through the resulting feelings, many autoheterosexuals prefer to conceive of their cross-gender embodiment as primarily a matter of identity. This leaves sexual shame buried deep within, unaddressed. On this unstable foundation of unresolved inner tension, they construct their cross-gender self.

It doesn't have to be this way.

I've talked to enough self-aware autohets to know it's possible to cut through that inner tension and truly accept oneself as autoheterosexual.

It's possible to directly face the sexual origins behind the cross-gender wish, work through those uncomfortable feelings, make peace with it, and ultimately come out the other side more emotionally grounded and comfortable with oneself.

This is the *based* path to self-acceptance, as proposed by rapper Lil B:

"Based means being yourself. Not being scared of what people think about you. Not being afraid to do what you wanna do. Being positive."[2]

A based autoheterosexual can think, "Yeah, it's ultimately sexual, but *so what?*". Rather than worrying that strangers are judging them, they can rest easy in the knowledge that there's nothing inherently wrong with them. They aren't hurting anyone.

By owning their situation and their response to it, self-aware, based autohets can avoid the mental gymnastics needed to view their cross-gender tendency as a function of gender identity instead of an outgrowth of autosexuality. They can understand why they behave and feel the way they do without having to rely on questionable gender metaphysics.

Although I have personally found this unapologetic, sex-positive approach liberating, I know it won't work for everyone. Not all of us have the chutzpah needed for this kind of brazen self-acceptance.

But enough of us do. It's time that more of us took the self-aware route by becoming informed about our orientations and accepting ourselves as we are, without apology.

HARNESSING THE CROSS-GENDER NORTH STAR

Beholden to technological society, people do what technology demands of them[3]. Drawn into a digital existence whose artifice falls short of meeting their emotional needs, their desire for love, connection, and meaning often goes unsatisfied. Further limited by innate ability, class, or other aspects of their lives, many never satisfy these deeper emotional needs.

On top of these challenges, we autoheterosexuals also have to address our longing to embody the other sex.

With no uniform solution for appeasing our inner cross-gender spirit, we must repeatedly decide the role our sexuality will play in our lives: will we fully repress, pursue transsexualism, or choose something between these two extremes?

Technology to change sexual orientation does not yet exist, so there's no way of escaping these decisions. We must decide the degree to which we incorporate our sexuality into our lives.

One way to chart our path through this gender cosmos is to treat the cross-gender traits we admire as a source of guidance— a personal North Star.

The gravity of this cross-gender North Star attracts us, drawing us closer. And although we may not be able to fly outside the range of its pull, we can choose to fall toward it with style by embodying traits we associate with the gender we admire and to which we aspire.

Those of us attracted to being men can cultivate masculine virtues such as strength, competence, courage, tenacity, discipline, ambition, confidence, independence, assertiveness, loyalty, mastery, or honor.

Those of us attracted to being women can nurture feminine virtues such as beauty, empathy, care, compassion, flexibility, love, gentleness, tolerance, sensitivity, kindness, cooperation, or grace.

By integrating valuable character traits, we can better see the value in ourselves. By tapping into this source of meaning, we can feel we matter. By guiding our lives with this inner light, we can carry our love within us, wherever we go.

HOW YOU CAN HELP

There are currently millions of pre-transition autoheterosexuals who privately grapple with gender issues but don't know why. Many feel confused, ashamed, or alone in their struggle.

In addition, many autoheterosexuals began medical transition before they understood the sexual orientation behind their cross-gender wish, so the consent they gave for such treatment cannot be considered informed.

Thus, widespread ignorance of autoheterosexuality continues to harm autoheterosexuals across the gender transition spectrum. These costs are unacceptable. This epistemic injustice must end.

To end this catastrophic ignorance, *autoheterosexuality must be destigmatized and its existence made common knowledge.* These twin goals must happen in tandem.

Unfortunately, I can't achieve this alone. I'll need help from other self-aware autoheterosexuals.

If you are autoheterosexual and want to help destigmatize our orientation, you can 1) *come out* and 2) *spread knowledge.*

By repurposing the strategies and tactics that destigmatized homosexuality and legalized gay marriage, we can destigmatize autoheterosexuality and improve the overall well-being of our kind.

And this time, change will come much faster: we have the internet.

COME OUT

For our orientations to be destigmatized, we must come out.

By coming out, we can be better seen and understood by others. Merely by existing openly as ourselves, we can demonstrate that it's fine to be autohet and that it's no cause for alarm.

It's often easiest to start with a close friend who you expect to be supportive. If that goes well, you can expand from there. It's okay to take your time with this process: coming out slowly is still far better than staying fully closeted.

If you weigh the risks and decide it's worth coming out as autoandrophilic, autogynephilic, or autoheterosexual, please do so.

SPREAD KNOWLEDGE

If we are to understand ourselves and be understood by those we love, we must spread knowledge about our orientations.

To achieve epistemic justice, we must seize the memes of production—starting with the single most influential source of knowledge: Wikipedia.

Wikipedia is the first place most people check when they want to learn about something. As a result, knowledge there tends to diffuse outward and find its way into articles, podcasts, social media posts, and other forms of media.

Creating, maintaining, and improving Wikipedia articles pertaining to our sexuality is one of the most accessible and effective ways to spread knowledge about our orientations. By enhancing Wikipedia articles with factual edits that incorporate knowledge from the sexology literature, we can end denial of our existence and help other autosexuals comprehend their experiences.

Each autosexual orientation deserves its own Wikipedia page. For English pages, the titles should adhere to scientific naming conventions (i.e., "auto-X-philia"). Overarching concepts such as "autosexual orientation", "allosexual orientation", and "autoheterosexuality" deserve their own pages as well.

The English pages are the most crucial. They are also where we will face the greatest resistance. To bypass this obstacle and diversify our campaign beyond the Anglosphere, autosexuals who speak other languages can create and edit Wikipedia pages in those languages.

Due to the huge demographic overlap between autists and autosexuals, quite a few of us have the capacity to develop a special interest in particular topics. This single-minded focus often yields a deep, detailed understanding of the subjects we love. In addition, many of us have a stubborn insistence on accuracy and truth. Thus, many of us have what it takes to be excellent Wikipedia contributors.

As important as Wikipedia is, however, not all of us have the inclination or temperament to be effective there, and that's okay. There are many other ways you can help spread knowledge of our orientations.

Do you ever make comments or posts on the internet? Do you have a podcast, make videos, or do live streams?

No matter what medium you work in, you can help by speaking of autoheterosexuality in a calm, accepting, matter-of-fact manner that treats it as an obviously real phenomenon.

When you feel ready to speak about your personal experience with autoheterosexuality, please do. Speaking of your direct experience will help other autohets feel less alone. It'll also help humanize the autohet experience for people who don't experience cross-gender attraction themselves.

Be unapologetic: you have nothing to apologize for. Nobody gets to choose their sexual orientation, and autoheterosexuality is a perfectly fine orientation to have. Like any orientation, there are acceptable and unacceptable ways to express it, but simply having the orientation is itself morally neutral.

We will sometimes get pushback from trans people and those who consider themselves allies. We will also get pushback from conservatives and certain types of feminists. Although these groups have drastically different ideologies and beliefs, all of them will use the twin tactics of shame and disgust.

Do not let this knock you off-center. Remain calm. Take some deep breaths. When possible, be kind.

By keeping your cool while others are losing their shit, the ideas you share are more likely to take root in the brains of others.

When engaged in online discourse, it isn't important to convince your conversation partners that you are right. On all social media platforms, the vast majority of users are lurkers. Thus, what matters most is creating the impression among these unseen witnesses that you are comparatively more knowledgeable, reasonable, and thoughtful. Always consider the lurker: they are the true target of your persuasion efforts.

To make your good intentions apparent, make it clear up front that you accept trans people regardless of what etiology they are. If you think both types of trans people should have access to gender-affirming medical care, say so. If you think both types of trans people should be treated respectfully and protected from discrimination, say so.

You will likely find that some messages play better with different audiences. Once you notice these patterns, consider the social context you're in and adjust accordingly.

Connect with other self-aware autoheterosexuals and signal boost each other. This will help us find each other and build community. By keeping an open line of communication among ourselves and having each other's backs, we will surmount the obstacles that lie ahead.

We will undoubtedly succeed at mainstreaming awareness of our orientations: ideas that accurately describe reality tend to persist and spread, and autoheterosexuality is obviously real.

If anything, the real challenge lies in destigmatizing it. But we will succeed at this too. By sharing our experiences and speaking to the romantic and sentimental side of autoheterosexuality, we can teach people not to fear the love that underlies our commitment to the cross-gender path.

ACKNOWLEDGMENTS

When reading the acknowledgments sections of books, I've sometimes thought that authors were just buttering the toast of their friends and colleagues by saying they couldn't have done it without them. While crafting this girthy tome, I realized I was probably wrong about that: without help from others, I wouldn't have even *started* this book, let alone finished it.

This book wouldn't exist without material and intellectual help from self-aware autoheterosexuals. I literally couldn't have done it without you.

Andrew Conru: thank you for sponsoring this project and giving helpful guidance when needed. I truly appreciate you helping out our kind by taking a chance on me.

Tailcalled: thank you for relentlessly seeking truth in matters of sexuality and transgenderism. Your sexology work is important. Thank you for lending your expertise whenever I had questions and for curating online spaces that help us collectively gain deeper knowledge of ourselves. I am less wrong about autogyne-philia because of your influence.

Zack M. Davis: your writing helped me feel sane when I struggled with being gaslit about my sexual orientation. It made a massive difference, as did you putting me in touch with Sophia. Thank you for putting so much careful thought into writing about autogynephilia and for looking over the manuscript.

Sophia: thank you for taking the time to speak with me. Your honesty markedly increased my sanity.

Pasha: thank you for starting and running r/askAGP, the largest online community of self-aware autoheterosexuals. The discourse there helped me realize it would be good if there were more of us.

Anne Lawrence: thank you for courageously seeking truth and spreading it despite intense pushback from the transgender community. Your work helped me understand not only my sexuality, but also the scientific evidence for its existence.

This book also wouldn't exist without emotional and social support from kith and kin.

Skylark Macadamia: thank you for being such a solid friend. You're amazing. I love you. Thank you for listening to my autistic ramblings, helping me write better, and demonstrating through your actions that coming out to you first was a good idea. Thank you for leaving such extensive, useful feedback on my manuscript. This book is better because of all your help.

Monel, beautiful queer ambassador: I met you just a couple weeks after I accepted that I was autogynephilic. Your loving support helped me become at peace with my orientation, and your patient ear helped me feel heard. I love you. Thank you for being you.

Mom and Dad: I love you. Thank you for skillfully combining your gametes and putting so much effort into creating a stable home throughout my childhood. Hearing about other people's childhoods throughout my adult life has made me realize how good y'all did.

My roommates: thank you for providing the supportive home environment that helped me deal with the hostile ignorance I faced elsewhere.

Women: thank you for existing. I love you.

To the hundreds of people who have spoken with me about autoheterosexuality and transgenderism: thank you for taking the time to communicate with me. It greatly improved my ability to share what I've learned with others.

To the trans women who told me I was wrong: thank you for the gift of doubt. Without it, I wouldn't have plunged deep into the sexology literature and realized how absolutely essential it was for a book like this to exist. I sincerely hope you can make peace with the fact that sexuality underlies your cross-gender wish.

Scientists: thank you for pursuing truth and knowledge so that humans can be less wrong over time.

Ray Blanchard: thank you for characterizing autogynephilia and figuring out the two-type MTF model. You truly did a kick-ass job. Thank you for responding when I had questions.

Michael Bailey: thank you for pursuing truth into the headwinds of controversy. Thank you for researching autosexual orientations, adding me to the listserv, pointing me toward funding, and responding when I had questions.

Kevin Hsu: thank you for researching autosexual orientations, corresponding with me, and letting me share your research findings with a wider audience. That furry correlation matrix will never not be amazing.

I also want to thank all the other scientists who took the time to answer my questions, share PDFs of their papers, or share their data with me. I don't want you to get burnt by the hellfire of controversy this book is likely to ignite, so I won't name names, but you have my sincere gratitude.

Alexandra Elbakyan: you advance science more than any other human alive. Even if you were awarded every single Nobel Prize, it still wouldn't properly account for your immense contribution to science. Without your website, I wouldn't have had a chance of writing this book. But thanks to your brave work, I could. Thank you.

Scribe: thank you for helping me put together such a solid book. I know it's customary for authors to individually thank publishing staff who had a hand in making the book, but I will leave y'all unnamed to shield you from controversy. None of you deserve to face social sanctions just for doing your job.

A. Sinner: thank you for working so hard to create graphics for this book—it's far better because of your graphical assistance. Thank you for accommodating my countless contradictory whims. It was a pleasure to work with you.

Michael A. Lombardi-Nash: thank you for helping my kind by translating the book that put the T in LGBT. It was by reading your wonderful English translation of Hirschfeld's *Die Transvestiten* that I became convinced I was on the right track. Thank you for granting permission to use several quotes from it in this book.

Transrace Community: thank you for letting me survey you. I appreciate how open-minded you are. Don't let the haters stop you. Remember: if it's okay to be transgender, it's also okay to be transrace. You aren't harming anyone by being a version of yourself that you can love, relate to, and take pride in.

Finally, I'd like to acknowledge some inanimate entities that have enriched my life.

Hoops: you are the best flow prop. I love arting with you. I have enjoyed your circular embrace over the past decade and hope to for many years to come.

Blue: you are the best color. Whether neon, light, or with a tinge of green, you improve the aesthetics just about anywhere you are found.

Dextroamphetamine: thank you for granting me the executive functioning needed to carry out this long, complicated project.

SORTING BY ETIOLOGY IN TRANSGENDER RESEARCH

To conduct transgenderism studies within the etiological paradigm, it's necessary to determine which study participants are autoheterosexual, which are homosexual, and which, if any, are seemingly neither.

To quicken the transition to an etiological paradigm of transgenderism, I'd like to offer some guidance to researchers about sorting technique and the type of data needed to sort in this manner.

Autoheterosexual study participants can be identified through direct and indirect means:

1. *Direct*—ask about indicators of autoheterosexuality (cross-gender arousal, gender euphoria, and nongenital physiologic arousal)
2. *Indirect*—ask about gender-based allosexuality to enable sorting with the two-type typology

Ideally, both direct and indirect lines of questioning will be used in tandem. This is more thorough, and it tests the replicability of the two-type typology.

As a standard approach, I recommend using a two-step sorting process:

1. Sort with the two-type typology
2. Recategorize those in the homosexual group who report prior cross-gender arousal into the autohet group

STEP ONE: SORT WITH THE TWO-TYPE TYPOLOGY

To sort trans study participants with the two-type typology, use their reported gender-based allosexuality:

* Trans people who report current or prior nonhomo-sexuality (K0–5)[1] go into the autoheterosexual group
* Trans people who report lifelong homosexuality (K6) go into the homosexual group

If you collect data on multiple sexuality measures such as attraction, behavior, and fantasy, it may be hard to decide where to draw the line between homosexuality and nonhomosexuality in participants with a mixture of K5 and K6 responses and no K0–4 responses.

For example, consider a participant who reports K6 fantasy, K6 behavior, and K5 attraction. Where should this participant go?

One option is picking a single measure as the discriminant for all participants. If you choose attraction, this participant would be sorted into the nonhomosexual group. But if you choose fantasy, they would be sorted into the homosexual group.

Another option is sorting based on the plurality of responses, or a composite score created from them. Since this participant had two K6 responses and one K5 response, this method would sort them into the homosexual group.

This procedure alone—typological sorting based on gender-based allosexuality—should properly sort most study participants. However, some autohet trans people report a strict homosexual preference and are thus improperly sorted with the two-type typology. To find some of them, do a second sorting step that utilizes participants' reported history of cross-gender arousal.

STEP TWO: RECATEGORIZE USING PRIOR CROSS-GENDER AROUSAL

Locate participants in the homosexual group who report prior history of cross-gender arousal from core, anatomic, or sartorial cross-gender embodiment. Also look for those who report prior arousal from interpersonal embodiment unrelated to meta-homosexuality.

Recategorize those who report such history into the autoheterosexual group.

At this point, the vast majority of study participants have been properly sorted. It's okay to stop here. Perfect sorting is impossible.

Further scrutiny of the homosexual group in the search for autoheterosexuals may generate some false positives.

On the other hand, stopping here will also miss some autoheterosexuals whose responses to questions about allosexuality and cross-gender arousal were influenced by social desirability bias or other, unknown factors. To find these participants, you could try further sorting with a third step that uses proxy indicators of autoheterosexuality to spot participants who are likely of autohet etiology.

OPTIONAL THIRD STEP: SORTING WITH PROXY INDICATORS OF AUTOHETEROSEXUALITY

Epistemic status: experimental. Enhanced typological sorting that utilizes proxy indicators of autoheterosexuality has not yet been tested, to my knowledge.

To check for autohet participants remaining in the homosexual group, you can use proxy indicators of autoheterosexuality that participants may not recognize as such:

* Nongenital Physiologic Arousal: piloerection, butterflies in the stomach, or increased heart rate in association with cross-gender embodiment or gender euphoria
* Attraction to Androgyny: gynandromorphophilia and androgynemorphophilia
* Gender Euphoria (mild): joy, relaxation, comfort, connectedness, or serenity
* Gender Euphoria (strong): excitement, twitterpation, or crying from joy

Nongenital physiologic arousal associated with cross-gender embodiment is likely the best proxy indicator of autohetero-sexuality to use: like genital arousal, these physiologic responses to stimuli are hard to fake. Piloerection (goose bumps) might be the best nongenital physiologic response to ask about simply because it's visually apparent, unambiguous, and easy to notice.

Attraction to androgyny is likely a good proxy indicator of autoheterosexuality because these types of attractions are much more common among autoheterosexuals than homosexuals.

Strong gender euphoria is likely a reliable indicator of auto-heterosexuality. Mild gender euphoria is probably less reliable, but you can make up for this by asking about their total life-time number of gender euphoria experiences—if they report hundreds, you can be more certain their feelings originate in autoheterosexuality.

One way to collect data on gender euphoria is to straightfor-wardly ask about "gender euphoria"—many trans people are familiar with this term. But you can also ask about the types of feelings they've had from cross-gender embodiment, such as the examples listed above.

Since enhanced typological sorting with proxy indicators is experimental, it's not clear what the cutoff lines should be for recategorizing participants, so I'll provisionally suggest cutoffs I consider conservative.

Recategorize as autoheterosexual those participants who report any of the following:

* Nongenital Physiologic Arousal: three or more prior instances
* Attraction to Androgyny: attraction to MTFS or FTMS which equals or exceeds their androphilia or gynephilia
* Gender Euphoria: three or more prior instances of strong euphoria; a hundred or more prior instances of mild euphoria

If possible, compare this recategorized group to the autoheterosexual and homosexual groups created by the two-step typological and arousal-based sorting method. If this recategorized group more closely resembles the autohet group than the homosexual group, this method of enhanced sorting via proxy measures likely improved the purity of the homosexual group. However, if it seems this enhanced sorting did not selectively identify autohets, revert to using the autohet and homosexual groups created by the two-step sorting process.

BEAUTY: EAT, FLEX, SLEEP

Many autoheterosexuals measure their attractiveness by the standards of the other sex. Predictably, they often feel as though they don't measure up.

However, beauty goes beyond sex traits and gender. Much of beauty attainment is about signaling good health. Being fit, trim, and healthy tends to be attractive regardless of sex or gender. Luckily, these nongendered aspects of beauty are things over which we typically have more control.

By changing how we use our bodies and what we put in them, we can change our body composition. Based on the signals we send to our bodies through these actions, it will build different levels of fat and muscle. Although our body's response to these stimuli depends on genetics, hormones, and other factors, much is still under our control.

EATING TO LOOK GOOD

As a general guideline, eat food that you can tell used to be alive just by looking at it. If you can't visually tell that a given food was once part of a living organism, it may be too processed. For example, foods like oil, bread, and candy don't show visible signs of former life in the way that meat, vegetables, nuts, and fruits do. Less-processed food will generally have more nutrients and fewer environmental contaminants.

Protein is the most satiating macronutrient. Carbs are the least. Fat is somewhere in between. If you eat enough good protein and fat, the satiation from these will help you make better decisions about the carbs you eat.

The ratio between protein, fat, and carbohydrates in your diet will impact your physique. To start with, aim for an even mix of energy from protein, fat, and carbs. With time and practice, you'll find the ratio that works best for you.

If you have more muscle, you will need higher amounts of protein. A conventional fitness benchmark for protein is one gram per pound of lean body mass per day.

The basics of eating to look good are pretty simple: eat meat and vegetables. If you need more energy or carbs, then eat fruit or beans too. If the food on your plate is 1/3 meat, 1/3 vegetables, and 1/3 beans, you're on the right track.

Figure out which meat, vegetables, fruit, and beans you are comfortable eating repeatedly. Become comfortable with eating the same foods from meal to meal. Your ancestors did it; so can you.

When you enter a grocery store, the path you walk should start with vegetables and fruit, lead to meat, then continue to eggs/nuts/cheese before heading to check out with the food you grabbed. It's best to avoid most of the aisles. They are full of processed temptations that take willpower to resist. Make it easy on yourself by not entering them in the first place.

Medicinal versus Recreational Eating

Because you are human, you will sometimes eat in a way that doesn't fit in with your long-term goals. Accept that this will happen and don't make a big deal out of it. This inner conflict between the long-term desire for well-being and the short-term desire for emotional satisfaction is common.

I've personally found it helpful to distinguish between medicinal and recreational eating in a way that resembles the distinction between medicinal and recreational drug usage. Medicinal eating is for function and form. Recreational eating is for feelings. It's okay to eat for feelings sometimes; just be aware that feelings are your motivator when this is the case.

Having a predetermined cheat day once a week is a great way to stick to medicinal eating while also allowing you to experience the emotional rewards from recreational eating. I recommend having a cheat day; it will help you create good habits the other six days of the week. Cheat days also give you a chance to feel the stark difference between eating for feelings versus eating for function, making the benefits of functional eating more apparent.

Another way to moderate your recreational eating is to constrain it to one part of the day. For example, if you eat three meals a day, make the first two medicinal and allow the final one to be recreational if that's how you're feeling that day. This is what I usually do.

WORKING OUT

Based on the stresses your body experiences, it will adapt in different ways. Short, intense outputs of force through weight lifting, gymnastics, or acrobatics will increase your power and strength. Outputting force over a longer period of time through running, swimming, or biking will increase your endurance and cardiovascular fitness.

It's common for fitness enthusiasts to do these different forms of exercise on alternating days to give the body a day to rest before it undergoes the same type of stress again. For example, someone may alternate between weight lifting and running by lifting weights on Mondays, Wednesdays, and Fridays, running on Tuesdays, Thursdays, and Saturdays, and resting on Sundays.

Another way to rest between strength training sessions is to alternate between leg days and arm days. This lets you strength train six days a week while also resting enough to recover properly.

No matter what fitness regimen you settle on, you must rest at least one day a week (this is nonnegotiable).

Experiment and find what works for you.

Symmetry

Use symmetry as a guiding principle.

If your top is strong, make your bottom strong too. If your front is strong, make your back strong too. If your left side is strong, make your right side strong too.

Muscles work together as a group—not in isolation. At the same time that some muscles contract and shorten, opposing muscles lengthen and provide stability. This antagonistic quality of muscle groups means it's possible to develop imbalances that compromise your form and can lead to injury. To restore balance, stretch the short, tight muscles and strengthen the long, loose ones.

Fitness newbies often focus on "mirror muscles" such as biceps, pecs, shoulders, and abs, but muscles on the back side can't be seen in the same way, so they are often neglected in comparison. Doing lifts such as dead lifts, squats, and rows can help strengthen the back side of the body, keeping the front and back in proper balance.

Likewise, focusing just on upper body exercises will make the upper body stronger and bigger but will leave the lower body underdeveloped in comparison, leaving it to shoulder the extra weight without being properly conditioned to accommodate it. For symmetry, make sure to strengthen your lower body as well (don't skip leg day).

Symmetry is important. Balance is protective. Fitness is a long-term pursuit. Be on the lookout for muscle imbalances so you don't get hurt.

WALK DOWN HABIT ROAD TO BEAUTY TOWN

Consistency is what gets results, so focus on building habits that will help in the long run. Habits are behavioral routines that can be trained over time through reinforcement. If you can make desired behaviors happen more and unwanted behaviors happen less, your trajectory will point toward a version of yourself that brings you greater satisfaction.

Even if you have big plans, start with tiny steps. If you plan on working out six days a week but currently don't work out at all, don't try to start with six days a week—you'll get hurt physically, emotionally, or both. Start with three days a week, and don't worry about doing full-fledged workouts. Just make sure you show up.

If you want to make a habit of exercising at the gym after work, you can start by going to the gym before or after work with the goal of doing just a single pushup or a few pullups. When you do this, consider it a success. The point is to develop a habit of showing up at the gym. With time, you'll probably add more exercises (you might as well...you're already at the gym!).

If you want to start a running habit, do something similar on the days you plan on running. Put on your running clothes, then jog or walk to the end of the street or around the block. Consider this a success so that you feel good about it, and the habit grows stronger. Add to your distance over time until you hit the distance that works for you.

SLEEP

Sleep is when you repair tissues. Sleep is when learning solidifies. If you neglect sleep, physical and mental decay will follow.

Ideally, you'll spend about a third of your life sleeping. Get a good bed. Few purchases have as high of a return on investment as a proper mattress.

Regular timing makes sleep more effective. Strive to sleep in a consistent time window. In the hour preceding bedtime, don't look at screens. If you want to read, read a book instead. Don't binge on food right before sleep either. Your guts need rest too.

Block outer stimuli. Minimize light, sound, and other vibrations.

Get blackout curtains. Cover or remove *all* light sources in your room. Avoid blue light at night. Wear an eye mask if it helps.

For quiet, minimize undesired noises. Turn off electronics and machines. Ear plugs can help guarantee restful sleep. If you sleep better with white noise, use your white noise of choice.

If you sleep better while cool, get a water-circulating cooling pad. If heavy covers bring you comfort, get a weighted blanket. For any sleep preference you have, there is a product for it.

Diet, sleep, and exercise are interdependent. Be vigilant about maintaining this health trinity. Improvement or degradation in any one of these domains is contagious and can spread to the others.

Autohet gender dysphoria can make it hard to see the point of taking care of yourself. To counteract this, stubbornly insist on maintaining your physical and mental health: it demonstrates through action that you are worth caring about.

FURTHER READING

Readers who want to learn more can start with some of the studies, papers, and books listed here.

If you aren't a college student or professor with institutional access to academic journals, it can sometimes be hard to access particular articles or books. If you are in this situation, find the raven with the red key and give it the DOI number. If you need a book, pop into the library named after the first book of the Bible.

You can also find books through your local library system or an interlibrary loan if they don't have it. To obtain papers, you can email one of the authors to request a PDF or check their ResearchGate page to see if it's hosted there.

BOOKS ABOUT AUTOGYNEPHILIA

Transvestites: The Erotic Drive to Cross-Dress
Magnus Hirschfeld (1910)
English translation by Michael A. Lombardi-Nash (1991)
German (1910): hosted on Digital Transgender Archive
English, E-book (2020): sold in 3 parts on Amazon
English, Hardcover (1991): ISBN: 0879756659

Men Trapped in Men's Bodies: Narratives of Autogynephilic Transsexualism
Anne Lawrence (2013)
DOI: 10.1007/978-1-4614-5182-2

Transvestites and Transsexuals: Toward a Theory of Cross-Gender Behavior
Richard F. Docter (1988)
DOI: 10.1007/978-1-4613-0997-0

"Eonism". First chapter in *Studies in the Psychology of Sex, Volume VII: Eonism and Other Supplementary Studies*
Havelock Ellis (1928)
Can be found on archive.org: *archive.org/details/b30010172/page/n11/mode/2up*.

RAY BLANCHARD

Empirical Typology Studies

Typology of Male-to-Female Transsexualism
Ray Blanchard (1985)
DOI: 10.1007/BF01542107

Nonhomosexual Gender Dysphoria
Ray Blanchard (1988)
DOI: 10.1080/00224498809551410

The Concept of Autogynephilia and the Typology of Male Gender Dysphoria
Ray Blanchard (1989)
DOI: 10.1097/00005053-198910000-00004

Reviews and Theorizing

The Classification and Labeling of Nonhomosexual Gender Dysphorias
Ray Blanchard (1989)
DOI: 10.1007/BF01541951

Clinical Observations and Systematic Studies of Autogynephilia
Ray Blanchard (1991)
DOI: 10.1080/00926239108404348

Erotic Target Location Errors in Male Gender Dysphorics, Paedophiles, and Fetishists
Kurt Freund & Ray Blanchard (1993)
DOI: 10.1192/bjp.162.4.558

Early History of the Concept of Autogynephilia
Ray Blanchard (2005)
DOI: 10.1007/s10508-005-4343-8

ANNE LAWRENCE

Becoming What We Love: Autogynephilic Transsexualism Conceptualized as an Expression of Romantic Love
Anne Lawrence (2007)
DOI: 10.1353/pbm.2007.0050

Erotic Target Location Errors: An Underappreciated Paraphilic Dimension
Anne Lawrence (2009)
DOI: 10.1080/00224490902747727

Sexual Orientation versus Age of Onset as Bases for Typologies (Subtypes)
  for Gender Identity Disorder in Adolescents and Adults
Anne Lawrence (2010)

DOI: 10.1007/s10508-009-9594-3

Autogynephilia and the Typology of Male-to-Female Transsexualism
Anne Lawrence (2017)

DOI: 10.1027/1016-9040/a000276

AUTOANDROPHILIC TRANSGENDERISM

Information for the Female-to-Male Crossdresser and Transsexual
Louis Sullivan (1985)
Can be found on Digital Transgender Archive

Coming Out for a Third Time: Transmen, Sexual Orientation,
  and Identity
Stefan Rowniak & Catherine Chesla (2013)

DOI: 10.1007/s10508-012-0036-2

Female-to-Male Transsexualism, Heterosexual Type: Two Cases
Robert Dickey & Judith Stephens (1995)

DOI: 10.1007/BF01541857

Gay and Bisexual Identity Development Among Female-to-Male
  Transsexuals in North America: Emergence of a Transgender
  Sexuality
Walter Bockting, Autumn Benner, & Eli Coleman (2009)

DOI: 10.1007/s10508-009-9489-3

Homosexual and Bisexual Identity in Sex-Reassigned Female-to-Male
  Transsexuals
Eli Coleman, Walter Bockting, & Louis Gooren (1993)

DOI: 10.1007/bf01552911

Make Me Feel Mighty Real: Gay Female-to-Male Transgenderists
   Negotiating Sex, Gender, and Sexuality
David Schleifer (2006)
DOI: 10.1177/1363460706058397

IN-DEPTH ACCOUNTS OF AUTOANDROPHILIA
Elsa B.

"Analysis of a Case of Transvestitism" by Emil Gutheil
Found in Chapter 16 (pp. 281–318) of the English translation of *Sexual
   Aberrations, Vol. 2* by Wilhelm Stekel (1930)
Hosted on *archive.org*

Mr. G

Splitting: A Case of Female Masculinity
Robert Stoller (1974)
Original Hardcover (1974): ISBN: 0701203943
Paperback Re-release (1997): ISBN: 0300065728
Note: Mr. G is *wild*

Lou Sullivan

We Both Laughed in Pleasure: The Selected Diaries of Lou Sullivan
Edited by Ellis Martin & Zach Ozma (2019)
ISBN: 1643620177
Note: Diary entries from 1961–1991

Lou Sullivan Diaries (1970–1980) and *Theories of Sexual Embodiment:
   Making Sense of Sensing*
Lanei Rodemeyer (2018)
DOI: 10.1007/978-3-319-63034-2

KEVIN HSU AND MICHAEL BAILEY
Empirical AGP and GAMP studies

Sexual Arousal Patterns of Autogynephilic Male Cross-Dressers
Kevin Hsu, A. M. Rosenthal, D. I. Miller, & J. Michael Bailey (2017)
DOI: 10.1007/s10508-016-0826-z

The Psychometric Structure of Items Assessing Autogynephilia
Kevin Hsu, A. M. Rosenthal, & J. Michael Bailey (2015)
DOI: 10.1007/s10508-014-0397-9

Who Are Gynandromorphophilic Men? An Internet Survey of Men with
  Sexual Interest in Transgender Women
A. M. Rosenthal, Kevin Hsu, & J. Michael Bailey (2017)
DOI: 10.1007/s10508-016-0872-6
Note: this is "the NU GAMP survey" from Chapter 4.1

How Autogynephilic Are Natal Females?
J. Michael Bailey & Kevin Hsu (2022)
DOI: 10.1007/s10508-022-02359-8

Empirical Studies on Other Autosexual Orientations

Autopedophilia: Erotic-Target Identity Inversions in Men Sexually
  Attracted to Children
Kevin Hsu & J. Michael Bailey (2017)
DOI: 10.1177/0956797616677082

The "Furry" Phenomenon: Characterizing Sexual Orientation, Sexual
  Motivation, and Erotic Target Identity Inversions in Male Furries
Kevin Hsu & J. Michael Bailey (2019)
DOI: 10.1007/s10508-018-1303-7

"Erotic Target Identity Inversions"
Chapter 20 (pp. 589–612) in *Gender and Sexuality Development:*
Contemporary Theory and Research, Edited by Doug P. VanderLaan
& Wang Ivy Wong (2022)
Kevin J. Hsu & J. Michael Bailey (2022)
Book ISBN: 9783030842734
Chapter DOI: 10.1007/978-3-030-84273-4_20
Preprint version hosted on Bailey's ResearchGate page

THE DISSENTING POINT OF VIEW

Blanchard's Autogynephilia Theory: A Critique
Charles Moser (2010)
DOI: 10.1080/00918369.2010.486241

Autogynephilia in Women
Charles Moser (2009)
DOI: 10.1080/00918360903005212

The Case Against Autogynephilia
Julia Serano (2010)
DOI: 10.1080/15532739.2010.514223

Autogynephilia: A Scientific Review, Feminist Analysis, and Alternative
'Embodiment Fantasies' Model
Julia Serano (2020)
DOI: 10.1177/0038026120934690

Evidence Against a Typology: A Taxometric Analysis of the Sexuality of
Male-to-Female Transsexuals
Jaimie Veale (2014)
DOI: 10.1007/s10508-014-0275-5

GLOSSARY

Acrotomophilia: attraction to amputees.

Adult Baby: an adult who embodies an extremely youthful state through the use of objects such as diapers, pacifiers, and stuffed animals, or through roleplay with someone who takes on the adult role of caregiver.

Adoptive Transracialism: transracialism associated with transracial adoption.

Age Regression: autosexual or autoromantic youthful embodiment.

Allo-: "other".

Alloandrophilia: attraction to others as men.

Allogynephilia: attraction to others as women.

Alloheterosexuality (allohet): attraction to others of the other sex; externally directed heterosexuality.

Allosexuality: attraction to others; externally directed sexual attraction.

Allosexual Orientation: an externally oriented, enduring, preferential sexual or romantic interest in a particular type of entity.

Alterhuman: an internal identity that is beyond the scope of what is traditionally considered human.

Ambiheterosexuality: attraction both *to* and *to being* the other sex; co-occurring alloheterosexuality and autoheterosexuality.

Anatomic Autoheterosexuality: sexual or romantic interest in having the body of the other sex; sexual or romantic interest in having physical features of the other sex.

Anatomic Autosexuality: sexual or romantic interest in having the physical form or physical features associated with a particular type of entity.

Androgynemorphophilia (AGMP): attraction to masculinized females with intact vulva; attraction to FTMs with intact vulva.

Androphilia: attraction to men; attraction to masculinity; attraction to adult human males.

Apotemnophilia: attraction to being an amputee; see *Autoacrotomophilia*.

Auto-: "self".

Autoabasiophilia: attraction to having impaired mobility.

Autoacrotomophilia: attraction to being an amputee; synonym for apotemnophilia.

Autoandrophilia (AAP): "love of self as a man"; attraction to being a man; attraction to oneself as a man; masculinity-based autosexual attraction.

Autochronophilia: attraction to being a particular age; attraction to being at a particular stage of sexual development; autosexual age-based attraction.

Autoexophilia: attraction to being a form of extraterrestrial life.

Autofictophilia: attraction to being a fictional character.

Autoandrogynemorphophilia (AAGMP): attraction to being a masculinized female; attraction to being a man with a vulva; attraction to being an FTM.

Autoanthrozoophilia: attraction to being an anthropomorphic animal; attraction to being a furry.

Autogynandromorphophilia (AGAMP): attraction to being a feminized male; attraction to being a woman with a penis; attraction to being an MTF.

Autogynephilia (AGP): "love of self as a woman"; attraction to being a woman; attraction to oneself as a woman; femininity-based autosexual attraction.

Autohebephilia: attraction to being a pubescent adolescent (Tanner stage 2–3, early puberty).

Autohet: abbreviation for *Autoheterosexual* or *Autoheterosexuality*.

Autoheterosexuality: attraction to being the other sex; attraction to being the gender associated with the other sex; attraction to cross-gender embodiment; internally directed heterosexuality; umbrella term for female autoandrophilia and male autogynephilia.

Autohomosexuality: attraction to being one's own sex; attraction to being the gender associated with one's sex; attraction to default-gender embodiment; internally directed homosexuality; umbrella term for female autogynephilia and male autoandrophilia.

Automythophylophilia: attraction to being a mythical humanoid race (elves, faeries, vampires, etc.).

Automythozoophilia: attraction to being a mythical nonhuman animal.

Autoobjectophilia: attraction to being a nonliving object.

Autopedophilia: attraction to being a prepubescent child (Tanner stage 1, roughly ages 3–11); umbrella term for attraction to being a prepubescent or peripubescent child.

Autophilia: "love of self"; see *Autosexuality*.

Autophylophilia: autosexual race-based attraction; attraction to being a particular race; attraction to being a particular human race.

Autosexuality: attraction to oneself; attraction to being; self-attraction; embodiment-based sexuality; internally-directed sexuality.

Autosexual Orientation: an enduring, preferential sexual or romantic interest in being a particular type of entity; attraction to being a particular type of entity.

Autosexual Theory of Trans Identity: for each attraction to, there exists a corresponding attraction to being, and for each attraction to being, there exists a corresponding type of trans identity—each with its own flavor of embodiment subtypes, euphoria/dysphoria, and shifts.

Autozoophilia: attraction to being an animal; attraction to being a nonhuman animal.

Behavioral Autoheterosexuality: interest in adopting behaviors associated with the other sex; interest in acting like the other sex.

Behavioral Autosexuality: interest in adopting behaviors associated with a particular type of entity.

Body Integrity Dysphoria: negative body integrity–related feelings; the type of dysphoria associated with transabled identity.

Bottom: a sexual partner who plays a receptive, responsive, or passive sexual role; to play a receptive, responsive, or passive sexual role.

Caregiver: someone who roleplays as the adult caretaker of an age regressor.

Chronophilia: an age-based sexual attraction; attraction to people of a particular age.

Cis-: "on this side of"; "on the same side of"; antonym of *Trans*.

Cisgender: when someone's gender identity corresponds to the gender associated with their sex.

Cisvestism: dressing in clothing associated with one's sex; dressing in clothing associated with one's default gender.

Core Autoheterosexuality: sexual or romantic interest in the idea of being the other sex.

Core Autosexuality: sexual or romantic interest in the idea of being a particular type of entity.

Cross-: crossing to the other side of a dimension of being; on the other side of a dimension of being; see *Trans*.

Cross-Embodiment: embodiment which signifies crossing to, or being on the other side of, a dimension of being.

Cross-Gender Embodiment: embodying a gender associated with the other sex; embodiment which signifies crossing gender; embodiment which signifies belonging to the other sex or the gender associated with it.

Cross-Gender Identity: identifying as a gender associated with the other sex; identifying as the other sex; internal sensation of belonging to the other sex or the gender associated with it.

Cross-Identity: identification as a type of entity that is incongruent with one's default physical form; see *Trans Identity*.

Cross-Sex Hormones: hormonal medications taken to approximate the hormone levels of the other sex.

Crossdreaming: cross-gender ideation; when an autoheterosexual person thinks of, imagines, or pictures themselves as the other sex or a gender associated with it; cross-embodiment ideation; when an autosexual person thinks of, imagines, or pictures themselves as a particular type of entity.

Desistance: when someone intends to transition gender but ultimately decides against it before beginning social or medical transition; deciding against gender transition before starting it.

Detransition: when someone who has socially or medically transitioned decides to socially or medically revert to living as their birth sex; deciding against gender transition after starting it.

Devotee: someone who is sexually attracted to amputees or people with other disabilities.

Disorder of Sexual Development (DSD): a congenital condition associated with atypical development of internal and external genital structures.

Dimension (sexual orientation): the dimension of attraction along which a sexual orientation acts (gender, race, age, species, disability, etc.).

Dimension (sexuality): a manifestation of sexuality that can be measured by researchers to gauge the presence of a sexual interest (e.g., arousal, attraction, preference, porn use, behavior, fantasy, etc.).

Dream Shift: dreaming about being the type of entity one is autosexually attracted to being; embodying one's erotic target in a dream.

Dysphoria (autosexual): downward mood shifts in response to perceived shortcomings of cross-embodiment; negative embodiment-related feelings; the opposite of *Euphoria*.

Enby: a nonbinary person; see *Nonbinary*.

Eonism: embodying traits associated with the other sex as an expression of the wish to be that sex; an archaic term for autoheterosexual transgenderism.

Epistemic Injustice: injustice pertaining to knowledge; knowledge-based injustice.

Erotic Target Identity Inversion (ETII): attraction to being the same type of entity that one is attracted to; an autosexual orientation.

Erotic Target Location Error (ETLE): nonallosexual erotic target locations (attractions to nonliving objects or oneself instead of other people); an etiological theory which proposes that autosexual orientations come about due to developmental errors in locating erotic targets in the environment.

Erotic Target: the type of entity to which a person is attracted; object of attraction; love object.

Etiological Paradigm of Transgenderism: a scientific framework for understanding transgenderism as a phenomenon with distinct ultimate causes such as homosexuality and autoheterosexuality.

Etiology: the study of causation or origin; the ultimate cause underlying a condition.

Euphoria (autosexual): good embodiment-related feelings; positive feelings associated with the perception of cross-embodiment; the opposite of *Dysphoria*.

Facial Feminization Surgery (FFS): a group of surgical procedures intended to feminize the face.

Female: of or denoting the sex that can bear offspring or produce ova.

Femdom: a genre of erotic media in which females or MTFs dominate males.

Feminine: qualities traditionally associated with females; femaleness.

Follicle Stimulating Hormone (LSH): hormone which stimulates the growth of ovarian follicles in females and plays a key role in sperm production in males.

Forced Feminization: a genre of erotic media in which males are forcibly feminized, often by females.

Fraternal Birth Order Effect (FBOE): the observation that the more sons a female has, the more likely each successive son is to be homosexual.

Furry: an anthropomorphic animal; a fan of anthropomorphic animals.

Fursona: a form of anthropomorphic identity adopted by fans of anthropomorphic animals.

Gamete: reproductive cells such as sperm or ova that combine to create a new organism.

Gender: sexness; the social and cultural domain of sex; a euphemism for sex that avoids conflation with sexual intercourse.

Gender Dysphoria: bad gender-related feelings; downward mood shifts in response to perceived shortcomings of cross-gender embodiment; the opposite of *Gender Euphoria*.

Gender Euphoria: good gender-related feelings; upward mood shifts in response to the perception of cross-gender embodiment; the opposite of *Gender Dysphoria*.

Gender Expression: how we outwardly embody masculinity and femininity through our appearance or behavior.

Gender Identity: sense of ourselves as masculine, feminine, in between the two, or somewhere outside of the gender binary.

Gender Identity Paradigm of Transgenderism: a scientific framework for understanding transgenderism in which transgender people are understood to have a gender identity incongruent with their biological sex. This paradigm does not incorporate the two known transgender etiologies.

Gender Incongruence: mismatch between an individual's sex or sex traits and their gender identity.

Gender Issues: continuous underlying liability toward a preference for gender transition; an umbrella term covering gender dysphoria and cross-gender ideation.

Gender Role: a social role associated with either males or females.

Gender Transition: socially and/or medically transitioning to live as a gender incongruent with one's sex; see *Social Transition* or *Medical Transition*.

Genderqueer: denoting or relating to an individual who does not subscribe to conventional gender distinctions but identifies with neither, both, or a combination of masculine and feminine genders; a gender identity or gender expression which challenges social constructions of binary gender; see *Nonbinary*.

Gonadotropin: a hormone that induces the gonads to produce sex hormones; category of hormones that includes luteinizing hormone (LH) and follicle stimulating hormone (FSH).

Gonadotropin-Releasing Hormone (GnRH): hormone released by the anterior pituitary gland that induces the release of luteinizing hormone and follicle stimulating hormone.

Gonadotropin-Releasing Hormone Agonist (GnRHa): a class of drugs that agonistically bind to the GnRH receptor; the drug category that puberty blockers belong to.

Gynandromorphophilia: attraction to feminized males with an intact penis; attraction to MTFs with an intact penis.

Gynephilia: attraction to women; attraction to femininity; attraction to adult human females.

Heritability: how much the variation of a trait within a population can be attributed to variation in genetic factors instead of the environment or random chance.

Heterosexual: other-sex attraction; an enduring sexual preference for people of the other sex (or the gender associated with it).

Homosexual: same-sex attraction; an enduring sexual preference for people of the same sex (or the gender associated with it).

Hormone Replacement Therapy (HRT): a euphemism for cross-sex hormones; see *Cross-Sex Hormones*.

Interpersonal Autoheterosexuality: sexual or romantic interest in socially being the other sex; sexual or romantic interest in being treated or seen as the other sex.

Interpersonal Autosexuality: sexual or romantic interest in embodying a social role associated with a particular type of entity; sexual or romantic interest in being seen or treated as a particular type of entity.

Intersex: an umbrella term for disorders of sexual development; see *Disorder of Sexual Development*.

Kintype: the type of entity or types of entities that an otherkin identifies as.

Little: an individual who engages in age regression; an individual with a youthful cross-age identity.

Littlespace: a mental shift associated with youthful embodiment; an autopedophilic mental shift.

Luteinizing Hormone (LH): a hormone produced in the anterior pituitary gland which induces gonadal hormone production.

Male: of or denoting the sex that produces sperm.

Masculine: qualities traditionally associated with males; maleness.

Maternal Immune Hypothesis: the hypothesis that maternal immune responses to the male proteins of male fetuses are the cause of the fraternal birth order effect.

Medical Transition: undergoing hormonal or surgical medical interventions in order to more closely resemble the other sex; getting body modifications or undergoing medical interventions in order to more fully embody a particular type of entity.

Mental Shift: a shift in mind state toward having thoughts, feelings, sensations, or perceptions associated with another type of entity; consciousness cross-embodiment.

Meta-Androphilia: sexual attraction to being a woman with a man; sexual attraction to men based in a desire to reinforce one's femininity.

Meta-Attraction: increased attraction to others based on what their traits imply about oneself; enhanced attraction to others because their traits affirm one's cross-gender self; gender-affirming attraction to others; enhanced attraction to others because their traits affirm one's sense of cross-embodiment.

Meta-Gynephilia: sexual attraction to being a man with a woman; sexual attraction to women based in a desire to reinforce one's masculinity.

Meta-Homosexuality: gender-affirming same-sex attraction; attraction to embodying the other sex with someone of the same sex.

Minority Stress Theory: theory positing that minorities are exposed to greater amounts of internal and external stressors, and that this increased exposure to stressors causes adverse health outcomes.

Mitochondria: organelles within cells that produce the chemical energy cells need to survive and function.

Mitochondrial Dysfunction: disordered functioning of mitochondria in which mitochondria become inefficient, misshapen, and/or produce increased amounts of oxidative molecules.

Nonalloheterosexual: sexualities aside from heterosexual attraction to others; see *Queer*.

Nonbinary: a gender identity which is neither fully feminine nor fully masculine, or which falls outside of the gender binary.

Nonvanilla: describes a sexual interest, behavior, or orientation which is not normophilic; see *Paraphilia*.

Normophilia: sexual interest in genital stimulation or preparatory fondling with phenotypically normal, physically mature, consenting human partners; see *Vanilla*.

Objectophilia: attraction to nonliving objects.

Organizational Hypothesis: the idea that sex hormone exposure in early development irreversibly alters the nervous system in ways that permanently alter later behavior in female-typical and male-typical ways.

Otherkin: an individual who identifies as a type of nonhuman entity.

Otherkith: an individual who identifies with a type of nonhuman entity.

Paradigm: a shared framework in which science is conducted.

Paraphilia: an enduring sexual preference that is not normophilic; see *Nonvanilla*.

Paraphilic Interest: a sexual interest which is not normophilic.

Persistence: the enduring desire to undergo social or medical gender transition.

Phalloplasty: a series of surgical procedures which result in the construction of a phallus.

Phantom Shift: sensing the presence of phantom anatomy associated with an erotic target; sensing the presence of phantom anatomy corresponding to a particular type of entity; proprioceptive cross-embodiment via phantom anatomy.

Philia: "love"; a sexual interest; a sexual or romantic attraction.

Phylophilia: race-based sexual attraction; attraction to a particular race; attraction to a particular human race.

Physiologic Autoheterosexuality: sexual or romantic interest in having the bodily functions of the other sex.

Physiologic Autosexuality: sexual or romantic interest in having the bodily functions of a particular type of entity.

Plushophilia: attraction to toy stuffed animals.

Pregnancy Transvestism: term used by Magnus Hirschfeld to describe the pregnancy embodiment of transfems; pregnancy embodiment associated with physiologic autogynephilia.

Pretender: an individual who temporarily embodies disability for sexual or emotional reasons.

Psyche Autoheterosexuality: sexual or romantic interest in having the thoughts, feelings, sensations, or perceptions of the other sex; sexual or romantic interest in embodying the consciousness of the other sex.

Psyche Autosexuality: sexual or romantic interest in having the thoughts, feelings, sensations, or perceptions of a particular type of entity; sexual or romantic interest in embodying the consciousness of a particular type of entity.

Puberty Blockers: drug administered to halt or delay puberty; see *Gonadotropin-Releasing Hormone Agonist.*

Queer: sexualities that are nonheterosexual, autoheterosexual, or based in nongendered dimensions of attraction; see *Nonalloheterosexual.*

Romance Hypothesis: the hypothesis that gender transition in autoheterosexuals can be motivated by a deep, long-term romantic attachment to the cross-gender self that persists even if overt cross-gender eroticism has waned.

Sartorial Autoheterosexuality: sexual or romantic interest in donning clothing or other body adornments associated with the other sex; sexual or romantic interest in adorning one's body with objects associated with the other sex.

Sartorial Autosexuality: sexual or romantic interest in donning clothing or other body adornments associated with a particular type of entity; sexual or romantic interest in adorning one's body with objects associated with a particular type of entity.

Sensory Shift/Perceptual Shift: a type of mental shift in which an individual feels themselves to have the sensory or perceptual abilities of an erotic target.

Sex: a method of reproduction in which two gametes fuse to create a new organism.

Sexual Dimorphism: when sexually reproducing species come in two main forms that correspond to the female and male reproductive strategies.

Sexual Fetishism: a sexual preference for nongenital body parts (partialism) or sexual interest in nonliving objects.

Sexual Identity: an identity pertaining to sexuality.

Sexual Inversion: an antiquated term for homosexuality that alludes to the psychosexual inversion associated with it.

Sexual Orientation: an enduring pattern of preferential sexual or romantic interest in a particular type of entity, embodiment, or method of interaction.

Sexual Preference: a sexual interest that is preferred over other sexual interests.

Shifting: when an autosexual person experiences phantom anatomy or a state of consciousness reminiscent of the type of entity they are attracted to being.

Sissification: eroticized feminization.

Sissy: an individual with erotic interest in feminizing themselves; a sexual identity held by some autogynephilic people.

Situational Transracialism: umbrella term for adoptive transracialism and other forms of transracialism associated with one's particular life circumstances.

Social Desirability Bias: a tendency to socially present oneself in ways that will garner approval from others; a bias toward presenting oneself in a socially desirable way.

Social Transition: changing one's name, stated identity, pronouns, dress, and other forms of gendered expression on a long-term basis in order to live as another gender; changing one's name, dress, speech, stated identity, or behavior on a long-term basis in order to socially embody a particular type of entity.

Suprabinary: beyond a binary; describes gender identities beyond those corresponding to the two sexes.

Teratophilia: attraction to monsters or deformed people.

Therian: an individual who identifies as a nonhuman animal; an individual with a deep integral or personal belief that they're a nonhuman animal.

Top: a sexual partner who plays an assertive, initiatory, or active sexual role; to play an assertive, initiatory, or active sexual role.

Trans: "across"; "on the other side of"; cross-.

Trans Identity: identification as a type of entity that is incongruent with one's default physical form; see *Cross-Identity*.

Transabled: an individual who identifies as, or socially/medically transitions to, having a disability that differs from their default ability; crossed in the dimension of disability.

Transage: an individual who identifies as, or socially/medically transitions to, an age that differs from their chronological age; crossed in the dimension of age.

Trans Man: a female-born individual who identifies as a man or socially/medically transitions to live as one.

Trans Woman: a male-born individual who identifies as a woman or socially/medically transitions to live as one.

Transfem: a male-born individual who has a feminine gender identity or has socially/medically transitioned to more fully embody femininity; an individual on the male-to-female (MTF) spectrum; an abbreviation for *Transfeminine*.

Transfeminine: a form of feminine gender identity held by some males; an individual on the male-to-female (MTF) spectrum.

Transgender: an individual who identifies as, or socially/medically transitions to, a gender that does not correspond to their sex; an individual with a nondefault gender identity; crossed in the dimension of gender.

Transgender Transformation: a genre of erotic media in which protagonists transform into the other sex or gain traits associated with it.

Transmasc: a female-born individual who has a masculine gender identity or has socially/medically transitioned to more fully embody masculinity; an individual on the female-to-male (FTM) spectrum; an abbreviation for *Transmasculine*.

Transmasculine: a form of masculine gender identity held by some females; an individual on the female-to-male (FTM) spectrum.

Transrace: an individual who identifies as, or socially/medically transitions to, a race that differs from their default race; crossed in the dimension of race.

Transsexual: an individual who has undergone medical interventions in order to more closely resemble the other sex; of or relating to medical gender transition.

Transsexualism: undergoing medical interventions in order to more closely resemble the other sex; medical gender transition.

Transspecies: an individual who identifies as, or socially/medically transitions to, a species that differs from their default species; crossed in the dimension of species.

Transvestism: wearing clothing or other body adornments associated with the other sex; donning body adornments to attain cross-embodiment.

Transvestite: an individual who wears clothing associated with the other sex as a symbol of inner personality; a crossdresser.

Trap: a slang term for an MTF individual with an intact penis which implies passability.

Two-Type Typology of Transgenderism: a categorization system for transgender people that sorts them into homosexual and autoheterosexual etiological groups based on whether their sexualities are homosexual or nonhomosexual with respect to their birth sex.

Underdressing: crossdressing beneath a cisvestic outer layer.

Vaginoplasty: a surgical procedure which results in the construction of a neovagina.

Vanilla: describes conventional sexual behavior; describes normative sexual behavior; see *Normophilia*.

Wannabe: an individual who admires amputees and wants to become one.

Zoophilia: "love of animals"; attraction to animals; attraction to nonhuman animals.

NOTES

1.0. Straight, Turned Inside Out

1   Doug P. VanderLaan, Zhiyuan Ren, and Paul L. Vasey, "Male Androphilia in the Ancestral Environment: An Ethnological Analysis," *Human Nature* 24, no. 4 (October 2013): 375–401, https://doi.org/10.1007/s12110-013-9182-z.

2   Ray Blanchard, "Early History of the Concept of Autogynephilia," *Archives of Sexual Behavior* 34, no. 4 (August 2005): 444, https://doi.org/10.1007/s10508-005-4343-8.

3   Wikipedia, s.v. "Autoandrophilia: Revision History," accessed September 27, 2022, https://en.wikipedia.org/w/index.php?title=Autoandrophilia&action=history; Wikipedia, s.v. "Autogynephilia: Revision History," accessed September 27, 2022, https://en.wikipedia.org/w/index.php?title=Autogynephilia&action=history.

4   Wikipedia, s.v. "Blanchard's Transsexualism Typology," last modified December 29, 2022, https://en.wikipedia.org/wiki/Blanchard%27s_transsexualism_typology.

5   E. Coleman et al., "Standards of Care for the Health of Transgender and Gender Diverse People, Version 8," *International Journal of Transgender Health* 23, no. 1 (September 6, 2022): S1–259, https://doi.org/10.1080/26895269.2022.2100644.

6   American Psychiatric Association, ed., *Diagnostic and Statistical Manual of Mental Disorders: DSM-5*, 5th ed. (Washington, DC: American Psychiatric Association Publishing, 2013), 457, https://doi.org/10.1176/appi.books.9780890425596; American Psychiatric Association, ed., *Diagnostic and Statistical Manual of Mental Disorders: DSM-5-TR*, 5th ed., text revision (Washington, DC: American Psychiatric Association Publishing, 2022), 517, https://doi.org/10.1176/appi.books.9780890425787.

7 Ozymandias, "Cis by Default," *Thing of Things* (blog), January 28, 2015, https://thingofthings.wordpress.com/2015/01/28/cis-by-default/.

8 David C. Geary, *Male, Female: The Evolution of Human Sex Differences*, 3rd ed. (Washington, DC: American Psychological Association, 2021), 26, https://doi.org/10.1037/0000181-000.

9 Jack Molay, "Crossdreaming Described," *Crossdreamers* (blog), August 3, 2014, https://www.crossdreamers.com/2014/08/crossdreaming-described.html.

10 Kevin J. Hsu, A. M. Rosenthal, and J. Michael Bailey, "The Psychometric Structure of Items Assessing Autogynephilia," *Archives of Sexual Behavior* 44, no. 5 (July 2015): 1301–12, https://doi.org/10.1007/s10508-014-0397-9.philia.

11 Lee Jussim et al., "Stereotype Accuracy: One of the Largest and Most Replicable Effects in All of Social Psychology," in *Handbook of Prejudice, Stereotyping, and Discrimination*, 2nd ed., ed. Todd D. Nelson (New York: Psychology Press, 2016), 31–63, https://doi.org/10.4324/9780203361993-8.

12 Jordan E. Rullo, "A Contemporary Review of the Distinct Conceptualizations of Bisexuality," unpublished research preliminary examination, (Salt Lake City: Department of Psychology, University of Utah, 2015).

13 Simon LeVay, "MTF Seeks MTF, Why?," *Transgender Tapestry* 93 (Spring 2001), 21, https://archive.org/details/transgendertapes9320unse/page/20/mode/2up.

1.1. Sex, Gender, and Transgender

1 Randy Thornhill and Craig T. Palmer, *A Natural History of Rape: Biological Bases of Sexual Coercion* (Cambridge, MA: MIT Press, 2000).

2 Lisa Allen, "Disorders of Sexual Development," *Obstetrics and Gynecology Clinics of North America* 36, no. 1 (March 2009): 25–45, https://doi.org/10.1016/j.ogc.2009.02.001.

3 Leonard Sax, "How Common is Intersex? A Response to Anne Fausto-Sterling," *The Journal of Sex Research* 39, no. 3 (August 1, 2002): 174–78, https://doi.org/10.1080/00224490209552139.

4 Melanie Blackless et al., "How Sexually Dimorphic Are We? Review and Synthesis," *American Journal of Human Biology* 12, no. 2 (March/April 2000): 151–66, https://doi.org/10.1002/(SICI)1520-6300(200003/04)12:2<151::AID-AJHB1>3.0.CO;2-F.

5 Tailcalled, "Why Do Trans Women Transition?," *Survey Anon's Gender Blog*, July 1, 2021, https://surveyanon.wordpress.com/2021/07/01/why-do-trans-women-transition/; Tailcalled, "Gender Issues: Continuous Underlying Liability towards Preference for Transitioning; an Umbrella Term Covering Gender Dysphoria and Cross-Gender Ideation, as Well as Possibly More Nebulous Things like 'Gender Identity,'" Hobbyist Sexologists, Discord, March 10, 2021.

6 Kenneth J. Zucker and Madison Aitken, "Sex Ratio of Transgender Adolescents: A Meta-Analysis" (Inside Matters: 3rd Meeting of the European Association for

Transgender Health, Rome, Italy, 2019), unpublished data; Sandy E. James et al., *The Report of the 2015 U.S. Transgender Survey* (Washington, DC: National Center for Transgender Equality, 2016), 245, https://www.ustranssurvey.org/reports/#2015report.

1.2. Sexual Orientation

1   Gary R. VandenBos, ed., *APA Dictionary of Psychology*, 2nd ed. (Washington, DC: American Psychological Association, 2015), 974, https://doi.org/10.1037/14646-000.

2   J. Michael Bailey et al., "Sexual Orientation, Controversy, and Science," *Psychological Science in the Public Interest* 17, no. 2 (September 2016): 45, https://doi.org/10.1177/1529100616637616.

3   American Psychiatric Association, ed., *Diagnostic and Statistical Manual of Mental Disorders: DSM-5*, 5th ed. (Washington, DC: American Psychiatric Association Publishing, 2013), 685, https://doi.org/10.1176/appi.books.9780890425596; American Psychiatric Association, ed., *Diagnostic and Statistical Manual of Mental Disorders: DSM-5-TR*, 5th ed., text revision (Washington, DC: American Psychiatric Association Publishing, 2022), 779, https://doi.org/10.1176/appi.books.9780890425787.

4   American Psychiatric Association, *Diagnostic and Statistical Manual of Mental Disorders*, 2013, 685.

5   Amy Marsh, "Love among the Objectum Sexuals," *Electronic Journal of Human Sexuality* 13 (March 2010), http://www.ejhs.org/volume13/ObjSexuals.htm.

6   Michael C. Seto, "The Puzzle of Male Chronophilias," *Archives of Sexual Behavior* 46, no. 1 (January 2017): 3–22, https://doi.org/10.1007/s10508-016-0799-y.

7   Bailey et al., "Sexual Orientation, Controversy, and Science," 48–49.

8   J. Michael Bailey, "Reply to Feinstein and Galupo and to Zivony: Sexual Arousal Pattern Is an Objective Although Imperfect Window on Sexual Orientation," *Proceedings of the National Academy of Sciences* 117, no. 50 (December 2020): 31579, https://doi.org/10.1073/pnas.2018065117.

9   Bailey et al., "Sexual Orientation, Controversy, and Science," 69–72.

10   Bailey et al., 70.

11   Marco Del Giudice, Tom Booth, and Paul Irwing, "The Distance Between Mars and Venus: Measuring Global Sex Differences in Personality," *PLoS ONE* 7, no. 1 (January 2012): e29265, https://doi.org/10.1371/journal.pone.0029265; Petri J. Kajonius and John Johnson, "Sex Differences in 30 Facets of the Five Factor Model of Personality in the Large Public (N = 320,128)," *Personality and Individual Differences* 129 (July 2018): 126–30, https://doi.org/10.1016/j.paid.2018.03.026; Alice H. Eagly and William Revelle, "Understanding the Magnitude of Psychological Differences Between Women and Men Requires Seeing the Forest and the Trees," *Perspectives on Psychological Science* 17, no. 5 (September 2022): 1339–58, https://doi.org/10.1177/17456916211046006.

12 Simon LeVay, *Gay, Straight, and the Reason Why: The Science of Sexual Orientation*, 2nd ed. (New York: Oxford University Press, 2017), 164.

13 Richard A. Lippa, "Interest, Personality, and Sexual Traits That Distinguish Heterosexual, Bisexual, and Homosexual Individuals: Are There Two Dimensions That Underlie Variations in Sexual Orientation?," *Archives of Sexual Behavior* 49, no. 2 (February 2020): 607–22, https://doi.org/10.1007/s10508-020-01643-9; Richard A. Lippa, "Sex Differences and Sexual Orientation Differences in Personality: Findings from the BBC Internet Survey," *Archives of Sexual Behavior* 37, no. 1 (February 2008): 173–87, https://doi.org/10.1007/s10508-007-9267-z; Richard A Lippa, "Sexual Orientation and Personality," *Annual Review of Sex Research* 16, no. 1 (2005): 119–53, https://www.tandfonline.com/doi/abs/10.1080/10532528.2005.10559831.

14 J. Michael Bailey and Kenneth J. Zucker, "Childhood Sex-Typed Behavior and Sexual Orientation: A Conceptual Analysis and Quantitative Review," *Developmental Psychology* 31, no. 1 (1995): 43–55, https://psycnet.apa.org/doi/10.1037/0012-1649.31.1.43; Mark S. Allen and Davina A. Robson, "Personality and Sexual Orientation: New Data and Meta-Analysis," *The Journal of Sex Research* 57, no. 8 (October 2020): 953–65, https://doi.org/10.1080/00224499.2020.1768204; Lippa, "Sex Differences and Sexual Orientation Differences in Personality"; Lippa, "Sexual Orientation and Personality"; Michael Peters, John T. Manning, and Stian Reimers, "The Effects of Sex, Sexual Orientation, and Digit Ratio (2D:4D) on Mental Rotation Performance," *Archives of Sexual Behavior* 36, no. 2 (April 2007): 251–60, https://doi.org/10.1007/s10508-006-9166-8.

15 Ivanka Savic and Per Lindström, "PET and MRI Show Differences in Cerebral Asymmetry and Functional Connectivity between Homo- and Heterosexual Subjects," *Proceedings of the National Academy of Sciences* 105, no. 27 (July 2008): 9403–8, https://doi.org/10.1073/pnas.0801566105.

16 Klára Bártová et al., "The Prevalence of Paraphilic Interests in the Czech Population: Preference, Arousal, the Use of Pornography, Fantasy, and Behavior," *The Journal of Sex Research* 58, no. 1 (2021): 86–96, https://doi.org/10.1080/00224499.2019.1707468; Samantha J. Dawson, Brittany A. Bannerman, and Martin L. Lalumière, "Paraphilic Interests: An Examination of Sex Differences in a Nonclinical Sample," *Sexual Abuse* 28, no. 1 (February 2016): 12, https://doi.org/10.1177/1079063214525645; Elena Baur et al., "Paraphilic Sexual Interests and Sexually Coercive Behavior: A Population-Based Twin Study," *Archives of Sexual Behavior* 45, no. 5 (July 2016): 1163–72, https://doi.org/10.1007/s10508-015-0674-2.

17 Ray Blanchard, "Fraternal Birth Order, Family Size, and Male Homosexuality: Meta-Analysis of Studies Spanning 25 Years," *Archives of Sexual Behavior* 47, no. 1 (January 2018): 10, https://doi.org/10.1007/s10508-017-1007-4.

18 Doug P. VanderLaan et al., "Birth Weight and Two Possible Types of Maternal Effects on Male Sexual Orientation: A Clinical Study of Children and Adolescents Referred to a Gender Identity Service," *Developmental Psychobiology* 57, no. 1 (January 2015): 26, https://doi.org/10.1002/dev.21254.

19   Anthony F. Bogaert et al., "Male Homosexuality and Maternal Immune Responsivity to the Y-Linked Protein NLGN4Y," *Proceedings of the National Academy of Sciences* 115, no. 2 (January 2018): 302–6, https://doi.org/10.1073/pnas.1705895114.

20   Ray Blanchard and Anthony F. Bogaert, "Proportion of Homosexual Men Who Owe Their Sexual Orientation to Fraternal Birth Order: An Estimate Based on Two National Probability Samples," *American Journal of Human Biology* 16, no. 2 (March/April 2004): 151–57, https://doi.org/10.1002/ajhb.20006; James M. Cantor et al., "How Many Gay Men Owe Their Sexual Orientation to Fraternal Birth Order?," *Archives of Sexual Behavior* 31, no. 1 (2002): 63–71, https://doi.org/10.1023/A:1014031201935.

21   Ray Blanchard, "Fertility in the Mothers of Firstborn Homosexual and Heterosexual Men," *Archives of Sexual Behavior* 41, no. 3 (June 2012): 555, https://doi.org/10.1007/s10508-011-9888-0.

22   Ray Blanchard, "A Possible Second Type of Maternal–Fetal Immune Interaction Involved in Both Male and Female Homosexuality," *Archives of Sexual Behavior* 41, no. 6 (December 2012): 1510, https://doi.org/10.1007/s10508-011-9896-0.

23   Christine Ablaza, Jan Kabátek, and Francisco Perales, "Are Sibship Characteristics Predictive of Same Sex Marriage? An Examination of Fraternal Birth Order and Female Fecundity Effects in Population-Level Administrative Data from the Netherlands," *The Journal of Sex Research* 59, no. 6 (July 2022): 671–83, https://doi.org/10.1080/00224499.2021.1974330.

24   Kurt Freund and Ray Blanchard, "Erotic Target Location Errors in Male Gender Dysphorics, Paedophiles, and Fetishists," *The British Journal of Psychiatry* 162, no. 4 (April 1993): 562, https://doi.org/10.1192/bjp.162.4.558.

2.0. Autogynephilia (AGP)

1   American Psychiatric Association, ed., *Diagnostic and Statistical Manual of Mental Disorders: DSM-5*, 5th ed. (Washington, DC: American Psychiatric Association Publishing, 2013), 818, https://doi.org/10.1176/appi.books.9780890425596.

2   Ray Blanchard, "The Concept of Autogynephilia and the Typology of Male Gender Dysphoria," *The Journal of Nervous and Mental Disease* 177, no. 10 (October 1989): 616, https://doi.org/10.1097/00005053-198910000-00004.

3   Kevin J. Hsu, A. M. Rosenthal, and J. Michael Bailey, "The Psychometric Structure of Items Assessing Autogynephilia," *Archives of Sexual Behavior* 44, no. 5 (July 2015): 1301–12, https://doi.org/10.1007/s10508-014-0397-9.

4   Havelock Ellis, "Sexo-Aesthetic Inversion," *Alienist and Neurologist* 34, no. 2 (May 1913): 156–67, https://babel.hathitrust.org/cgi/pt?id=mdp.39015067286420&view=1up&seq=176; Havelock Ellis, "Sexo-Aesthetic Inversion," *Alienist and Neurologist* 34, no. 3 (August 1913): 249–79, https://babel.hathitrust.org/cgi/pt?id=mdp.39015067286420&view=1up&seq=269.

5   Ellis, "Sexo-Aesthetic Inversion," May 1913, 164.

6   Ellis, "Sexo-Aesthetic Inversion," August 1913, 275.

7   "Fictionmania," accessed January 9, 2023, https://www.fictionmania.tv/.

8   Andrea Long Chu, *Females* (New York: Verso, 2019), 65.

9   Richard F. Docter, *Transvestites and Transsexuals: Toward a Theory of Cross-Gender Behavior*, Perspectives in Sexuality (New York: Plenum Press, 1988), 215, https://doi.org/10.1007/978-1-4613-0997-0.

10 Richard von Krafft-Ebing, *Psychopathia Sexualis,* 12th ed., trans. F. J. Rebman (Rebman Company, 1906), 313.

11 Von Krafft-Ebing, 317.

12 Von Krafft-Ebing, 317.

13 Magnus Hirschfeld, *Transvestites: The Erotic Drive to Cross-Dress*, trans. Michael A. Lombardi-Nash (Buffalo, NY: Prometheus Books, 1991), 184–96.

14 Von Krafft-Ebing, *Psychopathia Sexualis*, 309.

15 Von Krafft-Ebing, 314.

16 Von Krafft-Ebing, 314.

17 Von Krafft-Ebing, 312, 321.

18 Von Krafft-Ebing, 316.

19 Von Krafft-Ebing, 316.

20 Von Krafft-Ebing, 315.

21 Von Krafft-Ebing, 315.

22 Von Krafft-Ebing, 314.

23 Von Krafft-Ebing, 314.

24 Von Krafft-Ebing, 316.

25 Von Krafft-Ebing, 315.

26 Von Krafft-Ebing, 316.

27 Von Krafft-Ebing, 313.

2.1. Anatomic Autogynephilia

1   Kevin J. Hsu, A. M. Rosenthal, and J. Michael Bailey, "The Psychometric Structure of Items Assessing Autogynephilia," *Archives of Sexual Behavior* 44, no. 5 (July 2015): 1311–12, https://doi.org/10.1007/s10508-014-0397-9.

2   Magnus Hirschfeld, *Transvestites: The Erotic Drive to Cross-Dress*, trans. Michael A. Lombardi-Nash (Buffalo, NY: Prometheus Books, 1991), 183.

3   Havelock Ellis, "Eonism," in *Studies in the Psychology of Sex*, vol. 7, *Eonism and Other Supplementary Studies* (Philadelphia: F. A. Davis Company, 1928), 36, https://archive.org/details/b30010172/page/n11/mode/2up.

4   Ray Blanchard, "Partial versus Complete Autogynephilia and Gender Dysphoria," *Journal of Sex & Marital Therapy* 19, no. 4 (1993): 304, https://doi.org/10.1080/00926239308404373; Hsu, Rosenthal, and Bailey, "The Psychometric Structure," 7.

5 Ellis, "Eonism," 51, 82, 98; Hirschfeld, *Transvestites, 120.*

6 Ellis, "Eonism," 49.

7 Hirschfeld, *Transvestites, 183.*

8 Ellis, "Eonism," 66.

9 Ellis, 94.

10 Hirschfeld, *Transvestites, 122.*

11 Hirschfeld, 129.

12 Hirschfeld, 73.

13 Ellis, "Eonism," 50.

14 Hirschfeld, *Transvestites, 57.*

15 Hirschfeld, 62.

16 Magnus Hirschfeld, *Sexual Anomalies and Perversions: A Summary of the Works of the Late Professor Dr. Magnus Hirschfeld,* ed. Norman Haire (London: Encyclopaedic Press, 1966), 200.

17 Ellis, "Eonism," 49.

18 Ellis, 82.

19 Florence Ashley, "Surgical Informed Consent and Recognizing a Perioperative Duty to Disclose in Transgender Health Care," *McGill Journal of Law and Health* 73 (2020): 75, https://ssrn.com/abstract=3633573.

20 Katharina Dobs et al., "How Face Perception Unfolds over Time," *Nature Communications* 10, no. 1 (2019), https://doi.org/10.1038/s41467-019-09239-1.

2.2. Sartorial Autogynephilia

1 Magnus Hirschfeld, *Sexual Anomalies and Perversions: A Summary of the Works of the Late Professor Dr. Magnus Hirschfeld, ed. Norman Haire (London: Encyclopaedic Press, 1966),* 188.

2 Magnus Hirschfeld, *Transvestites: The Erotic Drive to Cross-Dress,* trans. Michael A. Lombardi-Nash (Buffalo, NY: Prometheus Books, 1991), 124.

3 Harry Benjamin, *The Transsexual Phenomenon,* electronic edition (Düsseldorf: Symposium Publishing, 1999).

4 Ray Blanchard, "Clinical Observations and Systematic Studies of Autogynephilia," *Journal of Sex & Marital Therapy* 17, no. 4 (1991): 237, https://doi.org/10.1080/00926239108404348; Kevin J. Hsu, A. M. Rosenthal, and J. Michael Bailey, "The Psychometric Structure of Items Assessing Autogynephilia," *Archives of Sexual Behavior* 44, no. 5 (July 2015): 1303, https://doi.org/10.1007/s10508-014-0397-9.

5 Hirschfeld, *Sexual Anomalies and Perversions, 221–22.*

6 Hirschfeld, *Transvestites, 127.*

7 Richard F. Docter, *Transvestites and Transsexuals: Toward a Theory of Cross-Gender Behavior,* Perspectives in Sexuality (New York: Plenum Press, 1988), 209, https://doi.org/10.1007/978-1-4613-0997-0.

8   Hirschfeld, *Transvestites, 60.*

9   Havelock Ellis, "Eonism," in *Studies in the Psychology of Sex,* vol. 7, *Eonism and Other Supplementary Studies* (Philadelphia: F. A. Davis Company, 1928), 62, https://wellcomecollection.org/works/njv7bbq7.

10   Hirschfeld, *Transvestites, 36.*

11   Hirschfeld, 105.

12   Hirschfeld, 69.

13   Hirschfeld, 75.

14   Hirschfeld, 66.

15   Hirschfeld, 127.

16   Hirschfeld, 39, 65.

17   Hirschfeld, 72.

18   Hirschfeld, 109.

19   Hirschfeld, *Sexual Anomalies and Perversions, 222.*

20   Hirschfeld, *Transvestites, 86, 109.*

21   Hirschfeld, 86.

22   Hirschfeld, 108.

23   Hirschfeld, 29, 61; Ellis, "Eonism," 87.

24   Hirschfeld, *Transvestites, 94.*

25   Ellis, "Eonism," 50.

26   Ellis, 46, 47.

27   Ellis, 52, 53.

28   Hirschfeld, *Transvestites, 94.*

29   Hirschfeld, 84.

30   Ellis, "Eonism," 89.

31   Ellis, 76.

32   Ellis, 74.

33   Ellis, 88–89.

34   Hirschfeld, *Transvestites, 65.*

35   Hirschfeld, 75.

36   Hirschfeld, 39.

37   Hirschfeld, 88–89.

38   Hirschfeld, 45.

39   Hirschfeld, 51, 129.

40   Hirschfeld, 73; Ellis, "Eonism," 85.

41   Hirschfeld, *Sexual Anomalies and Perversions, 218; Hirschfeld, Transvestites, 335.*

42   Hirschfeld, *Transvestites, 50.*

43   Hirschfeld, 55.

44   Hirschfeld, *Sexual Anomalies and Perversions, 221.*

45   Ellis, "Eonism," 88–89.

46   Hirschfeld, *Transvestites, 38.*

47 Hirschfeld, *Sexual Anomalies and Perversions, 221.*
48 Hirschfeld, *Transvestites, 24.*
49 Hirschfeld, *47.*
50 Hirschfeld, *39, 69, 105.*
51 Hirschfeld, *Sexual Anomalies and Perversions, 200.*
52 Ellis, "Eonism," *52.*
53 Hirschfeld, *Transvestites, 127.*
54 Hirschfeld, *42.*
55 Ellis, "Eonism," *67.*
56 Ellis, *52.*
57 Hirschfeld, *Transvestites, 69.*
58 Ellis, "Eonism," *43.*

2.3. Behavioral Autogynephilia

1   Mia Mulder (@Potatopolitics), "Trans women transition for one single, depraved sexual reason: Dress go spinny," Twitter, July 18, 2019, 11:10 a.m., https://twitter.com/Potatopolitics/status/1151886955187200001.

2   "Dress Go Spinny," Know Your Meme, accessed August 11, 2022, https://knowyourmeme.com/memes/dress-go-spinny.

3   Havelock Ellis, "Eonism," in *Studies in the Psychology of Sex*, vol. 7, *Eonism and Other Supplementary Studies* (Philadelphia: F. A. Davis Company, 1928), 71, https://wellcomecollection.org/works/njv7bbq7.

4   Magnus Hirschfeld, *Transvestites: The Erotic Drive to Cross-Dress*, trans. Michael A. Lombardi-Nash (Buffalo, NY: Prometheus Books, 1991), 37.

5   Hirschfeld, 20.

6   Hirschfeld, 20–21.

7   Hirschfeld, 60.

8   Hirschfeld, 62.

9   Ellis, "Eonism," 88.

10 Ellis, 85.

11 Hirschfeld, *Transvestites, 108.*

12 Hirschfeld, 106.

13 Hirschfeld, 91.

14 Hirschfeld, 129.

15 Hirschfeld, 73.

16 Hirschfeld, 77.

17 Hirschfeld, 24, 31, 51; Ellis, "Eonism," 65.

18 Hirschfeld, *Transvestites, 130.*

19 Hirschfeld, 179.

20 Hirschfeld, 117.

21 Hirschfeld, 59.

22 Richard von Krafft-Ebing, *Psychopathia Sexualis*, 12th ed., trans. F. J. Rebman (Rebman Company, 1906), 318.

2.4. *Physiologic Autogynephilia*

1 Richard von Krafft-Ebing, *Psychopathia Sexualis*, 12th ed., trans. F. J. Rebman (Rebman Company, 1906), 316.

2 Von Krafft-Ebing, 322.

3 Karl Abraham, "Über hysterische Traumzustände," *Jahrbuch* für *Psychoanalytische und Psychopathologische Forschung* 2, no. 1 (1910): 1–32, https://pep-web.org/search/document/JPPF.002.0001A?page=P0001; Karl Abraham, *Klinische Beiträge zur Psychoanalyse* (Leipzig: Internationaler Psychoanalytischer Verlag, 1921), 71–74, http://journals.lww.com/00005053-192203000-00084.

4 Havelock Ellis, "Eonism," in *Studies in the Psychology of Sex*, vol. 7, *Eonism and Other Supplementary Studies* (Philadelphia: F. A. Davis Company, 1928), 16, https://archive.org/details/b30010172/page/16/mode/2up.

5 Abraham, *Klinische Beiträge zur Psychoanalyse*, 74.

6 Magnus Hirschfeld, *Sexual Anomalies and Perversions: A Summary of the Works of the Late Professor Dr. Magnus Hirschfeld*, ed. Norman Haire (London: Encyclopaedic Press, 1966), 218.

7 Hirschfeld, 199.

8 Ellis, "Eonism," 96.

9 Hirschfeld, *Sexual Anomalies and Perversions*, 216.

10 Hirschfeld, 217.

11 Magnus Hirschfeld, *Transvestites: The Erotic Drive to Cross-Dress*, trans. Michael A. Lombardi-Nash (Buffalo, NY: Prometheus Books, 1991), 119–20.

12 Hirschfeld, *Sexual Anomalies and Perversions*, 216.

13 Hirschfeld, *Transvestites*, 89.

14 Hirschfeld, 31.

15 Von Krafft-Ebing, *Psychopathia Sexualis*, 311.

16 Von Krafft-Ebing, 317.

17 Ellis, "Eonism," 98.

18 Hirschfeld, *Transvestites*, 63–64.

19 Hirschfeld, 54.

20 Ceylan Yeginsu, "Transgender Woman Breast-Feeds Baby after Hospital Induces Lactation," *New York Times*, February 15, 2018, https://www.nytimes.com/2018/02/15/health/transgender-woman-breast-feed.html.

21 Tamar Reisman and Zil Goldstein, "Case Report: Induced Lactation in a Transgender Woman," *Transgender Health* 3, no. 1 (January 2018): 25, https://doi.org/10.1089/trgh.2017.0044.

22 Rachel Wamboldt, Shirley Shuster, and Bikrampal S. Sidhu, "Lactation Induction in a Transgender Woman Wanting to Breastfeed: Case Report," *The Journal of*

Clinical Endocrinology & Metabolism 106, no. 5 (May 2021): e2049, https://doi. org/10.1210/clinem/dgaa976.

23 Emily Trautner, Megan McCool-Myers, and Andrea Braden Joyner, "Knowledge and Practice of Induction of Lactation in Trans Women among Professionals Working in Trans Health," *International Breastfeeding Journal* 15, no. 1 (July 2020): 63, https://doi.org/10.1186/s13006-020-00308-6.

24 Trautner, McCool-Myers, and Joyner, 3.

25 Katelyn Burns, "Yes, Trans Women can Breastfeed—Here's How," Them, May 9, 2018, https://www.them.us/story/trans-women-breastfeed.

26 "6 Transgender Women Talk Menstruation," *Aisle* (blog), July 21, 2020, https:// periodaisle.com/blogs/all/6-transgender-women-talk-menstruation; Alaina Kailyn, "Trans Girl Periods. Yes, That's Right. No, I'm Being Serious. Just Read the Damn Article," *OnWednesdays* (blog), October 6, 2016, https://web.archive.org/ web/20200407165133/http://www.onwednesdays.net/trans-girl-periods/.

27 "6 Transgender Women Talk Menstruation."

28 "6 Transgender Women Talk Menstruation."

2.5. Interpersonal Autogynephilia

1 Richard F. Docter, *Transvestites and Transsexuals: Toward a Theory of Cross-Gender Behavior*, Perspectives in Sexuality (New York: Plenum Press, 1988), 76–77, https://doi.org/10.1007/978-1-4613-0997-0.

2 William J. Beischel, "Gender Pleasure: The Positive Affective Component of Gender/Sex" (PhD diss., University of Michigan, 2022), 44, https://hdl.handle. net/2027.42/174393.

3 Magnus Hirschfeld, *Transvestites: The Erotic Drive to Cross-Dress*, trans. Michael A. Lombardi-Nash (Buffalo, NY: Prometheus Books, 1991), 127.

4 Hirschfeld, 23.

5 Hirschfeld, 24.

6 Hirschfeld, 26.

7 Hirschfeld, 63, 143.

8 Havelock Ellis, "Eonism," in *Studies in the Psychology of Sex*, vol. 7, *Eonism and Other Supplementary Studies* (Philadelphia: F. A. Davis Company, 1928), 98, https://archive.org/details/b30010172/page/98/mode/2up.

9 Ellis, 80.

10 Magnus Hirschfeld, *Sexual Anomalies and Perversions: A Summary of the Works of the Late Professor Dr. Magnus Hirschfeld*, ed. Norman Haire (London: Encyclopaedic Press, 1966), 206.

11 Hirschfeld, *Transvestites*, 132.

12 Hirschfeld, 84.

13 Hirschfeld, 92–93.

14 Hirschfeld, 94.

15   Hirschfeld, 61.

16   Hirschfeld, 31.

17   Ellis, "Eonism," 49; Hirschfeld, *Transvestites,* 117.

18   Ellis, "Eonism," 67.

19   Richard von Krafft-Ebing, *Psychopathia Sexualis,* 12th ed., trans. F. J. Rebman (Rebman Company, 1906), 310.

20   Von Krafft-Ebing, 321.

21   Hirschfeld, *Transvestites,* 116.

22   Hirschfeld, 71.

23   Anne A. Lawrence, *Men Trapped in Men's Bodies: Narratives of Autogynephilic Transsexualism,* Focus on Sexuality Research (New York: Springer, 2013), 130, https://www.doi.org/10.1007/978-1-4614-5182-2; Ray Blanchard, "Clinical Observations and Systematic Studies of Autogynephilia," *Journal of Sex & Marital Therapy* 17, no. 4 (1991): 237, https://doi.org/10.1080/00926239108404348.

24   Lawrence, *Men Trapped in Men's Bodies,* 132.

25   Lawrence, 133.

26   Lawrence, 135.

27   Lawrence, 136.

28   Niklas Långström and Kenneth J. Zucker, "Transvestic Fetishism in the General Population," *Journal of Sex & Marital Therapy* 31, no. 2 (March–April 2005): 90, https://doi.org/10.1080/00926230590477934.

29   Ashley Brown, Edward D. Barker, and Qazi Rahman, "Erotic Target Identity Inversions Among Men and Women in an Internet Sample," *The Journal of Sexual Medicine* 17, no. 1 (January 2020): 99–110, https://doi.org/10.1016/j.jsxm.2019.10.018.

30   Ray Blanchard, "The Concept of Autogynephilia and the Typology of Male Gender Dysphoria," *The Journal of Nervous and Mental Disease* 177, no. 10 (October 1989): 621, https://doi.org/10.1097/00005053-198910000-00004.

31   Ray Blanchard, "Nonmonotonic Relation of Autogynephilia and Heterosexual Attraction," *Journal of Abnormal Psychology* 101, no. 2 (May 1992): 275, https://doi.org/10.1037/0021-843X.101.2.271.

32   Ray Blanchard, "Typology of Male-to-Female Transsexualism," *Archives of Sexual Behavior* 14, no. 3 (June 1985): 247–61, https://doi.org/10.1007/BF01542107.

33   Larry Nuttbrock et al., "A Further Assessment of Blanchard's Typology of Homosexual versus Non-Homosexual or Autogynephilic Gender Dysphoria," *Archives of Sexual Behavior* 40, no. 2 (April 2011): 247–57, https://doi.org/10.1007/s10508-009-9579-2.

34   Jaime M. Grant et al., *Injustice at Every Turn: A Report of the National Transgender Discrimination Survey* (Washington, DC: National Center for Transgender Equality and National Gay and Lesbian Task Force, 2011), 177, https://transequality.org/sites/default/files/docs/resources/NTDS_Report.pdf.

35   Grant et al., 174.

36 Sandy E. James et al., *The Report of the 2015 U.S. Transgender Survey* (Washington, DC: National Center for Transgender Equality, 2016), 59, https://transequality.org/sites/default/files/docs/usts/USTS-Full-Report-Dec17.pdf.

37 Blanchard, "The Concept of Autogynephilia," 622.

38 Kurt Freund, Robin Watson, and Robert Dickey, "The Types of Heterosexual Gender Identity Disorder," *Annals of Sex Research*, 4, no. 1 (1991): 96, https://doi.org/10.1007/BF00850141.

39 Ellis, "Eonism," 101.

40 Hirschfeld, *Transvestites, 130.*

41 Von Krafft-Ebing, *Psychopathia Sexualis, 322.*

42 Von Krafft-Ebing, 316.

43 Von Krafft-Ebing, 318.

44 Ellis, "Eonism," 53.

45 Ellis, 52.

46 Hirschfeld, *Transvestites, 51.*

47 Hirschfeld, 54.

48 Hirschfeld, 61.

49 Hirschfeld, 94.

3.0. Autoandrophilia (AAP)

1 Klára Bártová et al., "The Prevalence of Paraphilic Interests in the Czech Population: Preference, Arousal, the Use of Pornography, Fantasy, and Behavior," *The Journal of Sex Research* 58, no. 1 (January 2021): 86–96, https://doi.org/10.1080/00224499.2019.1707468.

2 Magnus Hirschfeld, *Transvestites: The Erotic Drive to Cross-Dress*, trans. Michael A. Lombardi-Nash (Buffalo, NY: Prometheus Books, 1991), 156.

3 Lou Sullivan, *We Both Laughed in Pleasure: The Selected Diaries of Lou Sullivan*, ed. Ellis Martin and Zach Ozma (New York: Nightboat Books, 2019); Lanei M. Rodemeyer, *Lou Sullivan Diaries (1970-1980) and Theories of Sexual Embodiment*, Crossroads of Knowledge (New York: Springer, 2018).

4 Rodemeyer, *Lou Sullivan Diaries*, 163.

5 Rodemeyer, 102, 146.

6 Rodemeyer, 102.

7 Wilhelm Stekel, *Sexual Aberrations: The Phenomena of Fetishism in Relation to Sex*, vol. 2 (London: John Lane, 1930), 304, https://archive.org/details/b29817043_0002.

8 Robert J. Stoller, *Splitting: A Case of Female Masculinity*, The International Psycho-Analytical Library, no. 97 (London: Hogarth Press, 1974).

9 Jamison Green, "Autoandrophilia?," *Transgender Tapestry* 93 (Spring 2001), 20, https://archive.org/details/transgendertapes9320unse/page/20/mode/2up.

10 Stekel, *Sexual Aberrations*, 299.

11 Stekel, 287.

12 Stekel, 286.

13 V. S. Ramachandran and Paul D. McGeoch, "Phantom Penises in Transsexuals," *Journal of Consciousness Studies* 15, no. 1 (January 2008): 9, https://philpapers.org/rec/RAMPPI-2.

14 Stoller, *Splitting, 37–38.*

15 Stoller, 13.

16 Stoller, 24.

17 Stoller, 16.

18 Stoller, 16–17.

19 Louis G. Sullivan, *Information for the Female-to-Male Crossdresser and Transsexual,* 2nd ed. (San Francisco: self-pub., 1985), 8, https://www.digitaltransgenderarchive.net/files/g158bh442.

20 Rodemeyer, *Lou Sullivan Diaries*, 36.

21 Robert J. Stoller, "Transvestism in Women," *Archives of Sexual Behavior* 11, no. 2 (April 1982): 104, https://doi.org/10.1007/BF01541978.

22 Rodemeyer, *Lou Sullivan Diaries*, 35.

23 Rodemeyer, 146.

24 Rodemeyer, 102.

25 Rodemeyer, 172.

26 Rodemeyer, 147.

27 Stekel, *Sexual Aberrations, 295.*

28 Stoller, "Transvestism in Women," 103.

29 Rodemeyer, *Lou Sullivan Diaries, 184.*

30 Walter Bockting, Autumn Benner, and Eli Coleman, "Gay and Bisexual Identity Development Among Female-to-Male Transsexuals in North America: Emergence of a Transgender Sexuality," *Archives of Sexual Behavior* 38, no. 5 (October 2009): 692, https://doi.org/10.1007/s10508-009-9489-3.

31 Robert J. Stoller, *Sex and Gender: The Development of Masculinity and Femininity* (London: Karnac Books, 1984), 194.

32 Stekel, *Sexual Aberrations, 302.*

33 Stekel, 284.

34 Stekel, 289.

35 Stekel, 294.

36 Stekel, 282.

37 Stekel, 302.

38 Stoller, "Transvestism in Women," 103.

39 Sullivan, *Female-to-Male Crossdresser and Transsexual, 7–8.*

40 Stoller, "Transvestism in Women," 105.

41 Stoller, 105.

42 Rodemeyer, *Lou Sullivan Diaries*, 14.

43 Rodemeyer, 24.

44 Rodemeyer, 27.

45   Richard A. Lippa, "Gender Differences in Personality and Interests: When, Where, and Why?," *Social and Personality Psychology Compass 4, no. 11 (November 2010): 1098–110, https://doi.org/10.1111/j.1751-9004.2010.00320.x.*

46   Jennifer Connellan et al., "Sex Differences in Human Neonatal Social Perception," *Infant Behavior and Development* 23, no. 1 (January 2000): 113–18, https://doi.org/10.1016/S0163-6383(00)00032-1.

47   Bártová et al., "Prevalence of Paraphilic Interests."

48   Stoller, *Splitting, 14.*

49   Stekel, *Sexual Aberrations, 286.*

50   Stekel, 281.

51   Stekel, 281.

52   Stekel, 287.

53   Stoller, "Transvestism in Women," 103–104.

54   Lou Sullivan, letter to Ray Blanchard, November 1, 1987, https://www.digitaltransgenderarchive.net/files/wh246s217.

55   Robert Dickey and Judith Stephens, "Female-to-Male Transsexualism, Heterosexual Type: Two Cases," *Archives of Sexual Behavior* 24, no. 4 (August 1995): 441, https://doi.org/10.1007/BF01541857.

56   David Schleifer, "Make Me Feel Mighty Real: Gay Female-to-Male Transgenderists Negotiating Sex, Gender, and Sexuality," *Sexualities* 9, no. 1 (February 2006): 67, https://doi.org/10.1177/1363460706058397.

57   Dickey and Stephens, "Female-to-Male Transsexualism," 443.

58   Rodemeyer, *Lou Sullivan Diaries, 36.*

59   Stoller, *Splitting, 64.*

60   Stoller, 54.

61   Stoller, 61.

62   Stoller, 63.

63   Stoller, 182.

64   Stoller, 60.

65   Stoller, 178.

66   Stoller, 67.

67   Stoller, 67.

3.1. Interpersonal Autoandrophilia

1   Lanei M. Rodemeyer, *Lou Sullivan Diaries (1970-1980) and Theories of Sexual Embodiment,* Crossroads of Knowledge (New York: Springer, 2018), 22.

2   Rodemeyer, 23.

3   Rodemeyer, 166.

4   Robert J. Stoller, "Transvestism in Women," *Archives of Sexual Behavior* 11, no. 2 (April 1982): 104, https://doi.org/10.1007/BF01541978.

5   Rodemeyer, *Lou Sullivan Diaries, 3.*

6   Wilhelm Stekel, *Sexual Aberrations: The Phenomena of Fetishism in Relation to Sex*, vol. 2 (London: John Lane, 1930), 284, https://archive.org/details/b29817043_0002.

7   Louis G. Sullivan, *Information for the Female-to-Male Crossdresser and Transsexual*, 2nd ed. (San Francisco: self-pub., 1985), 10, https://www.digitaltransgenderarchive.net/files/g158bh442.

8   J. H. Vogt, "Five Cases of Transsexualism in Females," *Acta Psychiatrica Scandinavica* 44, no. 1 (March 1968): 73, https://doi.org/10.1111/j.1600-0447.1968.tb07636.x.

9   Sullivan, *Female-to-Male Crossdresser and Transsexual*, 8.

10   Rodemeyer, *Lou Sullivan Diaries*, 106.

11   Rodemeyer, 163.

12   Rodemeyer, 178.

13   Lou Sullivan, letter to Ray Blanchard, November 1, 1987, https://www.digitaltransgenderarchive.net/files/wh246s217.

14   Robert J. Stoller, *Splitting: A Case of Female Masculinity*, The International Psycho-Analytical Library, no. 97 (London: Hogarth Press, 1974), 292.

15   Stoller, "Transvestism in Women," 106.

16   Stoller, 109.

17   Stoller, *Splitting, 276.*

18   Stoller, 285.

19   Stoller, 291.

20   Stoller, 277.

21   Stoller, 14.

22   Robert Dickey and Judith Stephens, "Female-to-Male Transsexualism, Heterosexual Type: Two Cases," *Archives of Sexual Behavior* 24, no. 4 (August 1995): 441, https://doi.org/10.1007/BF01541857.

23   Dickey and Stephens, 442.

24   Ray Blanchard, Leonard H. Clemmensen, and Betty W. Steiner, "Heterosexual and Homosexual Gender Dysphoria," *Archives of Sexual Behavior* 16, no. 2 (April 1987): 143, https://doi.org/10.1007/BF01542067.

25   Stoller, "Transvestism in Women," 104.

26   Walter Bockting, Autumn Benner, and Eli Coleman, "Gay and Bisexual Identity Development Among Female-to-Male Transsexuals in North America: Emergence of a Transgender Sexuality," *Archives of Sexual Behavior* 38, no. 5 (October 2009): 696, https://doi.org/10.1007/s10508-009-9489-3.

27   J. Michael Bailey and Ray Blanchard, "Gender Dysphoria is Not One Thing," *4thWaveNow* (blog), December 7, 2017, https://4thwavenow.com/2017/12/07/gender-dysphoria-is-not-one-thing/.

28   Rodemeyer, *Lou Sullivan Diaries*, 22.

29   Sullivan, letter to Ray Blanchard.

30   Dorothy Clare and Bryan Tully, "Transhomosexuality, or the Dissociation of Sexual Orientation and Sex Object Choice," *Archives of Sexual Behavior* 18, no. 6 (December 1989): 533, https://doi.org/10.1007/BF01541679.

31 David Schleifer, "Make Me Feel Mighty Real: Gay Female-to-Male Transgenderists Negotiating Sex, Gender, and Sexuality," *Sexualities* 9, no. 1 (February 2006): 67–68, https://doi.org/10.1177/1363460706058397.

32 Meredith L. Chivers and J. Michael Bailey, "Sexual Orientation of Female-to-Male Transsexuals: A Comparison of Homosexual and Nonhomosexual Types," *Archives of Sexual Behavior* 29, no. 3 (June 2000): 269, https://doi.org/10.1023/A:1001915530479.

33 Bockting, Benner, and Coleman, "Gay and Bisexual Identity Development," 694.

34 S. Colton Meier et al., "Measures of Clinical Health among Female-to-Male Transgender Persons as a Function of Sexual Orientation," *Archives of Sexual Behavior* 42, no. 3 (April 2013): 470, https://doi.org/10.1007/s10508-012-0052-2.

35 J. Defreyne et al., "Sexual Orientation in Transgender Individuals: Results from the Longitudinal ENIGI Study," *International Journal of Impotence Research* 33, no. 7 (2021): 694–702, https://doi.org/10.1038/s41443-020-00402-7.

36 Lisa M. Diamond, *Sexual Fluidity: Understanding Women's Love and Desire* (Cambridge, MA: Harvard University Press, 2008).

37 Diamond, 196.

38 Diamond, 200.

39 Joanna Russ, *Magic Mommas, Trembling Sisters, Puritans & Perverts: Feminist Essays*, The Crossing Press Feminist Series (Trumansburg, NY: The Crossing Press, 1985), 79–97.

40 "FanFiction," FanFiction.net, accessed September 29, 2022, https://www.fanfiction.net/.

41 Uli Meyer, "Hidden in Straight Sight: Trans*gressing Gender and Sexuality via BL," in *Boys' Love Manga: Essays on the Sexual Ambiguity and Cross-Cultural Fandom of the Genre*, ed. Antonia Levi, Mark McHarry, and Dru Pagliassotti (Jefferson, NC: McFarland & Company, 2008), 246.

42 Miyuki Hashimoto, "Visual Kei Otaku Identity—An Intercultural Analysis," *Intercultural Communication Studies* 16, no. 1 (2007): 92, https://www-s3-live.kent.edu/s3fs-root/s3fs-public/file/10-Miyuki-Hashimoto.pdf.

43 Akiko Mizoguchi, "Theorizing Comics/Manga Genre as a Productive Forum: Yaoi and Beyond," in *Comics Worlds and the World of Comics: Towards Scholarship on a Global Scale*, ed. Jaqueline Berndt, Global Manga Studies, vol. 1 (Kyoto: International Manga Research Center, Kyoto Seika University, 2010), 157.

44 Mizoguchi, 159.

45 Stefan Rowniak and Catherine Chesla, "Coming Out for a Third Time: Transmen, Sexual Orientation, and Identity," *Archives of Sexual Behavior* 42, no. 3 (April 2013): 449–61, https://doi.org/10.1007/s10508-012-0036-2.

46 Eli Coleman, Walter O. Bockting, and Louis Gooren, "Homosexual and Bisexual Identity in Sex-Reassigned Female-to-Male Transsexuals," *Archives of Sexual Behavior* 22, no. 1 (February 1993): 41–42, https://doi.org/10.1007/BF01552911; Bockting, Benner, and Coleman, "Gay and Bisexual Identity Development," 694.

47 Bockting, Benner, and Coleman, "Gay and Bisexual Identity Development," 694.

48   Raine Dozier, "Beards, Breasts, and Bodies: Doing Sex in a Gendered World," *Gender & Society* 19, no. 3 (June 2005): 312, https://doi.org/10.1177/0891243204272153.

49   Dozier, 312.

50   Rowniak and Chesla, "Coming Out for a Third Time," 457.

51   Bockting, Benner, and Coleman, "Gay and Bisexual Identity Development," 695.

52   Rowniak and Chesla, "Coming Out for a Third Time," 455.

4.0. Are Traps Gay?

1   K. J. Hsu et al., "Who are Gynandromorphophilic Men? Characterizing Men with Sexual Interest in Transgender Women," *Psychological Medicine* 46, no. 4 (March 2016): 819–27, https://doi.org/10.1017/S0033291715002317.

2   Hsu et al., 822.

3   Kevin J. Hsu et al., "Sexual Arousal Patterns of Autogynephilic Male Cross-Dressers," *Archives of Sexual Behavior* 46, no. 1 (January 2017): 247–253, https://doi.org/10.1007/s10508-016-0826-z.

4.1. Gynandromorphophilia (GAMP)

1   Christin Scarlett Milloy, "Beware the Chasers: 'Admirers' Who Harass Trans People," Slate, October 2, 2014, https://slate.com/human-interest/2014/10/trans-chasers-exploitive-admirers-who-harass-trans-people.html; Avery Brooks Tompkins, "'There's No Chasing Involved': Cis/Trans Relationships, 'Tranny Chasers,' and the Future of a Sex-Positive Trans Politics," *Journal of Homosexuality* 61, no. 5 (2014): 766–80, https://doi.org/10.1080/00918369.2014.870448.

2   Ray Blanchard and Peter I. Collins, "Men with Sexual Interest in Transvestites, Transsexuals, and She-Males," *The Journal of Nervous and Mental Disease* 181, no. 9 (September 1993): 570–75, https://doi.org/10.1097/00005053-199309000-00008.

3   Christian C. Joyal, Amélie Cossette, and Vanessa Lapierre, "What Exactly Is an Unusual Sexual Fantasy?," *The Journal of Sexual Medicine* 12, no. 2 (February 2015): 337, https://doi.org/10.1111/jsm.12734.

4   Ogi Ogas and Sai Gaddam, *A Billion Wicked Thoughts: What the Internet Tells Us about Sexual Relationships* (New York: Dutton, 2011), 308.

5   K. J. Hsu et al., "Who are Gynandromorphophilic Men? Characterizing Men with Sexual Interest in Transgender Women," *Psychological Medicine* 46, no. 4 (March 2016): 819–27, https://doi.org/10.1017/S0033291715002317.

6   Justin Lehmiller, email message to author, "Re: Fantasy Survey Stats Request- AGP/AAP, TV, + GAMP," October 13, 2021.

7   "The 2019 Year in Review," Pornhub Insights, December 11, 2019, https://www.pornhub.com/insights/2019-year-in-review.

8   A. M. Rosenthal, Kevin J. Hsu, and J. Michael Bailey, "Who are Gynandromorphophilic Men? An Internet Survey of Men with Sexual Interest in

Transgender Women," *Archives of Sexual Behavior* 46, no. 1 (January 2017): 255–64, https://doi.org/10.1007/s10508-016-0872-6.

9   Rosenthal, Hsu, and Bailey, 5.

10 Rosenthal, Hsu, and Bailey, 5.

11 Rosenthal, Hsu, and Bailey, 5.

12 Rosenthal, Hsu, and Bailey, 6.

13 Rosenthal, Hsu, and Bailey, 6.

14 Rosenthal, Hsu, and Bailey, 5–6.

15 Junko Mitsuhashi and Kazumi Hasegawa, "The Transgender World in Contemporary Japan: The Male to Female Cross-Dressers' Community in Shinjuku," *Inter-Asia Cultural Studies* 7, no. 2 (June 2006): 217, https://doi.org/10.1080/14649370600673847.

16 Rosenthal, Hsu, and Bailey, "Who are Gynandromorphophilic Men?," 5.

17 Rosenthal, Hsu, and Bailey, 6.

18 Rosenthal, Hsu, and Bailey, 6.

19 Martin S. Weinberg and Colin J. Williams, "Men Sexually Interested in Transwomen (MSTW): Gendered Embodiment and the Construction of Sexual Desire," *The Journal of Sex Research* 47, no. 4 (July 2010): 374–83, https://doi.org/10.1080/00224490903050568.

20 Weinberg and Williams, 380.

21 Weinberg and Williams, 380.

22 Mitsuhashi and Hasegawa, "The Transgender World in Contemporary Japan," 222.

23 Mitsuhashi and Hasegawa, 222.

24 "The REAL Reasons Men Like Trans Women," Kat Blaque, December 17, 2019, YouTube video, 40:27, https://www.youtube.com/watch?v=ysSVxrKVMyg&t=360s.

25 Rosenthal, Hsu, and Bailey, "Who are Gynandromorphophilic Men?," 5.

26 Rosenthal, Hsu, and Bailey, 6.

27 Don Kulick, "The Gender of Brazilian Transgendered Prostitutes," *American Anthropologist* 99, no. 3 (September 1997): 578, https://doi.org/10.1525/aa.1997.99.3.574.

28 Kulick, 584.

29 Rosenthal, Hsu, and Bailey, "Who are Gynandromorphophilic Men?," 6.

30 Ray Blanchard, "The Concept of Autogynephilia and the Typology of Male Gender Dysphoria," *The Journal of Nervous and Mental Disease* 177, no. 10 (October 1989): 623, https://doi.org/10.1097/00005053-198910000-00004.

31 Kevin J. Hsu, "email message to author, December 14, 2021; Blanchard, "The Concept of Autogynephilia," 621.

32 Rosenthal, Hsu, and Bailey, "Who are Gynandromorphophilic Men?," 6.

33 Rosenthal, Hsu, and Bailey, 6.

34 Rosenthal, Hsu, and Bailey, 6.

35 Rosenthal, Hsu, and Bailey, 7.

36 Kevin J. Hsu et al., "Sexual Arousal Patterns of Autogynephilic Male Cross-Dressers," *Archives of Sexual Behavior* 46, no. 1 (January 2017): 247–53, https://

doi.org/10.1007/s10508-016-0826-z; Hsu et al., "Who Are Gynandromorphophilic Men? Characterizing Men."

37   Hsu et al., "Sexual Arousal Patterns."

38   Hsu et al., "Sexual Arousal Patterns."

39   Rosenthal, Hsu, and Bailey, "Who are Gynandromorphophilic Men?," 5.

40   Paul L. Vasey and Doug P. VanderLaan, "Avuncular Tendencies and the Evolution of Male Androphilia in Samoan *Fa'afafine*," *Archives of Sexual Behavior* 39, no. 4 (August 2010): 821–30, https://doi.org/10.1007/s10508-008-9404-3.

41   Lanna J. Petterson et al., "Reconsidering Male Bisexuality: Sexual Activity Role and Sexual Attraction in Samoan Men Who Engage in Sexual Interactions with *Fa'afafine*," *Psychology of Sexual Orientation and Gender Diversity* 3, no. 1 (2016): 11–26, https://doi.org/10.1037/sgd0000160.

42   Paul L. Vasey and Doug P. VanderLaan, "Birth Order and Male Androphilia in Samoan *Fa'afafine*," *Proceedings of the Royal Society B: Biological Sciences* 274, no. 1616 (June 2007): 1437–42, https://doi.org/10.1098/rspb.2007.0120.

43   Lanna J. Petterson, "Male Sexual Orientation: A Cross-Cultural Perspective" (PhD diss., University of Lethbridge, 2020), https://hdl.handle.net/10133/5763.

44   Roland Imhoff et al., "Vicarious Viewing Time: Prolonged Response Latencies for Sexually Attractive Targets as a Function of Task- or Stimulus-Specific Processing," *Archives of Sexual Behavior* 41, no. 6 (December 2012): 1389–401, https://doi.org/10.1007/s10508-011-9879-1.

45   Lanna J. Petterson and Paul L. Vasey, "Samoan Men's Sexual Attraction and Viewing Time Response to Male-to-Feminine Transgender and Cisgender Adults," *Archives of Sexual Behavior* 50, no. 3 (April 2021): 879, https://doi.org/10.1007/s10508-020-01905-6.

46   Petterson and Vasey, 880–81.

47   Lanna J. Petterson et al., "Heterogeneity in the Sexual Orientations of Men Who Have Sex with *Fa'afafine* in Samoa," *Archives of Sexual Behavior* 49, no. 2 (February 2020): 517–29, https://doi.org/10.1007/s10508-020-01646-6; Petterson et al., "Reconsidering Male Bisexuality."

48   Petterson et al., "Heterogeneity in the Sexual Orientations"; Petterson et al., "Reconsidering Male Bisexuality," 8–11.

49   Petterson et al., "Reconsidering Male Bisexuality," 5.

50   Petterson et al., 19, 21.

51   Petterson et al., 18, 20.

52   Petterson et al., "Heterogeneity in the Sexual Orientations," 3.

53   Petterson et al., 7.

54   Weinberg and Williams, "Men Sexually Interested in Transwomen," 380.

55   Rosenthal, Hsu, and Bailey, "Who are Gynandromorphophilic Men?," 6.

56   Hsu et al., "Sexual Arousal Patterns."

57   Ray Blanchard, "The She-Male Phenomenon and the Concept of Partial Autogynephilia," *Journal of Sex & Marital Therapy* 19, no. 1 (Spring 1993): 69–76, https://doi.org/10.1080/00926239308404889.

58 Blanchard, 73.

59 Ray Blanchard, "Partial versus Complete Autogynephilia and Gender Dysphoria," *Journal of Sex & Marital Therapy* 19, no. 4 (Winter 1993): 305, https://doi.org/10.1080/00926239308404373.

60 Tompkins, "'There's No Chasing Involved.'"

61 Karen L. Blair and Rhea Ashley Hoskin, "Transgender Exclusion from the World of Dating: Patterns of Acceptance and Rejection of Hypothetical Trans Dating Partners as a Function of Sexual and Gender Identity," *Journal of Social and Personal Relationships* 36, no. 7 (July 2019): 2074–95, https://doi.org/10.1177/0265407518779139.

62 Petterson, "Male Sexual Orientation," 257.

4.2. Mental Health and Transgenderism

1 I. H. Meyer, "Prejudice, Social Stress, and Mental Health in Lesbian, Gay, and Bisexual Populations: Conceptual Issues and Research Evidence," *Psychological Bulletin* 129, no. 5 (2003): 674–97, https://doi.org/10.1037/0033-2909.129.5.674.

2 Ilan H. Meyer et al., "Minority Stress, Distress, and Suicide Attempts in Three Cohorts of Sexual Minority Adults: A U.S. Probability Sample," *PLoS ONE* 16, no. 3 (March 2021): e0246827, https://doi.org/10.1371/journal.pone.0246827.

3 Meyer et al.

4 Varun Warrier et al., "Elevated Rates of Autism, Other Neurodevelopmental and Psychiatric Diagnoses, and Autistic Traits in Transgender and Gender-Diverse Individuals," *Nature Communications* 11, no. 1 (August 2020), https://doi.org/10.1038/s41467-020-17794-1.

5 E. A. Pascoe and L. Smart Richman, "Perceived Discrimination and Health: A Meta-Analytic Review," *Psychological Bulletin* 135, no. 4 (2009): 538, https://doi.org/10.1037/a0016059.

6 Kenneth J. Zucker, Anne A. Lawrence, and Baudewijntje P. C. Kreukels, "Gender Dysphoria in Adults," *Annual Review of Clinical Psychology* 12 (March 2016): 230, https://doi.org/10.1146/annurev-clinpsy-021815-093034.

7 J. Michael Bailey, "The Minority Stress Model Deserves Reconsideration, Not Just Extension," *Archives of Sexual Behavior* 49, no. 7 (October 2020): 2265–68, https://doi.org/10.1007/s10508-019-01606-9.

8 Tinca J. C. Polderman et al., "Meta-Analysis of the Heritability of Human Traits Based on Fifty Years of Twin Studies," *Nature Genetics* 47, no. 7 (July 2015): 704, https://doi.org/10.1038/ng.3285.

9 Polderman et al., 704.

10 Heather M. Maranges and Tania A. Reynolds, "Heritability," in *The Wiley Encyclopedia of Personality and Individual Differences: Models and Theories*, ed. Bernardo J. Carducci and Christopher S. Nave (Hoboken, NJ: Wiley, 2020), 244, https://doi.org/10.1002/9781118970843.ch41.

11   Maranges and Reynolds, 243.

12   Thomas J. Bouchard, "Genetic Influence on Human Psychological Traits: A
      Survey," *Current Directions in Psychological Science* 13, no. 4 (August 2004): 150,
      https://doi.org/10.1111/j.0963-7214.2004.00295.x.

13   Bouchard, 150.

14   Y. E. Willems et al., "The Heritability of Self-Control: A Meta-Analysis,"
      *Neuroscience & Biobehavioral Reviews 100 (May 2019): 330, https://doi.org/10.1016/j.
      neubiorev.2019.02.012.*

15   Bouchard, "Genetic Influence," 150; Thomas J. Bouchard, "The Wilson Effect: The
      Increase in Heritability of IQ with Age," *Twin Research and Human Genetics 16, no.
      5 (2013): 924, https://doi.org/10.1017/thg.2013.54.*

16   Patrick F. Sullivan, Michael C. Neale, and Kenneth S. Kendler, "Genetic
      Epidemiology of Major Depression: Review and Meta-Analysis," *The American
      Journal of Psychiatry* 157, no. 10 (October 2000): 1552, https://doi.org/10.1176/appi.
      ajp.157.10.1552; Ana Maria Fernandez-Pujals et al., "Epidemiology and Heritability
      of Major Depressive Disorder, Stratified by Age of Onset, Sex, and Illness Course
      in Generation Scotland: Scottish Family Health Study (GS:SFHS)," *PLoS ONE* 10,
      no. 11 (November 2015), https://doi.org/10.1371/journal.pone.0142197; Kenneth
      S. Kendler et al., "A Swedish National Twin Study of Lifetime Major Depression,"
      The American Journal of Psychiatry 163, no. 1 (January 2006): 109, https://doi.
      org/10.1176/appi.ajp.163.1.109.

17   John M. Hettema, Michael C. Neale, and Kenneth S. Kendler, "A Review and
      Meta-Analysis of the Genetic Epidemiology of Anxiety Disorders," *The American
      Journal of Psychiatry* 158, no. 10 (October 2001): 1568, https://doi.org/10.1176/appi.
      ajp.158.10.1568.

18   Murray B. Stein, Kerry L. Jang, and W. John Livesley, "Heritability of Anxiety
      Sensitivity: A Twin Study," *The American Journal of Psychiatry* 156, no. 2
      (February 1999): 249, https://doi.org/10.1176/ajp.156.2.246; David Mataix-Cols et
      al., "Population-Based, Multigenerational Family Clustering Study of Obsessive-
      Compulsive Disorder," *JAMA Psychiatry* 70, no. 7 (2013): 709, https://doi.
      org/10.1001/jamapsychiatry.2013.3.

19   Svenn Torgersen et al., "The Heritability of Cluster B Personality Disorders
      Assessed Both by Personal Interview and Questionnaire," *Journal of Personality
      Disorders* 26, no. 6 (December 2012): 863, https://doi.org/10.1521/pedi.2012.26.6.848.

20   Sven Sandin et al., "The Heritability of Autism Spectrum Disorder," *JAMA*
      318, no. 12 (2017): 1183, https://doi.org/10.1001/jama.2017.12141; Beata Tick et al.,
      "Heritability of Autism Spectrum Disorders: A Meta-Analysis of Twin Studies," *The
      Journal of Child Psychology and Psychiatry* 57, no. 5 (May 2016): 585, https://doi.
      org/10.1111/jcpp.12499.

21   Peter McGuffin et al., "The Heritability of Bipolar Affective Disorder and the
      Genetic Relationship to Unipolar Depression," *Archives of General Psychiatry* 60,
      no. 5 (2003): 502, https://doi.org/10.1001/archpsyc.60.5.497.

22   Alastair G. Cardno et al., "Heritability Estimates for Psychotic Disorders: The Maudsley Twin Psychosis Series," *Archives of General Psychiatry* 56, no. 2 (1999): 166, https://doi.org/10.1001/archpsyc.56.2.162.

23   H. Larsson et al., "The Heritability of Clinically Diagnosed Attention Deficit Hyperactivity Disorder across the Lifespan," *Psychological Medicine* 44, no. 10 (2014): 2223, https://doi.org/10.1017/S0033291713002493.

24   Frederick L. Coolidge and Ari Stillman, "The Strong Heritability of Gender Dysphoria," in *The Plasticity of Sex*, ed. Marianne J. Legato (Cambridge, MA: Academic Press Elsevier, 2020), 76, https://doi.org/10.1016/B978-0-12-815968-2.00006-2.

25   B. P. Zietsch et al., "Do Shared Etiological Factors Contribute to the Relationship between Sexual Orientation and Depression?," *Psychological Medicine* 42, no. 3 (2012): 528, https://doi.org/10.1017/S0033291711001577.

26   Zietsch et al., 528.

27   Andrea Ganna et al., "Large-Scale GWAS Reveals Insights into the Genetic Architecture of Same-Sex Sexual Behavior," *Science 365, no. 6456 (August 2019): eaat7693, https://doi.org/10.1126/science.aat7693.*

28   Andrea Ganna et al., "Large-Scale GWAS Reveals Insights into the Genetic Architecture of Same-Sex Sexual Behavior," *Science* 365, no. 6456 (August 2019): table S19, https://doi.org/10.1126/science.aat7693.

29   Ganna et al., 63–64.

30   Bishoy Hanna et al., "Psychiatric Disorders in the U.S. Transgender Population," *Annals of Epidemiology 39 (November 2019): 1–7.e1, https://doi.org/10.1016/j.annepidem.2019.09.009.*

31   Varun Warrier et al., "Elevated Rates of Autism, Other Neurodevelopmental and Psychiatric Diagnoses, and Autistic Traits in Transgender and Gender-Diverse Individuals," *Nature Communications* 11, no. 1 (December 2020): supplementary table 8, https://www.nature.com/articles/s41467-020-17794-1#Sec36.

32   Warrier et al., "Elevated Rates of Autism," supplementary figure 2.

33   Warrier et al., supplementary figure 2.

34   Meng-Chuan Lai et al., "Prevalence of Co-Occurring Mental Health Diagnoses in the Autism Population: A Systematic Review and Meta-Analysis," *The Lancet Psychiatry 6, no. 10 (October 2019): 819–29, https://doi.org/10.1016/S2215-0366(19)30289-5.*

35   Jorge Lugo-Marín et al., "Prevalence of Psychiatric Disorders in Adults with Autism Spectrum Disorder: A Systematic Review and Meta-Analysis," *Research in Autism Spectrum Disorders 59 (March 2019): 31, https://doi.org/10.1016/j.rasd.2018.12.004.*

36   Niklas Långström and Kenneth J. Zucker, "Transvestic Fetishism in the General Population," *Journal of Sex & Marital Therapy* 31, no. 2 (2005): 91, https://doi.org/10.1080/00926230590477934.

37   Jaime M. Grant et al., *Injustice at Every Turn: A Report of the National Transgender Discrimination Survey* (Washington, DC: National Center for Transgender

Equality and National Gay and Lesbian Task Force, 2011), 82, https://transequality.
org/sites/default/files/docs/resources/NTDS_Report.pdf.

38   Sandy E. James et al., *The Report of the 2015 U.S. Transgender Survey* (Washington,
DC: National Center for Transgender Equality, 2016), 8, https://www.ustranssurvey.
org/reports/#2015report.

39   Ronald C. Kessler, Guilherme Borges, and Ellen E. Walters, "Prevalence of
and Risk Factors for Lifetime Suicide Attempts in the National Comorbidity
Survey," *Archives of General Psychiatry* 56, no. 7 (1999): 617, https://doi.
org/10.1001/archpsyc.56.7.617; Matthew K. Nock et al., "Cross-National
Prevalence and Risk Factors for Suicidal Ideation, Plans and Attempts," *The
British Journal of Psychiatry* 192, no. 2 (2008): 98–105, https://doi.org/10.1192/
bjp.bp.107.040113.

40   Elena García-Vega et al., "Suicidal Ideation and Suicide Attempts in Persons
with Gender Dysphoria," *Psicothema* 30, no. 3 (2018): 284, https://doi.org/10.7334/
psicothema2017.438.

41   Jessica Xavier, Julie A. Honnold, and Judith B. Bradford, *The Health, Health-
Related Needs, and Lifecourse Experiences of Transgender Virginians* (Virginia
Department of Health, 2007), 23, https://doi.org/10.1037/e544442014-001.

42   Larry Nuttbrock et al., "Psychiatric Impact of Gender-Related Abuse Across the
Life Course of Male-to-Female Transgender Persons," *The Journal of Sex Research*
47, no. 1 (2010): 16, https://doi.org/10.1080/00224490903062258.

43   Louis Bailey, Sonja J. Ellis, and Jay McNeil, "Suicide Risk in the UK Trans
Population and the Role of Gender Transition in Decreasing Suicidal Ideation and
Suicide Attempt," *Mental Health Review Journal* 19, no. 4 (December 2014): 213,
https://doi.org/10.1108/MHRJ-05-2014-0015; Stephen Whittle, Lewis Turner, and
Maryam Al-Alami, *Engendered Penalties: Transgender and Transsexual People's
Experiences of Inequality and Discrimination* (London: Press For Change, 2007),
78, http://www.pfc.org.uk/pdf/EngenderedPenalties.pdf.

44   Runsen Chen et al., "Suicidal Ideation and Attempted Suicide amongst Chinese
Transgender Persons: National Population Study," *Journal of Affective Disorders*
245 (February 2019): 1131, https://doi.org/10.1016/j.jad.2018.12.011.

45   Nock et al., "Cross-National Prevalence and Risk Factors."

46   Michael King et al., "A Systematic Review of Mental Disorder, Suicide, and
Deliberate Self Harm in Lesbian, Gay and Bisexual People," *BMC Psychiatry* 8
(2008), https://doi.org/10.1186/1471-244X-8-70.

47   Travis Salway et al., "A Systematic Review and Meta-Analysis of Disparities in
the Prevalence of Suicide Ideation and Attempt Among Bisexual Populations,"
Archives of Sexual Behavior 48, no. 1 (January 2019): 89–111, https://doi.org/10.1007/
s10508-018-1150-6.

48   Travis Salway Hottes et al., "Lifetime Prevalence of Suicide Attempts Among
Sexual Minority Adults by Study Sampling Strategies: A Systematic Review and
Meta-Analysis," *American Journal of Public Health* 106, no. 5 (May 2016): e5,

https://doi.org/10.2105/AJPH.2016.303088; Salway et al., "A Systematic Review and Meta-Analysis of Disparities," 14.

49 Kessler, Borges, and Walters, "Lifetime Suicide Attempts"; Matthew K. Nock et al., "Cross-National Analysis of the Associations among Mental Disorders and Suicidal Behavior: Findings from the WHO World Mental Health Surveys," ed. Rachel Jenkins, *PLoS Medicine* 6, no. 8 (2009): e1000123, https://doi.org/10.1371/journal.pmed.1000123; Lay San Too et al., "The Association between Mental Disorders and Suicide: A Systematic Review and Meta-Analysis of Record Linkage Studies," *Journal of Affective Disorders* 259 (December 2019): 302–313, https://doi.org/10.1016/j.jad.2019.08.054.

50 "What Does the Scholarly Research Say about the Effect of Gender Transition on Transgender Well-Being?," What We Know, accessed August 16, 2022, https://whatweknow.inequality.cornell.edu/topics/lgbt-equality/what-does-the-scholarly-research-say-about-the-well-being-of-transgender-people/.

51 N. A. Livingston et al., "Sexual Minority Stress and Suicide Risk: Identifying Resilience through Personality Profile Analysis," *Psychology of Sexual Orientation and Gender Diversity* 2, no. 3 (2015): 326, https://doi.org/10.1037/sgd0000116.

52 Bailey, Ellis, and McNeil, "Suicide Risk in the UK Trans Population," 213.

53 "What Does the Scholarly Research Say," What We Know.

54 Nuttbrock et al., "Psychiatric Impact of Gender-Related Abuse," 18.

55 Brian A. Rood et al., "Predictors of Suicidal Ideation in a Statewide Sample of Transgender Individuals," *LGBT Health* 2, no. 3 (September 2015): 273, https://doi.org/10.1089/lgbt.2013.0048.

56 Rood et al., 273.

57 Jody L. Herman, Taylor N. T. Brown, and Ann P. Haas, *Suicide Thoughts and Attempts Among Transgender Adults: Findings from the 2015 U.S. Transgender Survey* (UCLA School of Law Williams Institute, September 2019) 37, https://williamsinstitute.law.ucla.edu/publications/suicidality-transgender-adults/.

58 Herman, Brown, and Haas, 27.

59 Herman, Brown, and Haas, 28.

4.3. Autism

1 David M. Greenberg et al., "Testing the Empathizing–Systemizing Theory of Sex Differences and the Extreme Male Brain Theory of Autism in Half a Million People," *Proceedings of the National Academy of Sciences* 115, no. 48 (November 2018): 12154, https://doi.org/10.1073/pnas.1811032115.

2 John F. Strang et al., "Increased Gender Variance in Autism Spectrum Disorders and Attention Deficit Hyperactivity Disorder," *Archives of Sexual Behavior* 43, no. 8 (November 2014): 1529, https://doi.org/10.1007/s10508-014-0285-3.

3 R. George and M.A. Stokes, "Sexual Orientation in Autism Spectrum Disorder," *Autism Research* 11, no. 1 (January 2018): 133–141, https://doi.org/10.1002/aur.1892.

4   Daniel Schöttle et al., "Sexuality in Autism: Hypersexual and Paraphilic Behavior in Women and Men with High-Functioning Autism Spectrum Disorder," *Dialogues in Clinical Neuroscience* 19, no. 4 (2017): 386, https://doi.org/10.31887/DCNS.2017.19.4/dschoettle; J. Dewinter, H. De Graaf, and S. Begeer, "Sexual Orientation, Gender Identity, and Romantic Relationships in Adolescents and Adults with Autism Spectrum Disorder," *Journal of Autism and Developmental Disorders* 47, no. 9 (September 2017): 2927–34, https://doi.org/10.1007/s10803-017-3199-9; Laura A. Pecora et al., "Characterising the Sexuality and Sexual Experiences of Autistic Females," *Journal of Autism and Developmental Disorders* 49, no. 12 (December 2019): 4834–46, https://doi.org/10.1007/s10803-019-04204-9.

5   Rita George and Mark A. Stokes, "Gender Identity and Sexual Orientation in Autism Spectrum Disorder," *Autism* 22, no. 8 (November 2018): 970–82, https://doi.org/10.1177/1362361317714587.

6   Gene G. Abel and Candice Osborn, "The Paraphilias: The Extent and Nature of Sexually Deviant and Criminal Behavior," *Psychiatric Clinics of North America* 15, no. 3 (September 1992): 686, https://doi.org/10.1016/S0193-953X(18)30231-4.

7   Lucrecia Cabral Fernandes et al., "Aspects of Sexuality in Adolescents and Adults Diagnosed with Autism Spectrum Disorders in Childhood," *Journal of Autism and Developmental Disorders* 46, no. 9 (September 2016): 3155–3165, https://doi.org/10.1007/s10803-016-2855-9; Schöttle et al., "Sexuality in Autism," 389.

8   Rita George, "Sexual Orientation and Gender-Identity in High Functioning Individuals with Autism Spectrum Disorder" (PhD diss., Deakin University, 2016), 216, http://hdl.handle.net/10536/DRO/DU:30089386.

9   George and Stokes, "Gender Identity and Sexual Orientation," 6.

10   George and Stokes, 7.

11   George and Stokes, 10.

12   Rita George and Mark A. Stokes, "A Quantitative Analysis of Mental Health among Sexual and Gender Minority Groups in ASD," *Journal of Autism and Developmental Disorders* 48, no. 6 (June 2018): 2052–63, https://doi.org/10.1007/s10803-018-3469-1.

13   George and Stokes, 6–8.

14   George, "Sexual Orientation and Gender-Identity in High Functioning Individuals," 193–229.

15   George, 209.

16   Simon Baron-Cohen, "Autism: The Empathizing–Systemizing (E-S) Theory," *Annals of the New York Academy of Sciences* 1156, no. 1 (March 2009): 68–80, https://doi.org/10.1111/j.1749-6632.2009.04467.x.

17   R. Su, J. Rounds, and P. I. Armstrong, "Men and Things, Women and People: A Meta-Analysis of Sex Differences in Interests," *Psychological Bulletin* 135, no. 6 (2009): 891, https://doi.org/10.1037/a0017364; Richard A. Lippa, "Gender Differences in Personality and Interests: When, Where, and Why?," *Social and Personality Psychology Compass* 4, no. 11 (November 2010): 1098, https://doi.org/10.1111/j.1751-9004.2010.00320.x.

18 Greenberg et al., "Testing the Empathizing–Systemizing Theory," 12152.

19 Bonnie Auyeung et al., "Fetal Testosterone and Autistic Traits," *British Journal of Psychology* 100, no. 1 (February 2009): 1, https://doi.org/10.1348/000712608X311731.

20 Rebecca M. Jones et al., "Brief Report: Female-to-Male Transsexual People and Autistic Traits," *Journal of Autism and Developmental Disorders* 42, no. 2 (February 2012): 304–305, https://doi.org/10.1007/s10803-011-1227-8.

21 Erin Ingudomnukul et al., "Elevated Rates of Testosterone-Related Disorders in Women with Autism Spectrum Conditions," *Hormones and Behavior* 51, no. 5 (May 2007): 600–601, https://doi.org/10.1016/j.yhbeh.2007.02.001; Alexa Pohl et al., "Uncovering Steroidopathy in Women with Autism: A Latent Class Analysis," *Molecular Autism* 5, (2014), https://doi.org/10.1186/2040-2392-5-27.

22 Pohl et al., "Uncovering Steroidopathy in Women with Autism," 5.

23 Pohl et al., 5.

24 Ashley Brown, Edward D. Barker, and Qazi Rahman, "Erotic Target Identity Inversions among Men and Women in an Internet Sample," *The Journal of Sexual Medicine 17, no. 1 (January 2020): 99–110, https://doi.org/10.1016/j.jsxm.2019.10.018.*

25 Melissa Hines, Charles Brook, and Gerard S. Conway, "Androgen and Psychosexual Development: Core Gender Identity, Sexual Orientation, and Recalled Childhood Gender Role Behavior in Women and Men with Congenital Adrenal Hyperplasia (CAH)," *Journal of Sex Research* 41, no. 1 (2004): 78, https://doi.org/10.1080/00224490409552215; Rebecca Knickmeyer et al., "Androgens and Autistic Traits: A Study of Individuals with Congenital Adrenal Hyperplasia," *Hormones and Behavior* 50, no. 1 (June 2006): 150, https://doi.org/10.1016/j.yhbeh.2006.02.006.

26 Rachel Loomes, Laura Hull, and William Polmear Locke Mandy, "What Is the Male-to-Female Ratio in Autism Spectrum Disorder? A Systematic Review and Meta-Analysis," *Journal of the American Academy of Child & Adolescent Psychiatry* 56, no. 6 (June 2017): 469, https://doi.org/10.1016/j.jaac.2017.03.013.

27 Vickie Pasterski, Liam Gilligan, and Richard Curtis, "Traits of Autism Spectrum Disorders in Adults with Gender Dysphoria," *Archives of Sexual Behavior* 43, no. 2 (February 2014): 387–93, https://doi.org/10.1007/s10508-013-0154-5.

28 Pasterski, Gilligan, and Curtis, 1.

29 Pasterski, Gilligan, and Curtis, 5.

30 Pasterski, Gilligan, and Curtis, 4.

31 Jones et al., "Brief Report," 304.

32 "Center of Expertise on Gender Dysphoria," Amsterdam UMC, accessed September 14, 2022, https://www.vumc.com/departments/center-of-expertise-on-gender-dysphoria.htm.

33 Annelou L. C. de Vries et al., "Autism Spectrum Disorders in Gender Dysphoric Children and Adolescents," *Journal of Autism and Developmental Disorders* 40, no. 8 (August 2010): 932, https://doi.org/10.1007/s10803-010-0935-9.

34 De Vries et al., 932.

35 De Vries et al., 934.

5.0. How Common Is Autoheterosexuality?

1   Ethel S. Person et al., "Gender Differences in Sexual Behaviors and Fantasies in a College Population," *Journal of Sex & Marital Therapy* 15, no. 3 (1989): 187–98, https://doi.org/10.1080/00926238908403822; Bing Hsu et al., "Gender Differences in Sexual Fantasy and Behavior in a College Population: A Ten-Year Replication," *Journal of Sex & Marital Therapy* 20, no. 2 (1994): 103–118, https://doi.org/10.1080/00926239408403421.

2   Ashley Brown, Edward D. Barker, and Qazi Rahman, "Erotic Target Identity Inversions Among Men and Women in an Internet Sample," *The Journal of Sexual Medicine* 17, no. 1 (January 2020): 99–110, https://doi.org/10.1016/j.jsxm.2019.10.018.

3   Elena Baur et al., "Paraphilic Sexual Interests and Sexually Coercive Behavior: A Population-Based Twin Study," *Archives of Sexual Behavior* 45, no. 5 (July 2016): 1163–72, https://doi.org/10.1007/s10508-015-0674-2; Christian C. Joyal and Julie Carpentier, "The Prevalence of Paraphilic Interests and Behaviors in the General Population: A Provincial Survey," *The Journal of Sex Research* 54, no. 2 (2017): 161–71, https://doi.org/10.1080/00224499.2016.1139034; Christian C. Joyal, Amélie Cossette, and Vanessa Lapierre, "What Exactly Is an Unusual Sexual Fantasy?," *The Journal of Sexual Medicine* 12, no. 2 (February 2015): 328–40, https://doi.org/10.1111/jsm.12734; Niklas Långström and Kenneth J. Zucker, "Transvestic Fetishism in the General Population," *Journal of Sex & Marital Therapy* 31, no. 2 (2005): 87–95, https://doi.org/10.1080/00926230590477934; Samuel S. Janus and Cynthia L. Janus, *The Janus Report on Sexual Behavior* (Hoboken, NJ: Wiley, 1993); Halilu Abdullahi, Racheal Olayemi Jafojo, and Owoidoho Udofia, "Paraphilia Among Undergraduates in a Nigerian University," *Sexual Addiction & Compulsivity* 22, no. 3 (2015): 249–57, https://doi.org/10.1080/10720162.2015.1057662; Justin J. Lehmiller, *Tell Me What You Want: The Science of Sexual Desire and How It Can Help You Improve Your Sex Life* (New York: Hachette Books, 2018); Alfred Spira and Nathalie Bajos, *Sexual Behaviour and AIDS* (Avebury, 1994); Christoph Joseph Ahlers et al., "How Unusual Are the Contents of Paraphilias? Paraphilia-Associated Sexual Arousal Patterns in a Community-Based Sample of Men," *The Journal of Sexual Medicine* 8, no. 5 (May 2011): 1362–70, https://doi.org/10.1111/j.1743-6109.2009.01597.x.

4   Spira and Bajos, *Sexual Behaviour and AIDS*.

5   Lehmiller, *Tell Me What You Want*.

6   Justin Lehmiller, email message to author, "Re: Fantasy Survey Stats Request- AGP/AAP, TV, + GAMP," October 13, 2021.

7   Klára Bártová et al., "The Prevalence of Paraphilic Interests in the Czech Population: Preference, Arousal, the Use of Pornography, Fantasy, and Behavior," *The Journal of Sex Research* 58, no. 1 (January 2021): 86–96, https://doi.org/10.1080/00224499.2019.1707468.

8   Michael C. Seto, "The Puzzle of Male Chronophilias," *Archives of Sexual Behavior* 46, no. 1 (January 2017): 3–22, https://doi.org/10.1007/s10508-016-0799-y.

9   Bártová et al., "The Prevalence of Paraphilic Interests."

10   J. Michael Bailey et al., "Sexual Orientation, Controversy, and Science," *Psychological Science in the Public Interest* 17, no. 2 (September 2016): 55, https://doi.org/10.1177/1529100616637616.

11   Bártová et al., "The Prevalence of Paraphilic Interests," 3–4.

12   Bailey et al., "Sexual Orientation, Controversy, and Science," 55.

13   Bailey et al., 55.

14   Brown, Barker, and Rahman, "Erotic Target Identity Inversions," 5.

15   Brown, Barker, and Rahman, 6.

16   Jaime M. Grant et al., *Injustice at Every Turn: A Report of the National Transgender Discrimination Survey* (Washington, DC: National Center for Transgender Equality and National Gay and Lesbian Task Force, 2011), 18, https://transequality.org/sites/default/files/docs/resources/NTDS_Report.pdf; Sandy E. James et al., *The Report of the 2015 U.S. Transgender Survey* (Washington, DC: National Center for Transgender Equality, 2016), 246, https://www.ustranssurvey.org/reports/#2015report.

17   In order to estimate the proportion of bisexuality associated with autoheterosexuality, I applied the bisexual identification rates in people who reported any amount of behavioral or sartorial autoheterosexuality from Brown et al. 2020 (30% of females, 48% of males) to the proportion of Czech people who reported some degree of preference for autoheterosexuality from Bártová et al. 2021 (9.6% of males, 5.7% of females). I used the prevalence estimates of bisexual and mostly heterosexual attraction from Bailey et al. 2016 (4.5% of males, 11.5% of females) as the baseline rates found in the general population.

In line with the leading etiological theory that suggests the cause of autoheterosexuality is a variation in the "where" of sexual attraction rather than the "what" (see Chapter 7.0), I assumed that 1) autoheterosexuals have the same rate of non-autohet-related bisexuality as the general population, and 2) elevated rates of bisexuality among autoheterosexuals can be attributed to autoheterosexuality itself.

This approach has various methodological flaws because it compares studies with population-representative samples to one that doesn't, in addition to assuming that there aren't significant differences in autohet prevalence between Americans and Czechs. Those caveats aside, this was the least flawed approach I could think of with the resources available, and it's just a starting point.

18   Roi Jacobson and Daphna Joel, "An Exploration of the Relations Between Self-Reported Gender Identity and Sexual Orientation in an Online Sample of Cisgender Individuals," *Archives of Sexual Behavior* 47, no. 8 (November 2018): 2407–426, https://doi.org/10.1007/s10508-018-1239-y.

19   Brown, Barker, and Rahman, "Erotic Target Identity Inversions," 5.

20   Tailcalled, "Lesbian Autoandrophilia?," *Survey Anon's Gender Blog*, March 17, 2018, https://surveyanon.wordpress.com/2018/03/17/lesbian-autoandrophilia/.

21 Ray Blanchard, "Typology of Male-to-Female Transsexualism," *Archives of Sexual Behavior* 14, no. 3 (June 1985): 247–61, https://doi.org/10.1007/BF01542107; Larry Nuttbrock et al., "A Further Assessment of Blanchard's Typology of Homosexual versus Non-Homosexual or Autogynephilic Gender Dysphoria," *Archives of Sexual Behavior* 40, no. 2 (April 2011): 247–57, https://doi.org/10.1007/s10508-009-9579-2; Anne A. Lawrence, "Sexuality Before and After Male-to-Female Sex Reassignment Surgery," *Archives of Sexual Behavior* 34, no. 2 (April 2005): 147–66, https://doi.org/10.1007/s10508-005-1793-y.

5.1. Arriving at the Two-Type Model

1 Everett K. Rowson, "The Effeminates of Early Medina," *Journal of the American Oriental Society* 111, no. 4 (October–December 1991): 676, https://doi.org/10.2307/603399.

2 Rowson, 675.

3 Magnus Hirschfeld, *Sexualpathologie: Ein Lehrbuch für Aerzte und Studierende* (A. Marcus & E. Webers, 1921); Magnus Hirschfeld, *Sexual Anomalies and Perversions: A Summary of the Works of the Late Professor Dr. Magnus Hirschfeld*, ed. Norman Haire (London: Encyclopaedic Press, 1966), 197.

4 Aleksandra Djajic-Horváth, "Magnus Hirschfeld," in *Encyclopedia Britannica Online*, May 10, 2022, https://www.britannica.com/biography/Magnus-Hirschfeld.

5 Harry Benjamin, *The Transsexual Phenomenon*, electronic edition (Düsseldorf: Symposium Publishing, 1999).

6 N. M. Fisk, "Editorial: Gender Dysphoria Syndrome—The Conceptualization that Liberalizes Indications for Total Gender Reorientation and Implies a Broadly Based Multi-Dimensional Rehabilitative Regimen," *Western Journal of Medicine* 120, no. 5 (May 1974): 386–91, https://www.ncbi.nlm.nih.gov/pmc/articles/PMC1130142/.

7 Fisk, 388.

8 J. Money, "Sex Reassignment," *International Journal of Psychiatry* 9 (1970): 249–69, https://pubmed.ncbi.nlm.nih.gov/5482977/.

9 Anne A. Lawrence, "Sexual Orientation versus Age of Onset as Bases for Typologies (Subtypes) for Gender Identity Disorder in Adolescents and Adults," *Archives of Sexual Behavior* 39, no. 2 (April 2010): 517, https://doi.org/10.1007/s10508-009-9594-3.

10 Peter M. Bentler, "A Typology of Transsexualism: Gender Identity Theory and Data," *Archives of Sexual Behavior* 5, no. 6 (November 1976): 567–84, https://doi.org/10.1007/BF01541220.

11 Bentler, 570.

12 Bentler, 567.

13 N. Buhrich and N. McConaghy, "Two Clinically Discrete Syndromes of Transsexualism," *The British Journal of Psychiatry* 133, no. 1 (1978): 73–76, https://doi.org/10.1192/bjp.133.1.73.

14 Buhrich and McConaghy, 75.

15 Buhrich and McConaghy, 74.

16 Buhrich and McConaghy, 75.

17 Kurt Freund, Betty W. Steiner, and Samuel Chan, "Two Types of Cross-Gender Identity," *Archives of Sexual Behavior* 11, no. 1 (February 1982): 49–63, https://doi.org/10.1007/BF01541365.

18 Freund, Steiner, and Chan, 55.

19 Freund, Steiner, and Chan, 56.

20 Freund, Steiner, and Chan, 56.

21 Freund, Steiner, and Chan, 57.

22 Freund, Steiner, and Chan, 56.

23 Freund, Steiner, and Chan, 56.

24 Buhrich and McConaghy, "Two Clinically Discrete Syndromes of Transsexualism."

25 Freund, Steiner, and Chan, "Two Types of Cross-Gender Identity," 49.

26 Freund, Steiner, and Chan, 61.

27 Ray Blanchard, "Early History of the Concept of Autogynephilia," *Archives of Sexual Behavior* 34, no. 4 (August 2005): 443, https://doi.org/10.1007/s10508-005-4343-8.

28 Ray Blanchard, "Autogynephilia and the Taxonomy of Gender Identity Disorders in Biological Males" (talk, 26th Annual Meeting of the International Academy of Sex Research, Paris, France, June 2000).

29 Ray Blanchard, "Typology of Male-to-Female Transsexualism," *Archives of Sexual Behavior* 14, no. 3 (June 1985): 247–61, https://doi.org/10.1007/BF01542107.

30 Ray Blanchard, "Nonhomosexual Gender Dysphoria," *Journal of Sex Research* 24, no. 1 (1988): 188–93, https://doi.org/10.1080/00224498809551410.

31 Blanchard, 189, 190.

32 Blanchard, 191.

33 Blanchard, 191.

34 Bentler, "A Typology of Transsexualism"; Buhrich and McConaghy, "Two Clinically Discrete Syndromes of Transsexualism."

35 Ray Blanchard, "The Concept of Autogynephilia and the Typology of Male Gender Dysphoria," *The Journal of Nervous and Mental Disease* 177, no. 10 (October 1989): 616–23, https://doi.org/10.1097/00005053-198910000-00004.

36 Blanchard, 619.

37 Blanchard, 621.

38 Blanchard, 621.

39 Blanchard, 622.

40 Blanchard, 621.

41 Blanchard, 622.

42 Blanchard, 622.

43 Ray Blanchard, "The Classification and Labeling of Nonhomosexual Gender Dysphorias," *Archives of Sexual Behavior* 18, no. 4 (August 1989): 324, https://doi.org/10.1007/BF01541951.

44 Blanchard, 323.

45 Julia M. Serano, "The Case Against Autogynephilia," *International Journal of Transgenderism* 12, no. 3 (2010): 180–81, https://doi.org/10.1080/15532739.2010.514223.

46 Ray Blanchard, Leonard H. Clemmensen, and Betty W. Steiner, "Social Desirability Response Set and Systematic Distortion in the Self-Report of Adult Male Gender Patients," *Archives of Sexual Behavior* 14, no. 6 (December 1985): 505–16, https://doi.org/10.1007/BF01541751.

47 Blanchard, Clemmensen, and Steiner, 511.

48 Blanchard, Clemmensen, and Steiner, 511.

49 Blanchard, Clemmensen, and Steiner, 513.

50 Fisk, "Editorial: Gender Dysphoria Syndrome."

51 Ray Blanchard, I. G. Racansky, and Betty W. Steiner, "Phallometric Detection of Fetishistic Arousal in Heterosexual Male Cross-Dressers," *The Journal of Sex Research* 22, no. 4 (November 1986): 452–62, http://www.jstor.org/stable/3812291.

52 Blanchard, Racansky, and Steiner, 459.

53 Blanchard, Racansky, and Steiner, 459.

54 Anne A. Lawrence, "Sexuality Before and After Male-to-Female Sex Reassignment Surgery," *Archives of Sexual Behavior* 34, no. 2 (April 2005): 147–66, https://doi.org/10.1007/s10508-005-1793-y.

55 Lawrence, 151.

56 Lawrence, 152.

57 Lawrence, 162.

58 Lawrence, 153.

59 Lawrence, 154.

60 Lawrence, 154.

61 Lawrence, 160.

62 Lawrence, 160.

63 Yolanda L. S. Smith et al., "Transsexual Subtypes: Clinical and Theoretical Significance," *Psychiatry Research* 137, no. 3 (December 2005): 151–60, https://doi.org/10.1016/j.psychres.2005.01.008.

64 Smith et al., 155.

65 Smith et al., 156.

66 Smith et al., 158.

67 Anne A. Lawrence, "Male-to-Female Transsexual Subtypes: Sexual Arousal with Cross-Dressing and Physical Measurements," *Psychiatry Research* 157, no. 1–3 (January 2008): 319, https://doi.org/10.1016/j.psychres.2007.06.018.

68 Lawrence, 320.

69 Larry Nuttbrock et al., "A Further Assessment of Blanchard's Typology of Homosexual versus Non-Homosexual or Autogynephilic Gender Dysphoria," *Archives of Sexual Behavior* 40, no. 2 (April 2011): 252, 255, https://doi.org/10.1007/s10508-009-9579-2.

70 Nuttbrock et al., 247.

71 Nuttbrock et al., 249.

72 Nuttbrock et al., 249.

73 Nuttbrock et al., 255.

74 Nuttbrock et al., 255.

75 Smith et al., "Transsexual Subtypes."

76 Smith et al., 156.

77 Walter Bockting, Autumn Benner, and Eli Coleman, "Gay and Bisexual Identity Development Among Female-to-Male Transsexuals in North America: Emergence of a Transgender Sexuality," *Archives of Sexual Behavior* 38, no. 5 (October 2009): 692, https://doi.org/10.1007/s10508-009-9489-3.

78 Lawrence, "Sexuality Before and After"; Blanchard, "Typology of Male-to-Female Transsexualism."

79 Meredith L. Chivers and J. Michael Bailey, "Sexual Orientation of Female-to-Male Transsexuals: A Comparison of Homosexual and Nonhomosexual Types," *Archives of Sexual Behavior* 29, no. 3 (2000): 259–78, https://doi.org/10.1023/A:1001915530479.

80 Chivers and Bailey, 268.

81 Chivers and Bailey, 269.

82 Chivers and Bailey, 269.

83 Chivers and Bailey, 275.

84 J. Michael Bailey, "What Is Sexual Orientation and Do Women Have One?," in *Contemporary Perspectives on Lesbian, Gay, and Bisexual Identities*, ed. Debra A. Hope, vol. 54, Nebraska Symposium on Motivation (New York: Springer, 2009), 43–63, https://doi.org/10.1007/978-0-387-09556-1_3.

85 Meredith L. Chivers and J. Michael Bailey, "A Sex Difference in Features that Elicit Genital Response," *Biological Psychology* 70, no. 2 (October 2005): 118, https://doi.org/10.1016/j.biopsycho.2004.12.002; Meredith L. Chivers et al., "A Sex Difference in the Specificity of Sexual Arousal," *Psychological Science* 15, no. 11 (November 2004): 740, https://doi.org/10.1111/j.0956-7976.2004.00750.x; Bailey, "What Is Sexual Orientation," 56.

86 Lisa M. Diamond, *Sexual Fluidity: Understanding Women's Love and Desire* (Cambridge, MA: Harvard University Press, 2008).

87 Lisa Littman, "Parent Reports of Adolescents and Young Adults Perceived to Show Signs of a Rapid Onset of Gender Dysphoria," *PLoS ONE* 13, no. 8 (August 2018): e0202330, https://doi.org/10.1371/journal.pone.0202330.

5.2. Changing Identity, Changing Preferences

1 S. Colton Meier et al., "Measures of Clinical Health among Female-to-Male Transgender Persons as a Function of Sexual Orientation," *Archives of Sexual Behavior* 42, no. 3 (April 2013): 463–74, https://doi.org/10.1007/s10508-012-0052-2.

2 Meier et al., 470.

3   Stefan Rowniak and Catherine Chesla, "Coming Out for a Third Time: Transmen, Sexual Orientation, and Identity," *Archives of Sexual Behavior* 42, no. 3 (April 2013): 449–61, https://doi.org/10.1007/s10508-012-0036-2.

4   Matthias K. Auer et al., "Transgender Transitioning and Change of Self-Reported Sexual Orientation," *PLoS ONE* 9, no. 10 (October 2014): e110016, https://doi.org/10.1371/journal.pone.0110016.

5   Auer et al., 5.

6   Auer et al., 6.

7   Auer et al., 8–10.

8   Auer et al., 10.

9   Auer et al., 10.

10   J. Defreyne et al., "Sexual Orientation in Transgender Individuals: Results from the Longitudinal ENIGI Study," *International Journal of Impotence Research* 33, no. 7 (2021): 694–702, https://doi.org/10.1038/s41443-020-00402-7.

11   Defreyne et al., 3.

12   Defreyne et al., 6.

13   Defreyne et al., 8; Auer et al., "Transgender Transitioning."

5.3. Which Kind of Trans Is the Most Common?

1   Alex Iantaffi and Walter O. Bockting, "Views from Both Sides of the Bridge? Gender, Sexual Legitimacy and Transgender People's Experiences of Relationships," *Culture, Health & Sexuality* 13, no. 3 (2011): 355–70, https://doi.org/10.1080/13691058.2010.537770; Jaime M. Grant et al., *Injustice at Every Turn: A Report of the National Transgender Discrimination Survey* (Washington, DC: National Center for Transgender Equality and National Gay and Lesbian Task Force, 2011), https://transequality.org/sites/default/files/docs/resources/NTDS_Report.pdf; Sandy E. James et al., *The Report of the 2015 U.S. Transgender Survey* (Washington, DC: National Center for Transgender Equality, 2016), https://www.ustranssurvey.org/reports/#2015report.

2   J. Defreyne et al., "Sexual Orientation in Transgender Individuals: Results from the Longitudinal ENIGI Study," *International Journal of Impotence Research* 33, no. 7 (2021): 694–702, *https://doi.org/10.1038/s41443-020-00402-7*; Matthias K. Auer et al., "Transgender Transitioning and Change of Self-Reported Sexual Orientation," *PLoS ONE* 9, no. 10 (October 2014): e110016, *https://doi.org/10.1371/journal.pone.0110016*; Yolanda L. S. Smith et al., "Transsexual Subtypes: Clinical and Theoretical Significance," *Psychiatry Research* 137, no. 3 (December 2005): 151–60, https://doi.org/10.1016/j.psychres.2005.01.008; Katrien Wierckx et al., "Sexual Desire in Trans Persons: Associations with Sex Reassignment Treatment," *The Journal of Sexual Medicine* 11, no. 1 (January 2014): 107–118, https://doi.org/10.1111/jsm.12365; Rebecca M. Jones et al., "Brief Report: Female-to-Male Transsexual People and Autistic Traits," *Journal of Autism and Developmental Disorders* 42,

no. 2 (February 2012): 301–306, https://doi.org/10.1007/s10803-011-1227-8; Anne
A. Lawrence and J. Michael Bailey, "Transsexual Groups in Veale et al. (2008) are
'Autogynephilic' and 'Even More Autogynephilic,'" *Archives of Sexual Behavior* 38,
no. 2 (April 2009): 173–75, https://doi.org/10.1007/s10508-008-9431-0.

3   Kenneth J. Zucker and Madison Aitken, "Sex Ratio of Transgender Adolescents:
      A Meta-Analysis" (Inside Matters: 3rd Meeting of the European Association for
      Transgender Health, Rome, Italy, 2019), unpublished data.

4   Madison Aitken et al., "Evidence for an Altered Sex Ratio in Clinic-Referred
      Adolescents with Gender Dysphoria," *The Journal of Sexual Medicine* 12, no. 3
      (March 2015): 756–63, https://doi.org/10.1111/jsm.12817.

5   Larry Nuttbrock et al., "A Further Assessment of Blanchard's Typology of
      Homosexual versus Non-Homosexual or Autogynephilic Gender Dysphoria,"
      Archives of Sexual Behavior 40, no. 2 (April 2011): 253, https://doi.org/10.1007/
      s10508-009-9579-2.

6   Anne A. Lawrence, "Societal Individualism Predicts Prevalence of
      Nonhomosexual Orientation in Male-to-Female Transsexualism," *Archives of
      Sexual Behavior* 39, no. 2 (April 2010): 573–83, https://doi.org/10.1007/s10508-008-
      9420-3; Anne A. Lawrence, "More Evidence that Societal Individualism Predicts
      Prevalence of Nonhomosexual Orientation in Male-to-Female Transsexualism,"
      Archives of Sexual Behavior 42, no. 5 (July 2013): 693–95, https://doi.org/10.1007/
      s10508-013-0083-3.

7   Lawrence, "Societal Individualism Predicts," 573.

8   Lawrence, "Societal Individualism Predicts Prevalence"; Lawrence, "More
      Evidence that Societal Individualism Predicts Prevalence"; Iantaffi and
      Bockting, "Views from Both Sides of the Bridge?"; James et al., *The Report of the
      2015 U.S. Transgender Survey*; Grant et al., *Injustice at Every Turn*; Auer et al.,
      "Transgender Transitioning"; Wierckx et al., "Sexual Desire in Trans Persons";
      Jones et al., "Brief Report: Female-to-Male Transsexual People"; Anna Herman-
      Jeglińska, Anna Grabowska, and Stanisław Dulko, "Masculinity, Femininity, and
      Transsexualism," *Archives of Sexual Behavior* 31, no. 6 (2002): 527–34, https://
      doi.org/10.1023/A:1020611416035; Nuttbrock et al., "A Further Assessment of
      Blanchard's Typology"; Jochen Hess et al., "Change in Sexual Attraction and
      Sexual Partnership within the Individual Transition Process in Transwomen,"
      Journal of Urology 203, no. Supplement 4 (April 2020): e1269, https://doi.
      org/10.1097/JU.0000000000000976.012.

9   Grant et al., *Injustice at Every Turn*.

10   James et al., *The Report of the 2015 U.S. Transgender Survey*.

11   Sari L. Reisner et al., "Comparing In-Person and Online Survey Respondents
      in the U.S. National Transgender Discrimination Survey: Implications for
      Transgender Health Research," *LGBT Health* 1, no. 2 (June 2014): 101, https://doi.
      org/10.1089/lgbt.2013.0018.

12   Reisner et al., 102.

13   S. Colton Meier et al., "Measures of Clinical Health among Female-to-Male Transgender Persons as a Function of Sexual Orientation," *Archives of Sexual Behavior* 42, no. 3 (April 2013): 468, https://doi.org/10.1007/s10508-012-0052-2.

5.4. More Females Are Transitioning

1   Kenneth J. Zucker and Madison Aitken, "Sex Ratio of Transgender Adolescents: A Meta-Analysis" (Inside Matters: 3rd Meeting of the European Association for Transgender Health, Rome, Italy, 2019), unpublished data; Madison Aitken et al., "Evidence for an Altered Sex Ratio in Clinic-Referred Adolescents with Gender Dysphoria," *The Journal of Sexual Medicine* 12, no. 3 (March 2015): 756–63, https://doi.org/10.1111/jsm.12817.

2   Aitken et al., "Evidence for an Altered Sex Ratio," 759.

3   Zucker and Aitken, "Sex Ratio of Transgender Adolescents: A Meta-Analysis"; Jody Herman, "LGB within the T: Sexual Orientation in the National Transgender Discrimination Survey and Implications for Public Policy," in *Trans Studies: The Challenge to Hetero/Homo Normativities*, ed. Yolanda Martínez-San Miguel and Sarah Tobias (New Brunswick, NJ: Rutgers University Press, 2016), 172–88; Sandy E. James et al., *The Report of the 2015 U.S. Transgender Survey* (Washington, DC: National Center for Transgender Equality, 2016), https://www.ustranssurvey.org/reports/#2015report.

4   Zucker and Aitken, "Sex Ratio of Transgender Adolescents: A Meta-Analysis."

5   Jaime M. Grant et al., *Injustice at Every Turn: A Report of the National Transgender Discrimination Survey* (Washington, DC: National Center for Transgender Equality and National Gay and Lesbian Task Force, 2011), 25, https://transequality.org/sites/default/files/docs/resources/NTDS_Report.pdf; James et al., *The Report of the 2015 U.S. Transgender Survey*, 46.

6   Lisa Littman, "Parent Reports of Adolescents and Young Adults Perceived to Show Signs of a Rapid Onset of Gender Dysphoria," *PLoS ONE* 13, no. 8 (August 2018): e0202330, https://doi.org/10.1371/journal.pone.0202330; J. Michael Bailey and Ray Blanchard, "Gender Dysphoria is Not One Thing," *4thWaveNow* (blog), December 7, 2017, https://4thwavenow.com/2017/12/07/gender-dysphoria-is-not-one-thing/.

7   Gary R. VandenBos, ed., *APA Dictionary of Psychology*, 2nd ed. (Washington, DC: American Psychological Association, 2015), 993, https://doi.org/10.1037/14646-000.

8   Littman, "Parent Reports of Adolescents and Young Adults."

9   Littman, 7.

10   Littman, 13.

11   Littman, 16.

12   Littman, 16.

13   Littman, 16.

14   Littman, 7.

15   Grant et al., *Injustice at Every Turn*, 29.

16 James et al., *The Report of the 2015 U.S. Transgender Survey, 59.*

17 Meredith L. Chivers and J. Michael Bailey, "Sexual Orientation of Female-to-Male Transsexuals: A Comparison of Homosexual and Nonhomosexual Types," *Archives of Sexual Behavior* 29, no. 3 (2000): 259–60, https://doi.org/10.1023/A:1001915530479; Bailey and Blanchard, "Gender Dysphoria is Not One Thing"; Ray Blanchard, "The Classification and Labeling of Nonhomosexual Gender Dysphorias," *Archives of Sexual Behavior* 18, no. 4 (August 1989): 32–37, https://doi.org/10.1007/BF01541951.

18 R. Su, J. Rounds, and P. I. Armstrong, "Men and Things, Women and People: A Meta-Analysis of Sex Differences in Interests," *Psychological Bulletin* 135, no. 6 (2009): 891, https://doi.org/10.1037/a0017364; Richard A. Lippa, "Gender Differences in Personality and Interests: When, Where, and Why?," *Social and Personality Psychology Compass* 4, no. 11 (November 2010): 1098, https://doi.org/10.1111/j.1751-9004.2010.00320.x.

19 Klára Bártová et al., "The Prevalence of Paraphilic Interests in the Czech Population: Preference, Arousal, the Use of Pornography, Fantasy, and Behavior," *The Journal of Sex Research* 58, no. 1 (January 2021): 86–96, https://doi.org/10.1080/00224499.2019.1707468.

20 Magnus Hirschfeld, *Transvestites: The Erotic Drive to Cross-Dress*, trans. Michael A. Lombardi-Nash (Buffalo, NY: Prometheus Books, 1991), 183.

21 Havelock Ellis, "Eonism," in *Studies in the Psychology of Sex*, vol. 7, Eonism and Other Supplementary Studies (Philadelphia: F. A. Davis Company, 1928), 36, https://archive.org/details/b30010172/page/36/mode/2up.

22 Ray Blanchard, "The DSM Diagnostic Criteria for Transvestic Fetishism," *Archives of Sexual Behavior* 39, no. 2 (April 2010): 370, https://doi.org/10.1007/s10508-009-9541-3.

23 Blanchard, 370.

24 American Psychiatric Association, ed., *Diagnostic and Statistical Manual of Mental Disorders: DSM-5*, 5th ed. (Washington, DC: American Psychiatric Association Publishing, 2013), 702, https://doi.org/10.1176/appi.books.9780890425596.

25 D. P. Schmitt et al., "Why Can't a Man Be More like a Woman? Sex Differences in Big Five Personality Traits across 55 Cultures," *Journal of Personality and Social Psychology* 94, no. 1 (2008): 175, https://doi.org/10.1037/0022-3514.94.1.168.

26 Amanda J. Baxter et al., "Challenging the Myth of an 'Epidemic' of Common Mental Disorders: Trends in the Global Prevalence of Anxiety and Depression between 1990 and 2010," *Depression and Anxiety* 31, no. 6 (June 2014): 505–516, https://doi.org/10.1002/da.22230.

27 Y. Sasson et al., "Epidemiology of Obsessive-Compulsive Disorder: A World View," *The Journal of Clinical Psychiatry* 58, no. Supplement 12 (1997): 10, https://www.psychiatrist.com/read-pdf/6527/.

28 Marie Galmiche et al., "Prevalence of Eating Disorders over the 2000–2018 Period: A Systematic Literature Review," *The American Journal of Clinical Nutrition* 109, no. 5 (May 2019): 1402–1413, https://doi.org/10.1093/ajcn/nqy342.

29 Michael S. Boroughs, Ross Krawczyk, and J. Kevin Thompson, "Body Dysmorphic Disorder among Diverse Racial/Ethnic and Sexual Orientation Groups: Prevalence Estimates and Associated Factors," *Sex Roles* 63, no. 9–10 (2010): 732, https://doi.org/10.1007/s11199-010-9831-1.

30 Littman, "Parent Reports of Adolescents and Young Adults," 33.

31 Helen Joyce, *Trans: Gender Identity and the New Battle for Women's Rights* (London: Oneworld Publications, 2022).

32 Judith Butler, "Imitation and Gender Insubordination," in *Inside/Out: Lesbian Theories, Gay Theories*, ed. Diana Fuss (New York: Routledge, 1991), 21.

33 Allison Nobles, "The Social Construction of Gender and Sex," The Society Pages, November 26, 2018, https://thesocietypages.org/trot/2018/11/26/the-social-construction-of-gender-and-sex/.

34 "Sex and Gender Identity," Planned Parenthood, accessed August 18, 2022, https://www.plannedparenthood.org/learn/gender-identity/sex-gender-identity.

35 Larry Nuttbrock et al., "A Further Assessment of Blanchard's Typology of Homosexual versus Non-Homosexual or Autogynephilic Gender Dysphoria," *Archives of Sexual Behavior* 40, no. 2 (April 2011): 249, https://doi.org/10.1007/s10508-009-9579-2.

36 Sarah Blaffer Hrdy, *The Woman That Never Evolved: With a New Preface and Bibliographical Updates* (Cambridge, MA: Harvard University Press, 1999).

6.0. Autohet Cross-Gender Development

1 Jocelyn Badgley and other contributors, "The Gender Dysphoria Bible," 8, accessed August 18, 2022, https://genderdysphoria.fyi/gdb.pdf.

2 Richard F. Docter, *Transvestites and Transsexuals: Toward a Theory of Cross-Gender Behavior*, Perspectives in Sexuality (New York: Plenum Press, 1988), 3, https://doi.org/10.1007/978-1-4613-0997-0.

3 Havelock Ellis, "Eonism," in *Studies in the Psychology of Sex*, vol. 7, *Eonism and Other Supplementary Studies* (Philadelphia: F. A. Davis Company, 1928), 71, https://archive.org/details/b30010172/page/70/mode/2up.

4 Anne A. Lawrence, "Sexuality Before and After Male-to-Female Sex Reassignment Surgery," *Archives of Sexual Behavior* 34, no. 2 (April 2005): 154, https://doi.org/10.1007/s10508-005-1793-y.

5 Richard F. Docter and Virginia Prince, "Transvestism: A Survey of 1032 Cross-Dressers," *Archives of Sexual Behavior* 26, no. 6 (1997): 602–603, https://doi.org/10.1023/A:1024572209266.

6 Docter, *Transvestites and Transsexuals*, 209.

7 Jody Herman, "LGB within the T: Sexual Orientation in the National Transgender Discrimination Survey and Implications for Public Policy," in *Trans Studies: The Challenge to Hetero/Homo Normativities*, ed. Yolanda Martínez-San Miguel and Sarah Tobias (New Brunswick, NJ: Rutgers University Press, 2016), 177; Sandy E. James et al.,

The Report of the 2015 U.S. Transgender Survey (Washington, DC: National Center for Transgender Equality, 2016), 245, https://www.ustranssurvey.org/reports/#2015report.

8   Ellis, "Eonism," 93–94.

9   Magnus Hirschfeld, *Transvestites: The Erotic Drive to Cross-Dress*, trans. Michael A. Lombardi-Nash (Buffalo, NY: Prometheus Books, 1991), 37.

10 Magnus Hirschfeld, *Sexual Anomalies and Perversions: A Summary of the Works of the Late Professor Dr. Magnus Hirschfeld*, ed. Norman Haire (London: Encyclopaedic Press, 1966), 218.

11 Zack M. Davis, "Lesser-Known Demand Curves," *The Scintillating but Ultimately Untrue Thought* (blog), December 18, 2017, http://unremediatedgender.space/2017/Dec/lesser-known-demand-curves/.

6.1. Gender Euphoria

1   Havelock Ellis, "Eonism," in *Studies in the Psychology of Sex*, vol. 7, *Eonism and Other Supplementary Studies* (Philadelphia: F. A. Davis Company, 1928), 46–47, https://wellcomecollection.org/works/njv7bbq7.

2   Richard F. Docter, *Transvestites and Transsexuals: Toward a Theory of Cross-Gender Behavior, Perspectives in Sexuality* (New York: Plenum Press, 1988), 103, https://doi.org/10.1007/978-1-4613-0997-0.

3   Jocelyn Badgley and other contributors, "The Gender Dysphoria Bible," 9, accessed August 18, 2022, https://genderdysphoria.fyi/gdb.pdf.

4   William J. Beischel, "Gender Pleasure: The Positive Affective Component of Gender/Sex" (PhD diss., University of Michigan, 2022), 39, https://hdl.handle.net/2027.42/174393.

5   Adrian Silbernagel, "Gender Euphoria: The Bright Side of Trans Experience," Thinking Queerly, Queer Kentucky, accessed January 13, 2023, https://queerkentucky.com/gender-euphoria-the-bright-side-of-trans-experience/.

6   Ellis, "Eonism," 67.

7   Magnus Hirschfeld, *Transvestites: The Erotic Drive to Cross-Dress*, trans. Michael A. Lombardi-Nash (Buffalo, NY: Prometheus Books, 1991), 29.

8   Magnus Hirschfeld, *Sexual Anomalies and Perversions: A Summary of the Works of the Late Professor Dr. Magnus Hirschfeld*, ed. Norman Haire (London: Encyclopaedic Press, 1966), 200–201.

9   Anne A. Lawrence, ed., "Thirty-One New Narratives About Autogynephilia: Plus Five Revealing Fantasy Narratives," AnneLawrence.com, 1999, no. 50, accessed January 30, 2023, available at https://web.archive.org/web/20120208181716/http://www.annelawrence.com/31narratives.html.

10 Richard von Krafft-Ebing, *Psychopathia Sexualis*, 12th ed., trans. F. J. Rebman (Rebman Company, 1906), 312.

11 Von Krafft-Ebing, 312.

12 Lawrence, "Thirty-One New Narratives About Autogynephilia," no. 48.

13 Zhahai Stewart, "What's All This NRE Stuff, Anyway? Reflections 15 Years Later," Aphrodite's Web, 2001, http://aphroweb.net/articles/nre.htm.

14 Megan Haynes, "Transgender Toronto Actress Set to Take on L.A.," *Toronto Star*, February 1, 2017, https://www.thestar.com/life/2017/02/01/transgender-toronto-actress-takes-on-the-us.html.

15 Helen Fisher, *Anatomy of Love: A Natural History of Mating, Marriage, and Why We Stray* (New York: W. W. Norton & Company, 2016).

16 "(If Loving You Is Wrong) I Don't Want To Be Right," featuring Luther Ingram, produced by John Baylor, on vinyl, KoKo, 1972.

17 Tailcalled, "Response to Contrapoints on Autogynephilia," *Survey Anon's Gender Blog* (blog), January 26, 2019, https://surveyanon.wordpress.com/2019/01/26/response-to-contrapoints-on-autogynephilia/.

18 Anne A. Lawrence, "Becoming What We Love: Autogynephilic Transsexualism Conceptualized as an Expression of Romantic Love," *Perspectives in Biology and Medicine* 50, no. 4 (Autumn 2007): 518, https://doi.org/10.1353/pbm.2007.0050.

19 Lawrence, "Becoming What We Love."

20 Lawrence, 518.

21 Lanei M. Rodemeyer, *Lou Sullivan Diaries (1970-1980) and Theories of Sexual Embodiment*, Crossroads of Knowledge (New York: Springer, 2018), 163.

22 Julia M. Serano, "The Case Against Autogynephilia," *International Journal of Transgenderism* 12, no. 3 (2010): 182, https://doi.org/10.1080/15532739.2010.514223; "Autogynephilia," ContraPoints, February 1, 2018, YouTube video, 48:54, https://www.youtube.com/watch?v=6czRFLs5JQo.

23 Ray Blanchard, "Clinical Observations and Systematic Studies of Autogynephilia," *Journal of Sex & Marital Therapy* 17, no. 4 (1991): 248, https://doi.org/10.1080/00926239108404348.

24 H. Taylor Buckner, "The Transvestic Career Path," *Psychiatry* 33, no. 3 (1970): 381–89, https://doi.org/10.1080/00332747.1970.11023637.

25 Buckner, 386.

26 Buckner, 385.

27 Buckner, 385.

28 Buckner, 387.

29 Hirschfeld, *Transvestites*, 140.

30 Hirschfeld, 39.

6.2. Gender Dysphoria

1 Magnus Hirschfeld, *Transvestites: The Erotic Drive to Cross-Dress*, trans. Michael A. Lombardi-Nash (Buffalo, NY: Prometheus Books, 1991), 178.

2 Magnus Hirschfeld, *Sexual Anomalies and Perversions: A Summary of the Works of the Late Professor Dr. Magnus Hirschfeld*, ed. Norman Haire (London: Encyclopaedic Press, 1966), 216.

3   Richard F. Docter, *Transvestites and Transsexuals: Toward a Theory of Cross-Gender Behavior*, Perspectives in Sexuality (New York: Plenum Press, 1988), 90, https://doi.org/10.1007/978-1-4613-0997-0.

4   Kevin J. Hsu, A. M. Rosenthal, and J. Michael Bailey, "The Psychometric Structure of Items Assessing Autogynephilia," *Archives of Sexual Behavior* 44, no. 5 (July 2015): 1301–1312, https://doi.org/10.1007/s10508-014-0397-9.

5   American Psychiatric Association, ed., *Diagnostic and Statistical Manual of Mental Disorders: DSM-5*, 5th ed. (Washington, DC: American Psychiatric Association Publishing, 2013), 451, https://doi.org/10.1176/appi.books.9780890425596.

6   American Psychiatric Association, 452.

7   Hsu, Rosenthal, and Bailey, "The Psychometric Structure," 7; Ray Blanchard, "The Concept of Autogynephilia and the Typology of Male Gender Dysphoria," *The Journal of Nervous and Mental Disease* 177, no. 10 (October 1989): 619, https://doi.org/10.1097/00005053-198910000-00004.

8   Hirschfeld, *Transvestites*, 28.

9   Lanei M. Rodemeyer, *Lou Sullivan Diaries (1970-1980) and Theories of Sexual Embodiment*, Crossroads of Knowledge (New York: Springer, 2018), 25.

10   Rodemeyer, 156.

11   Rodemeyer, 184.

12   Hirschfeld, *Sexual Anomalies and Perversions*, 188.

13   Zinnia Jones, "Depersonalization in Gender Dysphoria: Widespread and Widely Unrecognized," Medium, February 27, 2018, https://zinniajones.medium.com/depersonalization-in-gender-dysphoria-widespread-and-widely-unrecognized-baaac395bcb0; Zinnia Jones, "In Our Own Words: Transgender Experiences of Depersonalization," September 1, 2017, https://www.academia.edu/34611836/In_our_own_words_transgender_experiences_of_depersonalization.

14   Jocelyn Badgley and other contributors, "The Gender Dysphoria Bible," 12–13, accessed August 18, 2022, https://genderdysphoria.fyi/gdb.pdf.

15   Jones, "Depersonalization in Gender Dysphoria."

16   Anette Kersting et al., "Dissociative Disorders and Traumatic Childhood Experiences in Transsexuals," *The Journal of Nervous and Mental Disease* 191, no. 3 (March 2003): 184, https://doi.org/10.1097/01.NMD.0000054932.22929.5D.

17   Kersting et al., 184–85.

18   Marco Colizzi, Rosalia Costa, and Orlando Todarello, "Dissociative Symptoms in Individuals with Gender Dysphoria: Is the Elevated Prevalence Real?," *Psychiatry Research* 226, no. 1 (March 2015): 176–77, https://doi.org/10.1016/j.psychres.2014.12.045.

19   Colizzi, Costa, and Todarello, 178.

20   Jessica Xavier, Julie A. Honnold, and Judith B. Bradford, *The Health, Health-Related Needs, and Lifecourse Experiences of Transgender Virginians* (Virginia Department of Health, 2007), 27, https://doi.org/10.1037/e544442014-001.

21 Havelock Ellis, "Eonism," in *Studies in the Psychology of Sex*, vol. 7, *Eonism and Other Supplementary Studies* (Philadelphia: F. A. Davis Company, 1928), 98, https://wellcomecollection.org/works/njv7bbq7.

22 Wilhelm Stekel, *Sexual Aberrations: The Phenomena of Fetishism in Relation to Sex*, vol. 2 (London: John Lane, 1930), 299, https://archive.org/details/b29817043_0002; Robert J. Stoller, *Splitting: A Case of Female Masculinity, The International Psycho-Analytical Library*, no. 97 (London: Hogarth Press, 1974), 37–38.

23 Ellis, "Eonism," 97.

24 Docter, *Transvestites and Transsexuals*, 88.

25 Hirschfeld, *Sexual Anomalies and Perversions*, 218.

26 Ellis, "Eonism," 71.

27 Ellis, 79.

28 Ellis, 85.

29 Ellis, 83.

30 Ira B. Pauly, "Female Transsexualism: Part I," *Archives of Sexual Behavior* 3, no. 6 (November 1974): 504, https://doi.org/10.1007/BF01541134.

31 Hirschfeld, *Sexual Anomalies and Perversions*, 188.

32 Docter, *Transvestites and Transsexuals*, 190.

33 Hirschfeld, *Transvestites*, 101.

34 Stekel, *Sexual Aberrations*, 282.

35 J. H. Vogt, "Five Cases of Transsexualism in Females," *Acta Psychiatrica Scandinavica* 44, no. 1 (March 1968): 79, https://doi.org/10.1111/j.1600-0447.1968.tb07636.x.

36 Vogt, 79.

37 Ellis, "Eonism," 87.

38 Vogt, "Five Cases of Transsexualism in Females," 79.

39 Vogt, 79.

40 Vogt, 77.

41 Vogt, 76.

42 Ellis, "Eonism," 84.

43 Vogt, "Five Cases of Transsexualism in Females," 76.

44 Vogt, 76.

45 Hirschfeld, *Transvestites*, 100.

46 Vogt, "Five Cases of Transsexualism in Females," 79.

47 Ellis, "Eonism," 87.

48 Aaron H. Devor, FTM: *Female-to-Male Transsexuals in Society* (Bloomington, IN: Indiana University Press, 2016), 195.

49 Hirschfeld, *Sexual Anomalies and Perversions*, 199–200.

50 Ellis, "Eonism," 96.

51 L. M. Lothstein, "The Aging Gender Dysphoria (Transsexual) Patient," *Archives of Sexual Behavior* 8, no. 5 (September 1979): 434, https://doi.org/10.1007/BF01541199.

52 Docter, *Transvestites and Transsexuals*, 189.

53 Docter, 189.

54 Stefan Rowniak and Catherine Chesla, "Coming Out for a Third Time: Transmen, Sexual Orientation, and Identity," *Archives of Sexual Behavior* 42, no. 3 (April 2013): 457, https://doi.org/10.1007/s10508-012-0036-2.

55 Vogt, "Five Cases of Transsexualism in Females," 79.

56 Ira B. Pauly, "Female Transsexualism: Part II," *Archives of Sexual Behavior* 3, no. 6 (November 1974): 512, https://doi.org/10.1007/BF01541135.

57 Anne A. Lawrence, ed., "Thirty-One New Narratives About Autogynephilia: Plus Five Revealing Fantasy Narratives," AnneLawrence.com, 1999, no. 41, accessed January 30, 2023, available at https://web.archive.org/web/20120208181716/http:/ www.annelawrence.com/31narratives.html.

58 Ellis, "Eonism," 62.

59 Hirschfeld, *Transvestites,* 69.

60 Niklas Långström and Kenneth J. Zucker, "Transvestic Fetishism in the General Population," *Journal of Sex & Marital Therapy* 31, no. 2 (2005): 90, https://doi. org/10.1080/00926230590477934.

61 Långström and Zucker, 90.

62 Anne A. Lawrence, ed., "Thirty-One New Narratives About Autogynephilia: Plus Five Revealing Fantasy Narratives," AnneLawrence.com, 1999, no. 19, accessed January 30, 2023, available at https://web.archive.org/web/20120208181716/http:/ www.annelawrence.com/31narratives.html.

63 Lawrence, no. 3.

64 Hirschfeld, *Transvestites,* 22.

65 Lawrence, "Twenty-Eight Narratives About Autogynephilia," no. 2.

66 Ellis, "Eonism," 67.

67 Anne Lawrence, "Sexuality and Transsexuality: A New Introduction to Autogynephilia," *Transgender Tapestry* 92 (Winter 2000), 17, https://archive. org/details/transgendertapes920unse/page/16/mode/2up; Anne Lawrence, "Narratives on Autogynephilia," *Transgender Tapestry* 92 (Winter 2000), https:// archive.org/details/transgendertapes920unse/page/22/mode/2up; Anne Lawrence, "Autogynephilia: Frequently-Asked Questions," *Transgender Tapestry* 92 (Winter 2000), 9, https://archive.org/details/transgendertapes920unse/page/24/mode/2up; "References and a Reading List on Autogynephilia," *Transgender Tapestry* 92 (Winter 2000), 13, https://archive.org/details/transgendertapes920unse/page/28/ mode/2up.

68 Lori Buckwalter, "Autogynephilia: All Dressed Up and No One To Be," *Transgender Tapestry* 93 (Spring 2001), https://archive.org/details/transgendertapes930unse/ page/22/mode/2up; Katherine K. Wilson, "Autogynephilia: New Medical Thinking or Old Stereotype?," *Transgender Tapestry* 93 (Spring 2001), https://archive.org/ details/transgendertapes930unse/page/20/mode/2up; Kate Barnes, "Some Observations on Autogynephilia," *Transgender Tapestry* 93 (Spring 2001), https:// archive.org/details/transgendertapes930unse/page/24/mode/2up.

69 Jessica Xavier, "Autogynephilia: What If It's All True?," *Transgender Tapestry* 93 (Spring 2001), https://archive.org/details/transgendertapes9320unse/page/22/mode/2up.

70 Xavier, 24.

71 Hirschfeld, *Sexual Anomalies and Perversions, 222.*

72 Docter, *Transvestites and Transsexuals, 189.*

73 Docter, 190.

74 Hirschfeld, *Transvestites, 72.*

75 Vogt, "Five Cases of Transsexualism in Females," 77.

76 Vogt, 77.

77 Lawrence, "Twenty-Eight Narratives About Autogynephilia," no. 4.

78 Hirschfeld, *Sexual Anomalies and Perversions, 138.*

79 Hirschfeld, 138.

80 Harry Benjamin, *The Transsexual Phenomenon*, electronic edition (Düsseldorf: Symposium Publishing, 1999), 22.

81 Lawrence, "Twenty-Eight Narratives About Autogynephilia," no. 15.

82 Lawrence, "Thirty-One New Narratives About Autogynephilia," no. 42; Hirschfeld, *Transvestites, 22.*

83 Hirschfeld, *Sexual Anomalies and Perversions, 199–200.*

84 Ellis, "Eonism," 60.

85 Viktor E. Frankl, *Man's Search for Meaning* (Boston: Beacon Press, 2006).

86 Heike Bauer, *The Hirschfeld Archives: Violence, Death, and Modern Queer Culture* (Philadelphia: Temple University Press, 2017), 39–40.

87 Hirschfeld, *Transvestites, 154.*

88 Rodemeyer, *Lou Sullivan Diaries, 165.*

89 Vogt, "Five Cases of Transsexualism in Females," 73.

90 Hirschfeld, *Sexual Anomalies and Perversions, 199.*

91 Ellis, "Eonism," 99.

92 Hirschfeld, *Sexual Anomalies and Perversions, 222–23.*

93 Hirschfeld, 223.

94 Hirschfeld, 200–201.

95 Richard von Krafft-Ebing, *Psychopathia Sexualis*, 12th ed., trans. F. J. Rebman (Rebman Company, 1906), 322.

96 Hirschfeld, *Transvestites, 109.*

6.3. Which Comes First: Sexuality or Identity?

1 Jack Molay, "Crossdreaming Described," *Crossdreamers* (blog), August 3, 2014, https://www.crossdreamers.com/2014/08/crossdreaming-described.html.

2 Jaimie F. Veale, Dave E. Clarke, and Terri C. Lomax, "Sexuality of Male-to-Female Transsexuals," *Archives of Sexual Behavior* 37, no. 4 (August 2008): 586–97, https://doi.org/10.1007/s10508-007-9306-9; Charles Moser, "Autogynephilia in Women," *Journal of Homosexuality* 56, no. 5 (2009): 539–47, https://

doi.org/10.1080/00918360903005212; Julia M. Serano, "The Case Against Autogynephilia," *International Journal of Transgenderism* 12, no. 3 (2010): 184, https://doi.org/10.1080/15532739.2010.514223.

3   Serano, "The Case Against Autogynephilia," 184.

4   Kevin J. Hsu and J. Michael Bailey, "Erotic Target Identity Inversions," in *Gender and Sexuality Development: Contemporary Theory and Research*, ed. Doug P. VanderLaan and Wang Ivy Wong (Cham, Switzerland: Springer, 2022), 589–612, https://www.researchgate.net/publication/353559193_Erotic_Target_Identity_Inversions.

5   Kurt Freund and Ray Blanchard, "Erotic Target Location Errors in Male Gender Dysphorics, Paedophiles, and Fetishists," *British Journal of Psychiatry* 162, no. 4 (April 1993): 558–63, https://doi.org/10.1192/bjp.162.4.558.

6   Veale, Clarke, and Lomax, "Sexuality of Male-to-Female Transsexuals"; Moser, "Autogynephilia in Women"; Scott Alexander, "Autogenderphilia is Common and Not Especially Related to Transgender," *Slate Star Codex* (blog), February 10, 2020, https://slatestarcodex.com/2020/02/10/autogenderphilia-is-common-and-not-especially-related-to-transgender/.

7   J. Michael Bailey and Kevin J. Hsu, "How Autogynephilic are Natal Females?," *Archives of Sexual Behavior* 51, no. 7 (October 2022): 3311–3318, https://doi.org/10.1007/s10508-022-02359-8.

8   Judith M. Glassgold et al., *Report of the American Psychological Association Task Force on Appropriate Therapeutic Responses to Sexual Orientation* (Washington, DC: American Psychological Association, August 2009), 83, https://www.apa.org/pi/lgbt/resources/therapeutic-response.pdf.

9   Anne A. Lawrence, *Men Trapped in Men's Bodies: Narratives of Autogynephilic Transsexualism, Focus on Sexuality Research* (New York: Springer, 2013), 169–71, https://www.doi.org/10.1007/978-1-4614-5182-2.

10   Lawrence, 75.

11   Lawrence, 76–77.

7.0. Autosexual Orientations

1   Kurt Freund and Ray Blanchard, "Erotic Target Location Errors in Male Gender Dysphorics, Paedophiles, and Fetishists," *British Journal of Psychiatry* 162, no. 4 (April 1993): 562, https://doi.org/10.1192/bjp.162.4.558.

2   Anne A. Lawrence, "Clinical and Theoretical Parallels Between Desire for Limb Amputation and Gender Identity Disorder," *Archives of Sexual Behavior* 35, no. 3 (June 2006): 263–78, https://doi.org/10.1007/s10508-006-9026-6.

3   Ray Blanchard, "Clinical Observations and Systematic Studies of Autogynephilia," *Journal of Sex & Marital Therapy* 17, no. 4 (1991): 246–48, https://doi.org/10.1080/00926239108404348.

4   Blanchard, 244.

5   Blanchard, 246–47.

6   Julia M. Serano, "The Case Against Autogynephilia," *International Journal of Transgenderism* 12, no. 3 (2010): 176–87, https://doi.org/10.1080/15532739.2010.514 223; Julia Serano, "Autogynephilia: A Scientific Review, Feminist Analysis, and Alternative 'Embodiment Fantasies' Model," *The Sociological Review* 68, no. 4 (2020): 763–78, https://doi.org/10.1177/0038026120934690.

7   "Autogynephilia," ContraPoints, February 1, 2018, YouTube video, 48:54, https:// www.youtube.com/watch?v=6czRFLs5JQo.

8   Jack Molay, "All You Need to Know about 'Autogynephilia,'" *Crossdreamers* (blog), July 5, 2014, https://www.crossdreamers.com/2014/07/the-autogynephilia-theory-again.html.

7.1. Transabled

1   John Money and Kent W. Simcoe, "Acrotomophilia, Sex and Disability: New Concepts and Case Report," *Sexuality and Disability* 7, no. 1–2 (1984): 43–50, https://doi.org/10.1007/BF01101829.

2   John Money, Russell Jobaris, and Gregg Furth, "Apotemnophilia: Two Cases of Self-Demand Amputation as a Paraphilia," *The Journal of Sex Research* 13, no. 2 (1977): 115–25, https://doi.org/10.1080/00224497709550967.

3   Dwight Dixon, "An Erotic Attraction to Amputees," *Sexuality and Disability* 6, no. 1 (1983): 10, https://doi.org/10.1007/BF01119844.

4   Michael B. First, "Desire for Amputation of a Limb: Paraphilia, Psychosis, or a New Type of Identity Disorder," *Psychological Medicine* 35, no. 6 (2005): 926, https://doi.org/10.1017/S0033291704003320; Rianne M. Blom et al., "Role of Sexuality in Body Integrity Identity Disorder (BIID): A Cross-Sectional Internet-Based Survey Study," *The Journal of Sexual Medicine* 14, no. 8 (August 2017): 1028–35, https://doi.org/10.1016/j.jsxm.2017.06.004.

5   Rianne M. Blom, Raoul C. Hennekam, and Damiaan Denys, "Body Integrity Identity Disorder," *PLoS ONE* 7, no. 4 (2012): e34702, https://doi.org/10.1371/journal. pone.0034702.

6   First, "Desire for Amputation of a Limb," 924.

7   First, 922.

8   First, 922.

9   First, 923.

10 First, 921, 925; Anne A. Lawrence, "Clinical and Theoretical Parallels Between Desire for Limb Amputation and Gender Identity Disorder," *Archives of Sexual Behavior* 35, no. 3 (June 2006): 265, https://doi.org/10.1007/s10508-006-9026-6.

11 First, "Desire for Amputation of a Limb," 926.

12 Blom, Hennekam, and Denys, "Body Integrity Identity Disorder," 3; Blom et al., "Role of Sexuality in Body Integrity Identity Disorder," 4; Leonie Maria Hilti et al., "The Desire for Healthy Limb Amputation: Structural Brain Correlates and Clinical Features of Xenomelia," *Brain* 136, no. 1 (January 2013): 318–29, https://doi.org/10.1093/

brain/aws316; Atsushi Aoyama et al., "Impaired Spatial-Temporal Integration of Touch in Xenomelia (Body Integrity Identity Disorder)," *Spatial Cognition & Computation* 12, no. 2–3 (2012): 99, https://doi.org/10.1080/13875868.2011.603773.

13   Blom et al., "Role of Sexuality in Body Integrity Identity Disorder," 4; Kayla D. Stone et al., "An Investigation of Lower Limb Representations Underlying Vision, Touch, and Proprioception in Body Integrity Identity Disorder," *Frontiers in Psychiatry* 11 (February 2020): 15, https://doi.org/10.3389/fpsyt.2020.00015.

14   Blom et al., "Role of Sexuality in Body Integrity Identity Disorder," 4; Olaf. Blanke et al., "Preliminary Evidence for a Fronto-Parietal Dysfunction in Able-Bodied Participants with a Desire for Limb Amputation," *Journal of Neuropsychology* 3, no. 2 (September 2009): 181–200, https://doi.org/10.1348/174866408X318653.

15   Blom, Hennekam, and Denys, "Body Integrity Identity Disorder," 4; Sarah Noll and Erich Kasten, "Body Integrity Identity Disorder (BIID): How Satisfied are Successful Wannabes," *Psychology and Behavioral Sciences* 3, no. 6 (December 2014): 222, https://doi.org/10.11648/j.pbs.20140306.17.

16   Noll and Kasten, "Body Integrity Identity Disorder," 225.

17   Noll and Kasten, 226.

18   Noll and Kasten, 227.

19   Noll and Kasten, 227.

20   Noll and Kasten, 227.

21   Helena De Preester, "Merleau-Ponty's Sexual Schema and the Sexual Component of Body Integrity Identity Disorder," *Medicine, Health Care and Philosophy* 16, no. 2 (2013): 177, https://doi.org/10.1007/s11019-011-9367-3.

22   Paul D. McGeoch et al., "Xenomelia: A New Right Parietal Lobe Syndrome," *Journal of Neurology, Neurosurgery & Psychiatry* 82, no. 12 (2011): 1314, https://doi.org/10.1136/jnnp-2011-300224.

23   Hilti et al., "The Desire for Healthy Limb Amputation," 327; McGeoch et al., "Xenomelia," 1314.

24   David Brang, Paul D. McGeoch, and Vilayanur S. Ramachandran, "Apotemnophilia: A Neurological Disorder," *NeuroReport* 19, no. 13 (August 2008): 1306, https://doi.org/10.1097/WNR.0b013e32830abc4d.

25   Blanke et al., "Preliminary Evidence for a Fronto-Parietal Dysfunction," 188.

7.2. *Transage*

1   Michael C. Seto, "The Puzzle of Male Chronophilias," *Archives of Sexual Behavior* 46, no. 1 (January 2017): 3–22, https://doi.org/10.1007/s10508-016-0799-y.

2   B. Terrance Grey, "What are Infantilism and Diaper Fetishes?," *Understanding Infantilism* (blog), last updated July 20, 2019, https://understanding.infantilism.org/what_is_infantilism.php.

3   "He's a Grown-Up Baby! | My Crazy Obsession (Full Episode)," TLC, August 15, 2019, YouTube video, 21:28, https://www.youtube.com/watch?v=yXugTKhysKM.

4 Stanley Thornton, biography, *Bedwetting ABDL* (blog), last modified May 6, 2020, https://web.archive.org/web/20210711084044/http://www.bedwettingabdl.com/Stanleys_personal_page.html.

5 "Is AB/DL a Fetish?," Riley Kilo, October 14, 2019, YouTube video, 11:36, https://www.youtube.com/watch?v=hesxIy7LEJI.

6 Kevin J. Hsu and J. Michael Bailey, "Autopedophilia: Erotic-Target Identity Inversions in Men Sexually Attracted to Children," *Psychological Science* 28, no. 1 (2017): 115–23, https://doi.org/10.1177/0956797616677082.

7 Hsu and Bailey, 5.

8 Hsu and Bailey, 6.

9 Cwis, "The 'Origins of ABDL' Survey," whyabdl.org, accessed September 12, 2022, https://www.whyabdl.org/surveyintro.

10 Cwis, "The 'Origins of ABDL' Survey."

11 Kevin J. Hsu, "Erotic Target Identity Inversions in Male Furries, Adult Baby/Diaper Lovers, and Eunuchs" (PhD diss., Northwestern University, 2019), 86, https://doi.org/10.21985/N2-4KWZ-PS97.

12 Hsu, 86.

13 Leah Beckmann, "An Interview with Stanley the Adult Baby," Gawker, May 22, 2012, https://www.gawker.com/5912292/an-interview-with-stanley-the-adult-baby.

14 Kaitlyn Hawkinson and Brian D. Zamboni, "Adult Baby/Diaper Lovers: An Exploratory Study of an Online Community Sample," *Archives of Sexual Behavior* 43, no. 5 (July 2014): 872, https://doi.org/10.1007/s10508-013-0241-7.

15 Hawkinson and Zamboni, 872.

16 B. Terrance Grey, "Primacy of Diapers among AB/DLs," *Understanding Infantilism* (blog), February 7, 2015, https://understanding.infantilism.org/surveys/primacy_of_diapers_among_abdls.php.

17 Hawkinson and Zamboni, "Adult Baby/Diaper Lovers," 869; Cwis, "The 'Origins of ABDL' Survey."

18 "Addicted To Living as an Adult Baby," My Strange Addiction, April 28, 2019, YouTube video, 7:36, https://www.youtube.com/watch?v=3FPkv4UvCvM.

19 Hawkinson and Zamboni, "Adult Baby/Diaper Lovers," 869.

20 B. Terrance Grey, "Why Want Diapers?," *Understanding Infantilism* (blog), September 15, 2001, https://understanding.infantilism.org/why_want_diapers.php.

21 Hsu, "Erotic Target Identity Inversions in Male Furries," 18.

22 Hsu and Bailey, "Autopedophilia," 5.

23 Hsu, "Erotic Target Identity Inversions in Male Furries," 82.

24 Hsu, 96.

25 Maggie Joyce, "The Adult Infant Identity," AB Discovery, 2019, https://abdiscover.files.wordpress.com/2020/06/the-adult-infant-identity.pdf.

26 James Giles, "Adult Baby Syndrome and Age Identity Disorder: Comment on Kise and Nguyen (2011)," *Archives of Sexual Behavior* 41, no. 2 (April 2012): 322, https://doi.org/10.1007/s10508-011-9884-4; Kurt Freund and Ray Blanchard, "Erotic Target

Location Errors in Male Gender Dysphorics, Paedophiles, and Fetishists," *British Journal of Psychiatry* 162, no. 4 (April 1993): 559, https://doi.org/10.1192/bjp.162.4.558.

27   Michael Bent, "The Identity Conflicts of the Adult Baby," June 2019, 4, https://abdiscover.files.wordpress.com/2019/06/subidentity.pdf.

28   Joyce, "The Adult Infant Identity," 4.

29   David Nordahl, *Michael*, accessed September 12, 2022, http://davidnordahl.com/images/links/6/246-Michael.jpg.

30   *Living with Michael Jackson: A Tonight Special*, directed by Julie Shaw, featuring Michael Jackson and Martin Bashir, 2003, https://www.imdb.com/title/tt0352524.

31   *Living with Michael Jackson.*

32   *Living with Michael Jackson.*

33   Michael Bailey, "Was Michael Jackson a Pedophile?," Science 2.0, July 1, 2009, https://www.science20.com/j_michael_bailey/was_michael_jackson_pedophile.

34   Michael Bailey, "Michael Jackson: Erotic Identity Disorder?," Science 2.0, July 1, 2009, https://www.science20.com/j_michael_bailey/michael_jackson_erotic_identity_disorder.

35   David Nordahl, online gallery, accessed September 12, 2022, http://davidnordahl.com/Michael_Jackson_Gallery/.

7.3. Furries

1   "FAQ," Alt+H, accessed September 12, 2022, https://www.alt-h.net/educate/faq.php.

2   S. E. Roberts et al., "Clinical Interaction with Anthropomorphic Phenomenon: Notes for Health Professionals about Interacting with Clients Who Possess This Unusual Identity," *Health & Social Work* 40, no. 2 (May 2015): e48, https://doi.org/10.1093/hsw/hlv020; Sharon E. Roberts et al., "The Anthrozoomorphic Identity: Furry Fandom Members' Connections to Nonhuman Animals," *Anthrozoös* 28, no. 4 (2015): 535, https://doi.org/10.1080/08927936.2015.1069993.

3   Courtney N. Plante et al., *FurScience! A Summary of Five Years of Research from the International Anthropomorphic Research Project* (Waterloo, Ontario: FurScience, 2016), 112, https://furscience.com/wp-content/uploads/2017/10/Fur-Science-Final-pdf-for-Website_2017_10_18.pdf.

4   "A Furry Glossary," Furry Grand Central, accessed January 18, 2023, https://web.archive.org/web/20190716000602/https://www.furcen.org/fgc/glossary.html.

5   "The Definition of the Furry Slang Word 'Yiff' and How It May Be Used," accessed January 18, 2023, https://web.archive.org/web/20050415121126/http:/www.cloudchasershaconage.furtopia.org/Yiff.txt.

6   Kyle Evans, "The Furry Sociological Survey," 2008, 8, https://www.gwern.net/docs/psychology/2008-evans.pdf; Plante et al., *FurScience! A Summary of Five Years of Research*, 43.

7   Plante et al., *FurScience! A Summary of Five Years of Research*, 93.

8   Plante et al., 84.

9   Kevin J. Hsu and J. Michael Bailey, "The 'Furry' Phenomenon: Characterizing Sexual Orientation, Sexual Motivation, and Erotic Target Identity Inversions in Male Furries," *Archives of Sexual Behavior* 48, no. 5 (July 2019): 1349–69, https://doi.org/10.1007/s10508-018-1303-7.

10   Evans, "The Furry Sociological Survey," 9.

11   Roberts et al., "Clinical Interaction with Anthropomorphic Phenomenon," e46.

12   Roberts et al., e48.

13   Plante et al., *FurScience! A Summary of Five Years of Research*, 38–42.

14   Hsu and Bailey, "The 'Furry' Phenomenon."

15   Hsu and Bailey, 4.

16   Hsu and Bailey, 14.

17   Hsu and Bailey, 15.

18   Thomas R. Brooks et al., "'Chasing Tail': Testing the Relative Strength of Sexual Interest and Social Interaction as Predictors of Furry Identity," *The Journal of Sex Research* (May 2022): 1–12, https://doi.org/10.1080/00224499.2022.2068180.

19   Brooks et al., 6.

20   Brooks et al., 6.

21   Ben Silverman, "Fursonas: Furries, Community, and Identity Online" (master's thesis, Massachusetts Institute of Technology, 2020), 52–67, https://cms.mit.edu/wp/wp-content/uploads/2021/01/477814762-Ben-Silverman-Fursonas-Furries-Community-and-Identity-Online.pdf.

22   Plante et al., *FurScience! A Summary of Five Years of Research*, 51.

23   Plante et al., 78.

24   Alexander Kranjec et al., *Illusory Body Perception and Experience in Furries* (Ottawa, Ontario: Social Sciences and Humanities Research Council of Canada, 2019), 600, https://cogsci.mindmodeling.org/2019/papers/0120/0120.pdf.

25   Kranjec et al., *Illusory Body Perception and Experience in Furries*.

26   Matthew R. Longo et al., "What Is Embodiment? A Psychometric Approach," *Cognition* 107, no. 3 (June 2008): 991, https://doi.org/10.1016/j.cognition.2007.12.004.

27   Kranjec et al., *Illusory Body Perception and Experience in Furries*, 599.

28   Kranjec et al., 600.

29   Kranjec et al., 600.

30   Kranjec et al., 600.

7.4. Therians

1   "Therianthropy," Therian Wiki, Fandom, accessed September 12, 2022, https://therian.fandom.com/wiki/Therianthropy.

2   Natalie Bricker, "Life Stories of Therianthropes: An Analysis of Nonhuman Identity in a Narrative Identity Model" (senior thesis, Lake Forest College, 2016), 1, https://core.ac.uk/download/pdf/48614354.pdf.

3 Courtney N. Plante et al., *FurScience! A Summary of Five Years of Research from the International Anthropomorphic Research Project* (Waterloo, Ontario: FurScience, 2016), 115, https://furscience.com/wp-content/uploads/2017/10/Fur-Science-Final-pdf-for-Website_2017_10_18.pdf; Lupa, *A Field Guide to Otherkin* (Stafford, England: Megalithica Books, 2007), 118.

4 Penny Bernstein et al., "Furries from A to Z (Anthropomorphism to Zoomorphism)," *Society & Animals* 16, no. 3 (2008): 216, https://doi.org/10.1163/156853008X323376.

5 Bricker, "Life Stories of Therianthropes," 1.

6 Bricker, 34.

7 Bricker, 10.

8 Venetia Laura Delano Robertson, "The Beast Within," *Nova Religio* 16, no. 3 (February 2013): 18, https://doi.org/10.1525/nr.2013.16.3.7.

9 Timothy Grivell, Helen Clegg, and Elizabeth C. Roxburgh, "An Interpretative Phenomenological Analysis of Identity in the Therian Community," *Identity* 14, no. 2 (2014): 125, https://doi.org/10.1080/15283488.2014.891999.

10 Grivell, Clegg, and Roxburgh, 122.

11 Bricker, "Life Stories of Therianthropes," 35.

12 Grivell, Clegg, and Roxburgh, "An Interpretative Phenomenological Analysis," 122.

13 Bricker, "Life Stories of Therianthropes," 41–42.

14 White Wolf, "Results of the 2013 Therian Census" (slideshow, 2013), 25, https://www.dropbox.com/s/y8vmmanknlvqpek/2013%20TSurvey.pptx.

15 Helen Clegg, Roz Collings, and Elizabeth C. Roxburgh, "Therianthropy: Wellbeing, Schizotypy, and Autism in Individuals Who Self-Identify as Non-Human," *Society & Animals* 27, no. 4 (2019): 407, https://doi.org/10.1163/15685306-12341540; Lupa, *A Field Guide to Otherkin*, 35, 280; White Wolf, "Results of the 2012 Therian Census" (slideshow, 2012), https://www.dropbox.com/s/ythgrrx7ez25f6l/TSurvey.pptx; White Wolf, "2013 Therian Census."

16 Clegg, Collings, and Roxburgh, "Therianthropy," 408; White Wolf, "2012 Therian Census"; White Wolf, "2013 Therian Census."

17 Jennifer W. Applebaum, Chuck W. Peek, and Barbara A. Zsembik, "Examining U.S. Pet Ownership Using the General Social Survey," *The Social Science Journal* (March 2020): 1–10, https://doi.org/10.1080/03623319.2020.1728507; Edwin Plotts, "Pet Ownership Statistics by State, and So Much More (Updated 2020)," Pawlicy Advisor, 2020, https://www.pawlicy.com/blog/us-pet-ownership-statistics/; Martin B. Marx et al., "Demographics of Pet Ownership among U.S. Adults 21 to 64 Years of Age," *Anthrozoös* 2, no. 1 (March 1988): 34, https://doi.org/10.2752/089279389787058262.

18 Plotts, "Pet Ownership Statistics by State."

19 The Utlah, "AHWw Poll'97 - The RESULTS!," alt.horror.werewolves, Google conversations, November 9, 1997, https://groups.google.com/g/alt.horror.werewolves/c/lYqSQB2DVQM/m/FGPjBFzqarQJ.

20 Robertson, "The Beast Within," 20.

21 Robertson, 20.

22 White Wolf, "2013 Therian Census," 38–42.

23 Bricker, "Life Stories of Therianthropes," 39–40.

24 Robertson, "The Beast Within," 20.

25 Bricker, "Life Stories of Therianthropes," 41.

26 "Mental Shift," Therian Wiki, Fandom, accessed September 12, 2022, https:// therian.fandom.com/wiki/Mental_Shift.

27 Lupa, *A Field Guide to Otherkin*, 128.

28 Lupa, 128.

29 Lupa, 128.

30 The Utlah, "AHWw Poll'97"; White Wolf, "2013 Therian Census."

31 The Utlah, "AHWw Poll'97."

32 "Vacillant Therianthropy," Therian Wiki, Fandom, accessed September 12, 2022, https://therian.fandom.com/wiki/Vacillant_Therianthropy.

33 White Wolf, "2012 Therian Census," 25, 26; White Wolf, "2013 Therian Census," 41, 42.

34 Asikaa, "The Great AHWw Survey!," alt.horror.werewolves, Google conversations, February 20, 1996, https://groups.google.com/g/alt.horror.werewolves/c/ OcrxF8eZxKQ/m/eIlC__URUvoJ; The Utlah, "AHWw Poll'97"; PinkDolphin, "Research: Fluid Identity & Experiences within Therianthropy 2020," survey results, April 2020, https://docs.google.com/forms/d/11dcX4zVEbG9xVK1nr mErYJlmmMNzkzXIqTbLPVZsaqs/viewanalytics; White Wolf, "2012 Therian Census"; White Wolf, "2013 Therian Census"; Reddit user: u/mithril-animal, "Therian Community Survey #1," January 2021, https://docs.google.com/forms/d/ e/1FAIpQLSfhV7jqm5znEoNQ-V6Uc9sIUBZ8RXF8xidHj-oMsDJOWKHxDw/ viewanalytics; PinkDolphin, "Therianthropy and Gender Experience," Survey Results, September 2020, https://docs.google.com/forms/d/1Eamup4muY5ir H1Zv9kxG18yM2yoezh_zosZP6agAtdk/viewanalytics; Citrakāyah, "Werelist Poll of 2013," 2013, https://citrakayah.ucoz.org/Werelist_Poll_of_2013.pdf; Reddit user: u/40-I-4-Z-Kalisza, "What Kind of Therian Are You?," May 2021, https://docs.google.com/forms/d/e/1FAIpQLSfl8KE1_oGz5qSrwi-4G7JDVDlMpiJnVtbvRDbErCtwMwefPQ/viewanalytics.

35 Reddit user: u/40-I-4-Z-Kalisza, "What Kind of Therian Are You?"; PinkDolphin, "Therianthropy and Gender Experience"; Reddit user: u/mithril-animal, "Therian Community Survey #1."

36 Christian C. Joyal, Amélie Cossette, and Vanessa Lapierre, "What Exactly Is an Unusual Sexual Fantasy?," *The Journal of Sexual Medicine* 12, no. 2 (February 2015): 334, https://doi.org/10.1111/jsm.12734.

37 Claude Crépault and Marcel Couture, "Men's Erotic Fantasies," *Archives of Sexual Behavior* 9, no. 6 (December 1980): 572, https://doi.org/10.1007/BF01542159.

38 Klára Bártová et al., "The Prevalence of Paraphilic Interests in the Czech Population: Preference, Arousal, the Use of Pornography, Fantasy, and Behavior,"

The Journal of Sex Research 58, no. 1 (January 2021): 86–96, https://doi.org/10.1080/00224499.2019.1707468.

39 Robertson, "The Beast Within," 17.

40 "F.A.Q.s," Therian-Guide, accessed September 12, 2022, https://www.therian-guide.com/index.php/7-FAQs.

41 Bricker, "Life Stories of Therianthropes," 28.

42 Clegg, Collings, and Roxburgh, "Therianthropy," 414.

43 Kevin J. Hsu and J. Michael Bailey, "The 'Furry' Phenomenon: Characterizing Sexual Orientation, Sexual Motivation, and Erotic Target Identity Inversions in Male Furries," *Archives of Sexual Behavior* 48, no. 5 (July 2019): 1349–69, https://doi.org/10.1007/s10508-018-1303-7.

7.5. Otherkin

1   Lupa, *A Field Guide to Otherkin* (Stafford, England: Megalithica Books, 2007), 31–33.

2   Lupa, 33.

3   Lupa, 33.

4   "Species Dysphoria," Otherkin Wiki, Fandom, accessed September 13, 2022, https://otherkin.fandom.com/wiki/Species_Dysphoria.

5   Lupa, *A Field Guide to Otherkin*, 40.

6   Arhuaine et al., "Otherkin FAQ v 4.0.1 (2/8/01)," accessed September 13, 2022, https://kinhost.org/res/Otherfaq.php.

7   Page Shepard (@who-is-page), "What is a Kinshift?," Tumblr, January 26, 2016, https://who-is-page.tumblr.com/post/138128500224/what-is-a-kinshift.

8   Page Shepard, "The Nonhumanity & Body Modification/Decoration Survey," February 2021, https://docs.google.com/forms/d/e/1FAIpQLSfAt2tZ9_dQ9wmZxqETg3WwCujLuOJfHNL9SoHubi2HVfL6qg/viewanalytics.

9   Page Shepard (@who-is-page), "The Nonhumanity & Body Modification/Decoration Survey," Tumblr, February 11, 2021, https://who-is-page.tumblr.com/post/642862756410834944/the-nonhumanity-body-modificationdecoration.

10 Shepard, "The Nonhumanity & Body Modification/Decoration Survey," February 2021.

11 Shepard.

12 Shepard.

13 Shepard.

14 Lupa, *A Field Guide to Otherkin*, 202; Reddit user: u/komondorok, "'KIN Survey," May 2015, https://drive.google.com/file/d/0Bz5ZHVD-qTcAVVl4OHMoR1JkeG8/view.

15 Reddit user: u/komondorok, "'KIN Survey."

16 "Therian Interviews Episode 2 : Dollkin [Objectkin/Otherkin] by 'L,'" PD, June 16, 2019, YouTube video, 1:54, https://www.youtube.com/watch?v=17UenvHYyqk.

17   Calico, "The Exact Definition of Being Other Hearted," The Other Hearts, January 9, 2015, https://theotherhearts.canadian-forum.com/t10-the-exact-definition-of-being-other-hearted.

18   Renata, "Otherhearted: What Exactly is Kith?," Therian-Guide, March 22, 2016, https://forums.therian-guide.com/Thread-Otherhearted-What-exactly-is-Kith--3337.

19   "Otherlink," Therian Wiki, Fandom, accessed September 13, 2022, https://therian.fandom.com/wiki/Otherlink.

20   Page Shepard (@who-is-page), "C'linkers and Copinglink," Tumblr, February 23, 2016, https://who-is-page.tumblr.com/post/139871297049/clinkers-and-copinglink.

21   Florentin Félix Morin, "Ego Hippo: The Subject as Metaphor," *Angelaki* 22, no. 2 (2017): 91, https://doi.org/10.1080/0969725X.2017.1322822; Christine Feraday, "For Lack of a Better Word: Neo-Identities in Non-Cisgender, Non-Straight Communities on Tumblr" (master's thesis, Toronto Metropolitan University, 2016), 55, https://doi.org/10.32920/ryerson.14648067.v1.

22   "The Truth about Trans," Stonewall UK, accessed September 13, 2022, https://web.archive.org/web/20211027010525/https://www.stonewall.org.uk/truth-about-trans.

23   Jody L. Herman, Andrew R. Flores, and Kathryn K. O'Neill, *How Many Adults and Youth Identify as Transgender in the United States?* (UCLA School of Law Williams Institute, June 2022), 1, https://williamsinstitute.law.ucla.edu/publications/trans-adults-united-states/.

24   Michelle M. Johns et al., "Transgender Identity and Experiences of Violence Victimization, Substance Use, Suicide Risk, and Sexual Risk Behaviors among High School Students — 19 States and Large Urban School Districts, 2017," *Morbidity and Mortality Weekly Report 68, no. 3 (January 25, 2019): 68, https://doi.org/10.15585/mmwr.mm6803a3.*

25   Jeffrey M. Jones, "LGBT Identification Rises to 5.6% in Latest U.S. Estimate," Gallup, February 24, 2021, https://news.gallup.com/poll/329708/lgbt-identification-rises-latest-estimate.aspx.

26   Asikaa, "The Great AHWW Survey!," alt.horror.werewolves, February 20, 1996, https://groups.google.com/g/alt.horror.werewolves/c/OcrxF8eZxKQ/m/eIlC__URUvoJ; The Utlah, "AHWw Poll'97 - The RESULTS!," alt.horror.werewolves, Google conversations, November 9, 1997, https://groups.google.com/g/alt.horror.werewolves/c/lYqSQB2DVQM/m/FGPjBFzqarQJ; Lopori, "Alterhumanity and Sexuality," January 2021, https://docs.google.com/forms/d/e/1FAIpQLScxRo-ZVSgHcReAksPIaGoOjbeQHEt3P9HF4ddeQ5JB7OzFxg/viewanalytics; PinkDolphin, "Research: Fluid Identity & Experiences within Therianthropy 2020," Survey Results, April 2020, https://docs.google.com/forms/d/11dcX4zVE bG9xVK1nrmErYJlmmMNzkzXIqTbLPVZsaqs/viewanalytics; Reddit user: u/komondorok, "'KIN Survey"; White Wolf, "Results of the 2012 Therian Census" (slideshow, 2012), https://www.dropbox.com/s/ythgrrx7ez25f6l/TSurvey.pptx; White Wolf, "Results of the 2013 Therian Census" (slideshow, 2013), https://www.

dropbox.com/s/y8vmmanknlvqpek/2013%20TSurvey.pptx; Tailcalled, "[Results] Otherkin Survey," imgur, July 21, 2018, https://imgur.com/a/dDlYEEu; Shepard, "The Nonhumanity & Body Modification/Decoration Survey"; Reddit user: u/mithril-animal, "Therian Community Survey #1," January 2021, https://docs.google.com/forms/d/e/1FAIpQLSfhV7jqm5znEoNQ-V6Uc9sIUBZ8RXF8xidHj-oMsDJOWKHxDw/viewanalytics; PinkDolphin, "Therianthropy and Gender Experience," Survey Results, September 2020, https://docs.google.com/forms/d/1Eamup4muY5irH1Zv9kxG18yM2yoezh_zosZP6agAtdk/viewanalytics; Citrakāyah, "Werelist Poll of 2013," 2013, https://citrakayah.ucoz.org/Werelist_Poll_of_2013.pdf; Reddit user: u/40-I-4-Z-Kalisza, "What Kind of Therian Are You?," May 2021, https://docs.google.com/forms/d/e/1FAIpQLSfl8KE1_0Gz5qSrwi-4G7JDVDlMpiJnVtbvRDbErCtwMwefPQ/viewanalytics.

27 "Therianthropy V.S. GENDER: Does It Influence Eachother?," PD, September 12, 2020, YouTube video, 10:46, https://www.youtube.com/watch?v=OF8iunTadYo.
28 PinkDolphin, "Therianthropy and Gender Experience."
29 PinkDolphin.
30 PinkDolphin.
31 PinkDolphin.
32 PinkDolphin.
33 PinkDolphin.
34 Lopori, "Alterhumanity and Sexuality."
35 Lopori.
36 PinkDolphin, "Therianthropy and Gender Experience."
37 Lopori, "Alterhumanity and Sexuality."
38 Lopori.
39 Lopori.
40 Lopori.
41 Lopori.
42 Lopori.
43 Lopori.
44 Lopori.
45 Lopori.
46 Lopori.
47 Lopori.
48 Lopori.
49 Lopori.
50 Lopori (@goddamnitlopori), "Alterhumanity and Sexuality Survey: The Results!," Tumblr, January 9, 2021, https://goddamnitlopori.tumblr.com/post/639799806560239616/alterhumanity-and-sexuality-survey-the-results.
51 Lopori.
52 Lopori.

7.6. Transrace

1   Rachel Doležal and Storms Reback, *In Full Color: Finding My Place in a Black and White World* (Dallas: BenBella Books, 2017), 11.

2   Doležal and Reback, 12.

3   Doležal and Reback, 23.

4   Doležal and Reback, 23.

5   Doležal and Reback, 59.

6   Doležal and Reback, 63.

7   Doležal and Reback, 63.

8   Doležal and Reback, 85.

9   Doležal and Reback, 93.

10   Doležal and Reback, 112.

11   Doležal and Reback, 115.

12   Emily Shapiro, "Rachel Dolezal is Asked about Father's Race in Interview with ABC's Spokane Affiliate," *ABC News*, June 12, 2015, https://abcnews.go.com/US/rachel-dolezal-asked-fathers-race-interview-abcs-spokane/story?id=31727573.

13   Richard Pérez-Peña, "Black or White? Woman's Story Stirs Up a Furor," *New York Times*, June 12, 2015, https://www.nytimes.com/2015/06/13/us/rachel-dolezal-naacp-president-accused-of-lying-about-her-race.html; Justin Wm. Moyer, "'Are You an African American?' Why an NAACP Official isn't Saying," Morning Mix, *Washington Post*, June 12, 2015, https://www.washingtonpost.com/news/morning-mix/wp/2015/06/12/spokane-naacp-president-rachel-dolezal-may-be-white/.

14   Robin Zheng, "Why Yellow Fever Isn't Flattering: A Case Against Racial Fetishes," *Journal of the American Philosophical Association* 2, no. 3 (2016): 400–419, https://doi.org/10.1017/apa.2016.25.

15   Anne A. Lawrence, *Men Trapped in Men's Bodies: Narratives of Autogynephilic Transsexualism*, Focus on Sexuality Research (New York: Springer, 2013), 186, https://www.doi.org/10.1007/978-1-4614-5182-2.

16   Lee Brown, "White Influencer 'Identifies as Korean' after Surgeries to Look Like BTS Singer," *New York Post*, June 28, 2021, https://nypost.com/2021/06/28/oli-london-identifies-as-korean-after-surgeries-to-look-like-bts-jimin/.

17   Zak Bennett and Erica Tempesta, "EXCLUSIVE: K-Pop Super Fan *marries* a Cardboard Cutout of His Singing Idol in a Bizarre Ceremony in Las Vegas – after Spending $165,000 on Surgery to Look Just Like the Star," Daily Mail, January 7, 2020, https://www.dailymail.co.uk/femail/article-7858307/K-pop-superfan-marries-cardboard-cutout-idol-Las-Vegas.html.

18   Kate Dennett, "EXCLUSIVE: 'I Have Become the Person I was Born to Be': Influencer Oli London Comes Out as a Transgender Woman after Causing Controversy by Saying They Identify as Korean Following Multiple Surgeries," Daily Mail, May 6, 2022, https://www.dailymail.co.uk/tvshowbiz/article-10789279/Influencer-Oli-London-claims-Korean-comes-transgender-woman.html.

19 Phil Illy, "Transracialism - Identity, Experiences, Embodiment, and Attraction," n.d.

20 Their "default" or "birth" race.

21 Christine Overall, "Transsexualism and 'Transracialism,'" *Social Philosophy Today* 20 (2004): 183–93, https://doi.org/10.5840/socphiltoday2004203; Rebecca Tuvel, "In Defense of Transracialism," *Hypatia* 32, no. 2 (2017): 263–78, https://doi.org/10.1111/hypa.12327.

22 Tuvel, "In Defense of Transracialism," 264.

23 John W. Loftus, *The Outsider Test for Faith: How to Know Which Religion Is True* (Amherst, NY: Prometheus Books, 2013).

24 Zinnia Jones, "Book Review: Alice Dreger, Autogynephilia, and the Misrepresentation of Trans Sexualities," April 1, 2016, https://www.academia.edu/80148791/Alice_Dreger_Autogynephilia_and_the_Misrepresentation_of_Trans_Sexualities; M. H. Wyndzen, "Autogynephilia & Ray Blanchard's Mis-Directed Sex-Drive Model of Transsexuality," *All Mixed Up* (blog), 2003, http://www.genderpsychology.org/autogynephilia/ray_blanchard/; "Autogynephilia," ContraPoints, February 1, 2018, YouTube video, 48:54, https://www.youtube.com/watch?v=6czRFLs5JQo; Julia Serano, "Autogynephilia: A Scientific Review, Feminist Analysis, and Alternative 'Embodiment Fantasies' Model," *The Sociological Review* 68, no. 4 (2020): 763–78, https://doi.org/10.1177/0038026120934690; Julia Serano, "Making Sense of Autogynephilia Debates," Medium, October 15, 2019, https://juliaserano.medium.com/making-sense-of-autogynephilia-debates-73d9051e88d3; Jack Molay, "The Autogynephilia Theory Debunked by New German Study," *Crossdreamers* (blog), May 21, 2020, https://www.crossdreamers.com/2020/05/the-autogynephilia-theory-debunked-by.html; Julia M. Serano, "The Case Against Autogynephilia," *International Journal of Transgenderism* 12, no. 3 (2010): 176–87, https://doi.org/10.1080/15532739.2010.514223; Zagria, "What Is Autogynephilia?," *A Gender Variance Who's Who* (blog), March 22, 2009, https://zagria.blogspot.com/2009/03/what-is-autogynephilia.html.

8.0. Culturally Integrating Autoheterosexuality

1 Bostock v. Clayton County, 590 U.S. (2020), 9, https://www.supremecourt.gov/opinions/19pdf/17-1618_hfci.pdf.

2 Richard L. Miller, "Public Displays of Affection," in *The Encyclopedia of Cross-Cultural Psychology*, ed. Kenneth D. Keith (Hoboken, NJ: Wiley, 2013), 1063–65, https://doi.org/10.1002/9781118339893.wbeccp443; Elizabeth Vaquera and Grace Kao, "Private and Public Displays of Affection among Interracial and Intra-Racial Adolescent Couples," *Social Science Quarterly* 86, no. 2 (June 2005): 484–508, https://doi.org/10.1111/j.0038-4941.2005.00314.x.

3 Dave Chapelle, "Dave Chappelle: The Closer (2021) | Transcript," Scraps from the Loft, October 6, 2021, https://scrapsfromtheloft.com/comedy/dave-chappelle-the-closer-transcript/.

4   Karen L. Blair and Rhea Ashley Hoskin, "Transgender Exclusion from the World of Dating: Patterns of Acceptance and Rejection of Hypothetical Trans Dating Partners as a Function of Sexual and Gender Identity," *Journal of Social and Personal Relationships* 36, no. 7 (2019): 2074–95, https://doi.org/10.1177/0265407518779139.

8.1. Juvenile Transsexualism

1   William Byne et al., "Report of the American Psychiatric Association Task Force on Treatment of Gender Identity Disorder," *Archives of Sexual Behavior* 41, no. 4 (August 2012): 763, https://doi.org/10.1007/s10508-012-9975-x.

2   Byne et al., 764.

3   E. Coleman et al., "Standards of Care for the Health of Transgender and Gender Diverse People, Version 8," *International Journal of Transgender Health* 23, no. sup1 (2022): S46, https://doi.org/10.1080/26895269.2022.2100644.

4   B. P. C. Kreukels et al., "A European Network for the Investigation of Gender Incongruence: The ENIGI Initiative," *European Psychiatry* 27, no. 6 (August 2012): 445–50, https://doi.org/10.1016/j.eurpsy.2010.04.009.

5   Bruce S. McEwen and Teresa A. Milner, "Understanding the Broad Influence of Sex Hormones and Sex Differences in the Brain," *Journal of Neuroscience Research* 95, no. 1–2 (January/February 2017): 24–39, https://doi.org/10.1002/jnr.23809; Michael J. Weiser, Chad D. Foradori, and Robert J. Handa, "Estrogen Receptor Beta in the Brain: From Form to Function," *Brain Research Reviews* 57, no. 2 (March 2008): 309–320, https://doi.org/10.1016/j.brainresrev.2007.05.013.

6   Elizabeth Murphy and Charles Steenbergen, "Estrogen Regulation of Protein Expression and Signaling Pathways in the Heart," *Biology of Sex Differences* 5, no. 1 (2014), https://doi.org/10.1186/2042-6410-5-6; Tao Luo and Jin Kyung Kim, "The Role of Estrogen and Estrogen Receptors on Cardiomyocytes: An Overview," *Canadian Journal of Cardiology* 32, no. 8 (August 2016): 1017–25, https://doi.org/10.1016/j.cjca.2015.10.021.

7   M. W. Pfaffl, I. G. Lange, and H. H. D. Meyer, "The Gastrointestinal Tract as Target of Steroid Hormone Action: Quantification of Steroid Receptor mRNA Expression (AR, ERα, ERβ and PR) in 10 Bovine Gastrointestinal Tract Compartments by Kinetic RT-PCR," *The Journal of Steroid Biochemistry and Molecular Biology* 84, no. 2–3 (February 2003): 159–66, https://doi.org/10.1016/S0960-0760(03)00025-6; Agata Mulak, Yvette Taché, and Muriel Larauche, "Sex Hormones in the Modulation of Irritable Bowel Syndrome," *World Journal of Gastroenterology* 20, no. 10 (2014): 2433, https://doi.org/10.3748/wjg.v20.i10.2433; Xin Yang et al., "Estrogen and Estrogen Receptors in the Modulation of Gastrointestinal Epithelial Secretion," *Oncotarget* 8, no. 57 (2017): 97683–92, https://doi.org/10.18632/oncotarget.18313.

8   Susan Kovats, "Estrogen Receptors Regulate Innate Immune Cells and Signaling Pathways," *Cellular Immunology* 294, no. 2 (April 2015): 63–69, https://doi.

org/10.1016/j.cellimm.2015.01.018; Iwona A. Buskiewicz, Sally A. Huber, and DeLisa Fairweather, "Sex Hormone Receptor Expression in the Immune System," in *Sex Differences in Physiology*, ed. Gretchen N. Neigh and Megan M. Mitzelfelt (Cambridge, MA; Academic Press Elsevier, 2016), 45–60, https://doi.org/10.1016/B978-0-12-802388-4.00004-5.

9   Ai Guo Wang et al., "The Expression of Estrogen Receptors in Hepatocellular Carcinoma in Korean Patients," *Yonsei Medical Journal* 47, no. 6 (December 2006): 811, https://doi.org/10.3349/ymj.2006.47.6.811.

10 P. D. Gupta et al., "Sex Hormone Receptors in the Human Eye," *Survey of Ophthalmology* 50, no. 3 (May–June 2005): 274–84, https://doi.org/10.1016/j.survophthal.2005.02.005.

11 Tolga Kirgezen et al., "Sex Hormone Receptor Expression in the Human Vocal Fold Subunits," *Journal of Voice* 31, no. 4 (July 2017): 476–82, https://doi.org/10.1016/j.jvoice.2016.11.005.

12 M. N. Dieudonné et al., "Evidence for Functional Estrogen Receptors α and β in Human Adipose Cells: Regional Specificities and Regulation by Estrogens," *American Journal of Physiology-Cell Physiology* 286, no. 3 (March 2004): C655–61, https://doi.org/10.1152/ajpcell.00321.2003; Steen B. Pedersen et al., "Demonstration of Estrogen Receptor Subtypes α and β in Human Adipose Tissue: Influences of Adipose Cell Differentiation and Fat Depot Localization," *Molecular and Cellular Endocrinology* 182, no. 1 (August 2001): 27–37, https://doi.org/10.1016/S0303-7207(01)00557-3.

13 J. A. Ruizeveld de Winter et al., "Androgen Receptor Expression in Human Tissues: An Immunohistochemical Study," *Journal of Histochemistry & Cytochemistry* 39, no. 7 (July 1991): 927–36, https://doi.org/10.1177/39.7.1865110.

14 C. Fede et al., "Hormone Receptor Expression in Human Fascial Tissue," *European Journal of Histochemistry* 60, no. 4 (November 2016): 2710, https://doi.org/10.4081/ejh.2016.2710; Martina Velders and Patrick Diel, "How Sex Hormones Promote Skeletal Muscle Regeneration," *Sports Medicine* 43, no. 11 (November 2013): 1089–100, https://doi.org/10.1007/s40279-013-0081-6; L. Ekenros et al., "Expression of Sex Steroid Hormone Receptors in Human Skeletal Muscle during the Menstrual Cycle," *Acta Physiologica* 219, no. 2 (February 2017): 486–93, https://doi.org/10.1111/apha.12757.

15 T. Ushiyama et al., "Expression of Genes for Estrogen Receptors α and β in Human Articular Chondrocytes," *Osteoarthritis and Cartilage* 7, no. 6 (November 1999): 560–66, https://doi.org/10.1053/joca.1999.0260; Paul Sciore, Cyril B. Frank, and David A. Hart, "Identification of Sex Hormone Receptors in Human and Rabbit Ligaments of the Knee by Reverse Transcription-Polymerase Chain Reaction: Evidence That Receptors are Present in Tissue from Both Male and Female Subjects," *Journal of Orthopaedic Research* 16, no. 5 (September 1998): 604–610, https://doi.org/10.1002/jor.1100160513; Wolf Dietrich et al., "Estrogen Receptor-β is the Predominant Estrogen Receptor Subtype in Normal Human Synovia," *Journal*

of the Society for Gynecologic Investigation 13, no. 7 (2006): 512–17, https://doi.org/10.1016/j.jsgi.2006.07.002.

16   Rosemary Bland, "Steroid Hormone Receptor Expression and Action in Bone," *Clinical Science* 98, no. 2 (2000): 217, https://pubmed.ncbi.nlm.nih.gov/10657279/; Aysha B. Khalid and Susan A. Krum, "Estrogen Receptors Alpha and Beta in Bone," *Bone* 87 (June 2016): 130–35, https://doi.org/10.1016/j.bone.2016.03.016.

17   K. Venken et al., "Sex Hormones, Their Receptors and Bone Health," *Osteoporosis International* 19, no. 11 (November 2008): 1521, https://doi.org/10.1007/s00198-008-0609-z.

18   Anna-Maria G. Psarra and Constantine E. Sekeris, "Steroid and Thyroid Hormone Receptors in Mitochondria," *IUBMB Life* 60, no. 4 (April 2008): 210–23, https://doi.org/10.1002/iub.37.

19   Michael T. Lin and M. Flint Beal, "Mitochondrial Dysfunction and Oxidative Stress in Neurodegenerative Diseases," *Nature* 443, no. 7113 (October 2006): 793, https://doi.org/10.1038/nature05292.

20   Yashika Bansal and Anurag Kuhad, "Mitochondrial Dysfunction in Depression," *Current Neuropharmacology* 14, no. 6 (2016): 610–18, https://doi.org/10.2174/1570159X14666160229114755; Josh Allen et al., "Mitochondria and Mood: Mitochondrial Dysfunction as a Key Player in the Manifestation of Depression," *Frontiers in Neuroscience* 12 (June 2018): 386, https://doi.org/10.3389/fnins.2018.00386; Gislaine T. Rezin et al., "Mitochondrial Dysfunction and Psychiatric Disorders," *Neurochemical Research* 34, no. 6 (June 2009): 1021–29, https://doi.org/10.1007/s11064-008-9865-8.

21   Dimitry A. Chistiakov et al., "The Role of Mitochondrial Dysfunction in Cardiovascular Disease: A Brief Review," *Annals of Medicine* 50, no. 2 (2018): 121–27, https://doi.org/10.1080/07853890.2017.1417631; Nageswara R. Madamanchi and Marschall S. Runge, "Mitochondrial Dysfunction in Atherosclerosis," *Circulation Research* 100, no. 4 (March 2007): 460–73, https://doi.org/10.1161/01.RES.0000258450.44413.96.

22   Carlos López-Otín et al., "The Hallmarks of Aging," *Cell* 153, no. 6 (June 2013): 1194–217, https://doi.org/10.1016/j.cell.2013.05.039.

23   Andrea Vasconsuelo, Lorena Milanesi, and Ricardo Boland, "Actions of 17β-Estradiol and Testosterone in the Mitochondria and Their Implications in Aging," *Ageing Research Reviews* 12, no. 4 (September 2013): 907–17, https://doi.org/10.1016/j.arr.2013.09.001.

24   Carolyn M. Klinge, "Estrogenic Control of Mitochondrial Function and Biogenesis," *Journal of Cellular Biochemistry* 105, no. 6 (December 2008): 1342–51, https://doi.org/10.1002/jcb.21936.

25   Consuelo Borrás et al., "Direct Antioxidant and Protective Effect of Estradiol on Isolated Mitochondria," *Biochimica et Biophysica Acta (BBA) - Molecular Basis of Disease* 1802, no. 1 (January 2010): 205–211, https://doi.org/10.1016/j.bbadis.2009.09.007.

26 Ronald W. Irwin et al., "Progesterone and Estrogen Regulate Oxidative
    Metabolism in Brain Mitochondria," *Endocrinology* 149, no. 6 (June 2008): 3167–75,
    https://doi.org/10.1210/en.2007-1227.

27 Yuko Hara et al., "Presynaptic Mitochondrial Morphology in Monkey Prefrontal
    Cortex Correlates with Working Memory and is Improved with Estrogen
    Treatment," *Proceedings of the National Academy of Sciences* 111, no. 1 (January
    2014): 486–91, https://doi.org/10.1073/pnas.1311310110.

28 Hara et al., 489.

29 Irwin et al., "Progesterone and Estrogen," 3167.

30 Venken et al., "Sex Hormones," 1521.

31 Giuseppe Saggese, Giampiero Igli Baroncelli, and Silvano Bertelloni, "Puberty
    and Bone Development," *Best Practice & Research Clinical Endocrinology &
    Metabolism* 16, no. 1 (March 2002): 53–64, https://doi.org/10.1053/beem.2001.0180.

32 S. Aubrey Stoch et al., "Bone Loss in Men with Prostate Cancer Treated
    with Gonadotropin-Releasing Hormone Agonists," *The Journal of Clinical
    Endocrinology & Metabolism* 86, no. 6 (June 2001): 2787–91, https://doi.org/10.1210/
    jcem.86.6.7558.

33 Marie Nolbert, Paulette Wells, and Gamal Hussein, "Impact of Leuprolide Acetate
    Disease Management Program on Patient Outcomes," *Clinical Research and
    Regulatory Affairs* 19, no. 1 (2002): 39, https://doi.org/10.1081/CRP-120004214.

34 Nolbert, Wells, and Hussein, 38–39.

35 Chandler Marrs, "Lupron Side Effects Survey Results Part One: Scope and
    Severity," Hormones Matter, October 4, 2017, https://www.hormonesmatter.com/
    lupron-side-effects-survey-results-scope-severity-side-effects/.

36 Nils R. Varney et al., "Neuropsychologic Dysfunction in Women Following
    Leuprolide Acetate Induction of Hypoestrogenism," *Journal of Assisted
    Reproduction and Genetics* 10, no. 1 (January 1993): 53–57, https://doi.
    org/10.1007/BF01204441; Miglena Grigorova, Barbara B. Sherwin, and Togas
    Tulandi, "Effects of Treatment with Leuprolide Acetate Depot on Working
    Memory and Executive Functions in Young Premenopausal Women,"
    Psychoneuroendocrinology 31, no. 8 (September 2006): 935–47, https://doi.
    org/10.1016/j.psyneuen.2006.05.004; Stefano Palomba et al., "Gonadotropin-
    Releasing Hormone Agonist with or without Raloxifene: Effects on Cognition,
    Mood, and Quality of Life," *Fertility and Sterility* 82, no. 2 (August 2004):
    480–82, https://doi.org/10.1016/j.fertnstert.2003.11.061.

37 Slawomir Wojniusz et al., "Cognitive, Emotional, and Psychosocial Functioning
    of Girls Treated with Pharmacological Puberty Blockage for Idiopathic Central
    Precocious Puberty," *Frontiers in Psychology* 7 (July 2016): 1053, https://doi.
    org/10.3389/fpsyg.2016.01053; D. Mul et al., "Psychological Assessments Before
    and After Treatment of Early Puberty in Adopted Children," *Acta Paediatrica*
    90, no. 9 (September 2001): 968–69, https://doi.org/10.1111/j.1651-2227.2001.
    tb01349.x.

38 Christina Jewett, "Women Fear Drug They Used to Halt Puberty Led to Health Problems," Kaiser Health News, February 2, 2017, https://khn.org/news/women-fear-drug-they-used-to-halt-puberty-led-to-health-problems/.

39 Chandler Marrs, "Lupron, Estradiol, and the Mitochondria: A Pathway to Adverse Reactions," Hormones Matter, January 16, 2015, https://www.hormonesmatter.com/lupron-estradiol-mitochondria-adverse-reactions/.

40 Lynne Millican, "They Say Lupron is Safe," Hormones Matter, August 31, 2022, https://www.hormonesmatter.com/they-say-lupron-safe/.

41 Sebastian E. E. Schagen et al., "Bone Development in Transgender Adolescents Treated with GnRH Analogues and Subsequent Gender-Affirming Hormones," *The Journal of Clinical Endocrinology & Metabolism* 105, no. 12 (December 2020): e4256, https://doi.org/10.1210/clinem/dgaa604; Janet Y. Lee et al., "Low Bone Mineral Density in Early Pubertal Transgender/Gender Diverse Youth: Findings from the Trans Youth Care Study," *Journal of the Endocrine Society* 4, no. 9 (September 2020): bvaa065, https://doi.org/10.1210/jendso/bvaa065.

42 Lee et al., "Low Bone Mineral Density," 6; Schagen et al., "Bone Development in Transgender Adolescents," e4256.

43 Mariska C. Vlot et al., "Effect of Pubertal Suppression and Cross-Sex Hormone Therapy on Bone Turnover Markers and Bone Mineral Apparent Density (BMAD) in Transgender Adolescents," *Bone* 95 (February 2017): 11–19, https://doi.org/10.1016/j.bone.2016.11.008; Schagen et al., "Bone Development in Transgender Adolescents," e4258, e4261.

44 Daniel Klink et al., "Bone Mass in Young Adulthood Following Gonadotropin-Releasing Hormone Analog Treatment and Cross-Sex Hormone Treatment in Adolescents with Gender Dysphoria," *The Journal of Clinical Endocrinology & Metabolism* 100, no. 2 (February 2015): e273, https://doi.org/10.1210/jc.2014-2439; Tobin Joseph, Joanna Ting, and Gary Butler, "The Effect of GnRH Analogue Treatment on Bone Mineral Density in Young Adolescents with Gender Dysphoria: Findings from a Large National Cohort," *Journal of Pediatric Endocrinology and Metabolism* 32, no. 10 (2019): 1077–81, https://doi.org/10.1515/jpem-2019-0046; Schagen et al., "Bone Development in Transgender Adolescents."

45 Maartje Klaver et al., "Early Hormonal Treatment Affects Body Composition and Body Shape in Young Transgender Adolescents," *The Journal of Sexual Medicine* 15, no. 2 (February 2018): 256, https://doi.org/10.1016/j.jsxm.2017.12.009.

46 Klaver et al., 256.

47 Schagen et al., "Bone Development in Transgender Adolescents"; Vlot et al., "Effect of Pubertal Suppression," 14.

48 Klink et al., "Bone Mass in Young Adulthood," e273.

49 Dorothy A. Nelson et al., "Comparison of Cross-Sectional Geometry of the Proximal Femur in White and Black Women from Detroit and Johannesburg," *Journal of Bone and Mineral Research* 19, no. 4 (April 2004): 560–65, https://doi.org/10.1359/JBMR.040104; B. Lawrence Riggs et al., "Population-Based Study of Age

and Sex Differences in Bone Volumetric Density, Size, Geometry, and Structure at Different Skeletal Sites," *Journal of Bone and Mineral Research* 19, no. 12 (December 2004): 1945–54, https://doi.org/10.1359/jbmr.040916.

50   Anne C. Looker, Thomas J. Beck, and Eric S. Orwoll, "Does Body Size Account for Gender Differences in Femur Bone Density and Geometry?," *Journal of Bone and Mineral Research* 16, no. 7 (July 2001): 1291–99, https://doi.org/10.1359/jbmr.2001.16.7.1291.

51   Madeleine S. C. Wallien and Peggy T. Cohen-Kettenis, "Psychosexual Outcome of Gender-Dysphoric Children," *Journal of the American Academy of Child & Adolescent Psychiatry* 47, no. 12 (December 2008): 1413–23, https://doi.org/10.1097/CHI.0b013e31818956b9; Thomas D. Steensma et al., "Factors Associated with Desistence and Persistence of Childhood Gender Dysphoria: A Quantitative Follow-Up Study," *Journal of the American Academy of Child & Adolescent Psychiatry* 52, no. 6 (June 2013): 582–90, https://doi.org/10.1016/j.jaac.2013.03.016.

52   K. D. Drummond et al., "A Follow-Up Study of Girls with Gender Identity Disorder," *Developmental Psychology* 44, no. 1 (2008): 34–45, https://doi.org/10.1037/0012-1649.44.1.34; Devita Singh, Susan J. Bradley, and Kenneth J. Zucker, "A Follow-Up Study of Boys with Gender Identity Disorder," *Frontiers in Psychiatry* 12 (March 2021): 632784, https://doi.org/10.3389/fpsyt.2021.632784.

53   Wallien and Cohen-Kettenis, "Psychosexual Outcome"; Steensma et al., "Factors Associated with Desistence and Persistence."

54   Wallien and Cohen-Kettenis, "Psychosexual Outcome"; Steensma et al., "Factors Associated with Desistence and Persistence."

55   Drummond et al., "A Follow-up Study of Girls."

56   Devita Singh, "A Follow-Up Study of Boys with Gender Identity Disorder" (PhD diss., University of Toronto, 2012), https://tspace.library.utoronto.ca/bitstream/1807/34926/1/Singh_Devita_201211_PhD_Thesis.pdf.

57   Drummond et al., "A Follow-up Study of Girls," 39.

58   Singh, "A Follow-Up Study of Boys."

59   This study of juvenile male gender dysphoria sorted bisexuals and homosexuals into the same group, so I used the list of individual cases provided in the supplementary materials to sort by homosexual and nonhomosexual instead. The study recorded sexual orientation using the Kinsey Scale, a 0–6 scale in which zero is fully heterosexual and six is fully homosexual. I sorted into the homosexual group those who were Kinsey sixes for sexual fantasy, as well as those who were Kinsey fives for sexual fantasy and Kinsey sixes for sexual behavior. All the rest were sorted into the nonhomosexual group.

60   Drummond et al., "A Follow-up Study of Girls," 40.

61   Singh, Bradley, and Zucker, "A Follow-Up Study of Boys."

62   Drummond et al., "A Follow-up Study of Girls," 39.

63   Devita Singh, Susan J. Bradley, and Kenneth J. Zucker, "A Follow-Up Study of Boys with Gender Identity Disorder," *Frontiers in Psychiatry* 12 (March 2021): appendix 2, https://doi.org/10.3389/fpsyt.2021.632784.

64   Byne et al., "Report of the American Psychiatric Association Task Force," 763.

65   P. T. Cohen-Kettenis and S. H. M. van Goozen, "Pubertal Delay as an Aid in Diagnosis and Treatment of a Transsexual Adolescent," *European Child & Adolescent Psychiatry* 7, no. 4 (December 1998): 246–48, https://doi.org/10.1007/s007870050073.

66   Annelou L. C. de Vries et al., "Puberty Suppression in Adolescents with Gender Identity Disorder: A Prospective Follow-Up Study," *The Journal of Sexual Medicine* 8, no. 8 (August 2011): 2277, https://doi.org/10.1111/j.1743-6109.2010.01943.x; Peggy T. Cohen-Kettenis, Henriette A. Delemarre-van de Waal, and Louis J. G. Gooren, "The Treatment of Adolescent Transsexuals: Changing Insights," *The Journal of Sexual Medicine* 5, no. 8 (August 2008): 1894, https://doi.org/10.1111/j.1743-6109.2008.00870.x.

67   Henriette A. Delemarre-van de Waal and Peggy T. Cohen-Kettenis, "Clinical Management of Gender Identity Disorder in Adolescents: A Protocol on Psychological and Paediatric Endocrinology Aspects," *European Journal of Endocrinology* 155, no. suppl_1 (2006): S136, https://doi.org/10.1530/eje.1.02231; de Vries et al., "Puberty Suppression in Adolescents," 2281.

68   Chantal M. Wiepjes et al., "The Amsterdam Cohort of Gender Dysphoria Study (1972–2015): Trends in Prevalence, Treatment, and Regrets," *The Journal of Sexual Medicine* 15, no. 4 (April 2018): 582–90, https://doi.org/10.1016/j.jsxm.2018.01.016.

69   Tessa Brik et al., "Trajectories of Adolescents Treated with Gonadotropin-Releasing Hormone Analogues for Gender Dysphoria," *Archives of Sexual Behavior* 49, no. 7 (October 2020): 2611–18, https://doi.org/10.1007/s10508-020-01660-8.

70   Tim Adams, "Transgender Children: The Parents and Doctors on the Frontline," *The Guardian*, November 13, 2016, https://www.theguardian.com/society/2016/nov/13/transgender-children-the-parents-and-doctors-on-the-frontline.

71   Johanna Olson, "Deciding When to Treat a Youth for Gender Re-Assignment," Kids in the House, accessed September 13, 2022, https://www.kidsinthehouse.com/teenager/sexuality/transgender/deciding-when-to-treat-a-youth-for-gender-re-assignment.

72   Polly Carmichael et al., "Gender Dysphoria in Younger Children: Support and Care in an Evolving Context" (talk, WPATH Symposium, Amsterdam, June 19, 2016), https://web.archive.org/web/20190803150242/http://wpath2016.conferencespot.org/62620-wpathv2-1.3138789/t001-1.3140111/f009a-1.3140266/0706-000523-1.3140268.

73   Carmichael et al.

74   Brik et al., "Trajectories of Adolescents," 5.

75   Steensma et al., "Factors Associated with Desistence and Persistence," 587.

76   Steensma et al., 584.

77   Kristina R. Olson et al., "Gender Identity 5 Years after Social Transition," *Pediatrics* 150, no. 2 (August 2022): e2021056082, https://doi.org/10.1542/peds.2021-056082.

78   Olson et al.retransition

79   Charles Pincourt and James Lindsay, *Counter Wokecraft: A Field Manual for Combatting the Woke in the University and Beyond* (Orlando, FL: New Discourses, 2021), 4–6; Helen Pluckrose and James Lindsay, *Cynical Theories: How Activist Scholarship Made Everything about Race, Gender, and Identity—and Why This Harms Everybody* (Durham, NC: Pitchstone Publishing, 2020), 14.

8.2. Ending the Cover-Up

1   Alice D. Dreger, "The Controversy Surrounding *The Man Who Would Be Queen*: A Case History of the Politics of Science, Identity, and Sex in the Internet Age," *Archives of Sexual Behavior* 37, no. 3 (June 2008): 366–421, https://doi.org/10.1007/s10508-007-9301-1.

2   Miranda Fricker, *Epistemic Injustice: Power and the Ethics of Knowing* (New York: Oxford University Press, 2007), 162.

3   James Lindsay, "Lived Experience," New Discourses, last modified April 17, 2020, https://newdiscourses.com/tftw-lived-experience/.

4   Zack M. Davis, "Psychology is about Invalidating People's Identities," *The Scintillating But Ultimately Untrue Thought* (blog), September 5, 2016, http://unremediatedgender.space/2016/Sep/psychology-is-about-invalidating-peoples-identities/.

5   Ray Blanchard (@BlanchardPhD), "Some years ago, I responded to a post on the closed listserv," Twitter, August 1, 2021, 3:02 p.m., https://twitter.com/BlanchardPhD/status/1421924355471200259.

6   Michael Bailey, "Questioning Sexual Identities," *Queer Majority*, no. 6: Identity, accessed September 13, 2022, https://www.queermajority.com/essays-all/questioning-sexual-identities.

8.3. A Call for Revolution

1   Thomas S. Kuhn, "The Structure of Scientific Revolutions," *American Journal of Physics* 31, no. 7 (1963): 554–55, https://doi.org/10.1119/1.1969660.

2   Antonio Guillamon, Carme Junque, and Esther Gómez-Gil, "A Review of the Status of Brain Structure Research in Transsexualism," *Archives of Sexual Behavior* 45, no. 7 (October 2016): 1615–48, https://doi.org/10.1007/s10508-016-0768-5.

3   J. Defreyne et al., "Sexual Orientation in Transgender Individuals: Results from the Longitudinal ENIGI Study," *International Journal of Impotence Research* 33, no. 7 (2021): 694–702, https://doi.org/10.1038/s41443-020-00402-7.

9.0. Closing Thoughts

1   Tina Fossella, "Human Nature, Buddha Nature: An Interview with John Welwood," *Tricycle: The Buddhist Review*, Spring 2011, https://tricycle.org/magazine/human-nature-buddha-nature/.

2   "Lil B Talks Getting Sucker Punched, Gay Rumors, & Drake Envy," Complex, June 9, 2010, https://www.complex.com/music/2010/06/lil-b-talks-getting-sucker-punched-gay-rumors-drake-envy.

3   Jacques Ellul, *The Technological Society: A Penetrating Analysis of Our Technical Civilization and of the Effect of an Increasingly Standardized Culture on the Future of Man* (New York: Vintage Books, 1964); Theodore John Kaczynski, *Technological Slavery: Enhanced Edition*, 4th ed. (Scottsdale, AZ: Fitch & Madison Publishers, 2022).

Appendix: Sorting by Etiology in Transgender Research

1   K=Kinsey Score (0=fully heterosexual, 3=evenly bisexual, 6=fully homosexual).

Printed in the USA
CPSIA information can be obtained
at www.ICGtesting.com
LVHW090227191123
764328LV00032B/1258/J

9 781544 541457